Praise for Dr. Tom Plaut's *Children With Asthma*

"*Children With Asthma* gives parents much needed information to help them take charge of asthma with their family's doctor."
T. BERRY BRAZELTON, M.D.
Author, *Infants and Mothers*

"The first user-friendly guide to asthma."
GUILLERMO R. MENDOZA, M.D.
Allergist, Los Angeles, California

"Asthma can be a frustrating, disruptive, and frightening condition, especially in children. But with the help of this wonderful aid, families can learn to manage symptoms and gain control. The need for parents, child, and physician to function as a management team is the keystone of Plaut's approach. He explains causes, complications, and intervention strategies in a clear, jargon-free manner."
Medical Self Care

"An excellent resource for parents, children, and physicians."
ELLIOTT ELLIS, M.D.
Past President, American Academy of Allergy and Immunology

"Enormous help as I educate myself. I feel grateful to find exactly what I need, exactly when I need it."
PAUL PAVESICH
Arlington, Virginia

"Your book helped me deal with the asthma and with finding a caring, supportive doctor. Many thanks."
DONNA CROWLEY
Pullman, Washington

"Reading the stories about families dealing with asthma made me feel like I was in a support group with them, going through the same thing they did."
JANICE DUDLEY
Britton, Michigan

"*Children With Asthma* not only helped me understand asthma but also calmed and educated both sets of grandparents. As I reread sections of the book I feel much more confident."
JULY LYNN
Carmichael, California

"Asthma ruled us, instead of us it, until I educated myself and found a doctor who was knowledgeable and aggressive in its treatment."
CYNTHIA WEBB
Prairieville, Louisiana

"No one, no book, was more helpful to me."
MINDY BUCEK
Houston, Texas

"We found your book the single most assuring source of information. You affirmed that our son could lead a normal, active, healthy life."
DENNIS J. OVITSKY, D.V.M.
Pittsfield, Massachusetts

"You gave me the confidence to talk to my child's doctor about better home management skills. We are doing much better as a team."
NANCY MORENO
Las Cruces, New Mexico

"Straightforward, informative and practical without talking down to its audience."
ELISE PECHTER MORSE
Cambridge, Massachussets

"If you want information to supplement what you have taught your patient—this is where it's all at! Tom Plaut's book is superb."
BERNARD BERMAN, M.D.
Past President,
American College of Allergy and Immunology

". . . comes as close as possible to changing the treatment of asthma from a mysterious illness guarded over by priest-like physicians dispensing magic potions to a condition that parents can treat (for the most part) confidently at home . . ."
LAWRENCE K. EPPLE JR., M.D.
Washington Post

"An important book for *all* families whose children have asthma."
JOANN BLESSING-MOORE, M.D.
Allergist, Palo Alto, California

". . . offers the information which educators and parents need to achieve asthma control at school."
ELLIE GOLDBERG, M.Ed.
Educational Rights Specialist

"Exactly what I needed to educate myself and learn about asthma in my two-year-old son."
ERICKA CLARK SHAW
San Francisco, California

Dr. Tom Plaut's

Asthma Guide for People
of All Ages

Other publications by Dr. Plaut

Children With Asthma: A Manual for Parents
One Minute Asthma: What You Need to Know
El asma in un minuto: lo que usted necesita saber
Asthma Peak Flow Diary
Asthma Signs Diary
Asthma Charts and Forms for the Physician's Office
Asthma Charts and Forms for the Physician's Office and Managed Care
Training Community Health Workers (co-editor)

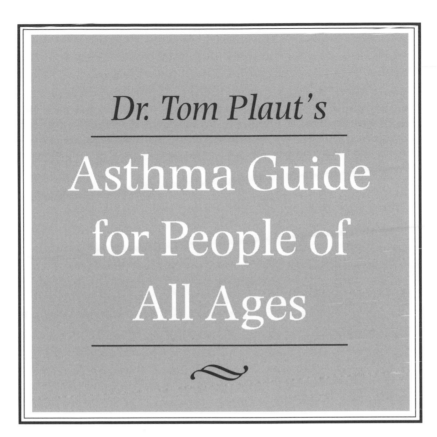

Dr. Tom Plaut's

Asthma Guide for People of All Ages

Thomas F. Plaut, M.D.

with Teresa B. Jones, M.A.

Pedipress, Inc.
Amherst, Massachusetts

NOTICE

The information in this book is not intended to serve as a replacement for medical advice. Any use of the information in this book is at the reader's discretion. The authors and publisher specifically disclaim any and all liability arising directly or indirectly from the use or application of any information contained in this book. Consult a health care professional regarding your specific situation.

For information address: Pedipress, Inc., 125 Red Gate Lane, Amherst, MA 01002

Library of Congress Cataloging-in-Publication Data

Plaut, Thomas F., 1933-
    [Asthma guide for people of all ages]
    Dr. Tom Plaut's asthma guide for people of all ages / Thomas F. Plaut, with Teresa B. Jones.
        p. cm.
    Include bibliographical references and index.
    ISBN 0-914625-22-5 (pbk.)
        1. Asthma — Popular works.   I. Title: Doctor Tom Plaut's asthma guide for people of all ages.   II. Title: Asthma guide for people of all ages.   III. Jones, Teresa B. (Teresa Bernadette), 1968-   IV. Title.

RC591 .P527 1999
616.2'38 — dc21   99-046826

LC99–046826

99   00   01   02   6   5   4   3   2   1

Designed by Barbara Werden Design

Illustrations by Carla Brennan

Printed in the United States of America

Dedicated to patients, parents, and professionals
who are willing to learn

Contents

Figures

Chapter 7 Asthma Treatment

Chapter 8 Working With Your Doctors

Resource Section

Tables and Sidebars

Acknowledgments

Patients and parents of children with asthma in my practice have contributed to this book in many ways. They challenged me to provide information in an understandable fashion. They helped improve my diaries and home treatment plans. The stories they wrote taught me about the many faces of asthma, the disruption it can cause in people's lives, and the determination needed to achieve excellent control over it.

I sought criticism and suggestions from many experts in the field of asthma, including physicians, nurses, respiratory therapists, and educators, to ensure that this book would be as accurate, clear, and current as possible. I want to express my gratitude to Peter Boggs, M.D., Myrna Dolovich, P. Eng., Elliot Ellis, M.D., David Stempel, M.D., Stanley Szefeler, M.D., and Larry Westby, R.R.T., who commented on individual chapters and were helpful and good-natured during our many conversations. Michael Welch, M.D. and Ellie Goldberg, M.Ed. were particulary generous with their time and comments.

I want also to thank Gary Brecher, M.D., Paul Ehrlich, M.D., Gilbert Friday, M.D., Anne Muñoz Furlong, Margo Harris, David Jamison, Emlen Jones, M.D., Ruben Manness, M.D., Guillermo Mendoza, M.D., Berri Mitchell, C.P.N.P., Nancy Sanker, O.T.R., Michael Schatz, M.D., Sheldon Specter, M.D., Richard Sveum, M.D., Jackie Trovato, Chris Wagner, C.P.N.P., Jeffrey Wald, M.D., and Maura Zazenski for reading individual chapters or sections and making suggestions that improved the book.

I greatly appreciate the work of Carla Brennan, whose lucid line drawings clarify the text. The artistry of Barbara Werden guides the reader smoothly through the book. Jo Landers produced the computer art, and Larry Gilman and Suzanne Plaut edited the manuscript with great skill. Stacey Velez cheerfully assisted me in the care of my office patients during this project. In addition to her writing and analysis, Teresa Jones's management skills and even temperament were essential factors in bringing this project to a timely conclusion.

Finally, I want to thank my son, David, for discussing asthma with me; my daughter, Rebecca, for her encouragement; and my wife, Johanna, for her support over the past thirty-six years.

Dr. Tom Plaut's

Asthma Guide for People
of All Ages

Introduction

You Can Control Asthma

You are probably aware of reports that asthma emergencies and hospitalizations are increasing. My patients and my readers rarely have these problems. They have learned to control their asthma and you can, too. By "controlling your asthma" I mean that you will have symptoms no more than two days per week, will rarely miss school or work because of asthma, will rarely require an urgent visit to the doctor or emergency room, will not be hospitalized, and will be able to exercise as long and as hard as everyone else. To achieve this control, you will need to learn:

- how to deliver inhaled medicines
- how to check your condition using peak flow or asthma signs
- how to follow a written plan based on asthma treatment zones

You could get the information in this book from your doctor, but it would take at least ten hours. It would be difficult for you to remember, and you would probably not want to pay for it. It makes more sense to use this book as a foundation that you and your doctor can build on. By doing so, you can become a skilled man-ager of your asthma care and continue your learning process.

My first book, *Children With Asthma: A Manual for Parents,* has helped hundreds of thousands of families since its publication in 1983. Many patients and health professionals asked me to expand my writing to include adults. This book outlines the blueprint for achieving excellent asthma control for people of all ages. It is consistent with the recommendations of the *Expert Panel Report 2: Guidelines for the Diagnosis and Management of Asthma,* a comprehensive report on asthma care published by the National Heart, Lung and Blood Institute in 1997.

Dr. Tom Plaut's Asthma Guide provides you with the basic information you need to communicate clearly with your doctor. It will help you understand asthma and its treatment so you can follow a plan designed by your doctor to control asthma. As you read, you will meet people who have overcome many of the problems you face. I am convinced that you, too, can improve your asthma control.

Most asthma books discuss the basics of asthma and the medicines used to treat it. You will find that important information here, but I believe that you need to learn more than that before you can fully control your asthma. So, I give serious attention to the following areas of asthma care:

• **The basics of asthma.** Understanding asthma starts with learning how the lungs work and how they change during the asthma reaction. Careful monitoring will tell you that an asthma episode is beginning and how severe it is. Allergens and other substances in your environment can trigger an asthma episode. It makes more sense to reduce triggers such as tobacco smoke, animal dander, or dust in your home than to increase your dose of medicines.

• **Asthma medicines.** We now understand how important it is to control and prevent long-term inflammation in the airways. We also know a lot more about asthma medicines, who is most likely to benefit from them, and what adverse effects to watch for. You will read about the medicines currently available to treat asthma, how they work, what they are supposed to do, how long they take to act, what adverse effects may occur, and the usual doses prescribed for home use.

• **Devices for inhaling asthma medicine.** Taking the right medicines, especially the ones needed daily to control persistent asthma, is an important part of your asthma treatment. Yet, many people who see me for an asthma consultation are taking the right medicines the wrong way. Their techniques for using a metered dose inhaler (alone or with a holding chamber), a dry powder inhaler, or a nebulizer are flawed. This prevents them from getting the full benefit from their medicines and may increase the adverse effects. You need specific instructions and demonstrations from a health professional to learn the proper use of each device. The descriptions and illustrations in this chapter will help.

• **Peak flow.** For patients five years of age and older, tracking airflow is the key to successful asthma treatment. The peak flow meter, a portable and inexpensive device, has revolutionized asthma care because you can use it at home to monitor your airflow. Once you know how to blow peak flow scores, you can learn to judge your asthma status and adjust treatment at home. You can also discuss specific numbers with your doctor, instead of using vague terms. As a result, you will receive better advice.

• **Using an asthma diary.** A well-designed asthma diary helps you collect information in an organized and useful fashion. It aids you in learning about your individual asthma situation, keeping track of medicines, and figuring out when to change your treatment. A diary that displays the asthma treatment zones also helps you communicate with health professionals and family members.

• **Treatment plans.** A one-page written treatment plan guides you in your daily routine and in care of an asthma episode. Based on peak flow scores or the four signs of asthma, it is easy to follow since the zones are identical to those in the asthma diaries. Once you have worked out an effective plan with your doctor, you will be able to manage most asthma problems at home.

An effective collaboration between you and your doctor requires that you do the day-to-day work of asthma management. It requires that your doctor guide you in learning how to use devices, diaries, and a treatment plan. He or she needs to prescribe the medicines and environmental changes that are essential for you to gain control over your asthma.

Using Dr. Tom Plaut's Asthma Guide

This is not a do-it-yourself book. It gives you the information you need to understand asthma and work with your health care provider. It does not give specific advice for your individual situation. If you were to read this book ten times, you would know more about asthma than most people. But you would still need the help of a health professional to manage your asthma effectively and safely. Your doctor will work out an asthma treatment plan based on all the individual information you collect, and will provide emergency care if you need it. The more knowledgeable and experienced you become, the more responsibility you can take on and the better care you will receive.

You will find clear explanations of the many areas of asthma management. Illustrations and first-person stories clarify the more complex aspects of asthma care. Step-by-step examples demonstrate how to use asthma management tools such as an asthma diary and a home treatment plan. Forms for your personal use are available at the back of the book. An extensive resource section and a medical bibliography can lead you to additional information.

No page in this book can stand alone. The facts, stories, diaries, and treatment plans are all woven together, each chapter building on what you have learned in earlier chapters. Chapter 7, "Asthma Treatment," and Chapter 8, "Working With Your Doctors," bring together the elements of asthma care and apply them to the practical task of controlling your asthma. "Asthma at School" focuses on issues more relevant to children under 18 years of age. The "Family and Travel" chapter provides information for a reader of any age.

The asthma stories you will read were written by many different patients and parents. All of these patients have been under my care except for Tori, Douglas, and Julie. I use patients' full names in long stories and first names in shorter selections. Some names have been changed, but all the stories are based on real people and the real details of their asthma care. None are composites.

The patient narratives in this book span a period of seventeen years. Since many changes in medicine treatment have taken place during that time, I have edited out most of the specific doses in the stories. Currently recommended doses are described thoroughly in Chapter 3, "Asthma Medicines."

For ease of reading and clarity, I have adopted a few conventions. My writing is addressed to "you" the reader. If you are the parent of a child with asthma, please read "your child" in its place. This information is appropriate for both children and adults, unless specifically stated otherwise. Similarly, I refer to your health care provider as "your doctor." However, nurses, nurse practitioners and respiratory therapists play an important role in providing asthma care. If you are receiving care from one of these health professionals, please substitute their title as you read "doctor." If you encounter terms or acronyms that are not familiar, please consult the glossary or index at the back of the book.

Finally, I have alternated the use of the pronouns "he" and "she" by chapter in referring to doctors and patients in general. The male pronoun is used for doctors in even-numbered chapters, and the female pronoun is used in odd-numbered chapters. This convention is reversed for patients.

Almost all of my patients gain excellent control over their asthma. There are no secrets or shortcuts and the day-to-day work is not exciting, but the results are dramatic. Once you achieve excellent asthma control, you should be able to maintain it throughout the year.

Read, learn, observe, analyze, discuss, act, and improve your asthma control.

THOMAS F. PLAUT, M.D.
Amherst, Massachusetts

Chapter One

Asthma Stories

The stories you will read here reveal how asthma has affected the lives of my patients. As you read their accounts, you will see the many steps parents and patients took to bring their asthma under control. These first-person accounts open windows into the fears, the trials, and the hard work of people searching to get the help they need. This chapter celebrates the successes of those who have done what is necessary to control their asthma.

Most of these stories were written by patients to prepare for our first consultation. Their writers recount a series of human events. You will learn from them and recognize yourself in their words, both rationally and intuitively. Readers of my previous book, *Children With Asthma: A Manual for Parents,* say they learned quickly because they connected with the experiences of my patients.

The first four stories were written in the early to mid-1980s by parents of asthma patients. At that time, I was a general pediatrician with a special interest in asthma but not yet an asthma specialist. Back then, I did not consider making an urgent visit to the doctor or missing a couple of days of school to be a sign that a

patient's asthma control was inadequate. I prescribed cromolyn or theophylline to prevent episodes, and metaproterenol as the primary quick relief medicine to treat episodes. Even then, most of my patients achieved results that were considered quite good.

Asthma care is much improved now. Knowledge, medicines, devices, educational tools, and expectations for asthma control have all changed. The stories of those earlier patients and their families provide both continuity with and contrast to the accounts written by patients who came to see me in the 1990s.

During the past ten years I have expanded my asthma consulting practice to include adults. Despite all of the advances in asthma care, new patients continue to come in for a consultation because they are not benefiting from their medicines, cannot live fully active lives, or feel at the mercy of their asthma. My treatment routines have become much more effective. I now prescribe the daily use of inhaled steroids for most of my patients. All of them monitor their asthma trends using a diary based on peak flow scores or asthma signs. (These terms are described in Chapter 2, "The

Basics of Asthma.") They adjust their treatment following a written home treatment plan that I have developed. Their stories show that most people with asthma can dramatically improve their condition within two weeks of starting an effective treatment plan.

Each one of my patients or their parents wrote an asthma narrative before their first visit; the age given refers to the time that they wrote the story. I follow the narrative with an account of their care and status over the years. You will meet some of these people again in later chapters of the book, and get to know many others through briefer stories. They will show you that there are no secrets in asthma care. It takes hard work in the early months of treatment to achieve excellent asthma control and continued attention to maintain it. But the results are worth the work.

STORIES FROM THE 1980s

■

Melissa, age 7
Jetta Pelak

Last year, my 7-year-old daughter, Melissa, had her first asthma attack. She had been rolling in the grass at a soccer field when she broke out in a red, blotchy rash. The next day she complained of a sore throat and not feeling well. By early afternoon she was in a deep sleep. She was breathing fifty times a minute and her chest pinched in with every breath.

It was a Sunday and my pediatrician was off-duty. The office of the pediatrician who was on call was forty-five minutes away, so I decided to go to an emergency clinic five minutes from my home. This proved to be a terrible experience. The doctor gave Missy an injection of epineph-

rine and an inhalation treatment. When we left the clinic she still had retractions. The doctor said there wasn't anything more he could do. It would go away. I certainly didn't know what to do and felt really helpless.

After an hour at home Missy had still not improved. I was shaking as I dialed the pediatrician who was on call for my doctor. He told me to come to his office immediately. He gave her two more injections and some liquid theophylline to be given every six hours. It took eight days until Missy felt well enough to return to school.

About five weeks later, Melissa had another attack after a field trip in the woods with her Brownie troop. We met her pediatrician in his office at 11:00 P.M. He gave her two injections of epinephrine and said Missy definitely had asthma. He prescribed liquid theophylline to be taken for seven days. After that, she was to take long-acting theophylline every eight hours and cromolyn by metered dose inhaler (MDI) three times a day. Missy improved slowly and returned to school after six days.

Six weeks ago we moved to western Massachusetts and into a very old and damp house. Since the move, Missy has had a cough at night and wakes up with terrible nasal congestion. She recently saw a doctor for her school physical. He said she was in good health. I mentioned her asthma symptoms and he suggested that I consider discontinuing the theophylline. He also recommended that I use a metaproterenol inhaler along with the cromolyn and that I read a book called *Children With Asthma*.

I couldn't consider any of these changes since it seemed to me that Melissa needed the theophylline more than ever. I did buy the book that week and began to read it, and at the same time made an appointment with an asthma specialist. Four weeks before the scheduled appointment Melissa woke up on a Sunday with a very bad cough. She complained of chest pain, shortness of breath, and a sore throat. I took her to the pediatrician, who prescribed an albuterol inhaler. Somehow I had the same helpless feeling as I left that office. It just didn't seem like enough.

That night was horrible. She went into that deep sleep again as she had with her first attack. She was breathing thirty-six times per minute and her stomach pushed out with each breath. It was an effort for her to breathe in and out. I sat on her bed with a flashlight all night and counted her respirations every hour, praying that we could make it until morning.

Several times I got up to wake my husband to take us to the emergency room at the hospital. But I was afraid to go there, too. The albuterol inhaler proved useless to Melissa. Her chest hurt too much to take a deep breath. When she needed it the most (during the middle of the night) I couldn't wake her enough to sit up, let alone coordinate her breathing with the inhaler puff.

Finally morning came. I called the asthma specialist's office and arranged to see him. I was sure he would give her an injection to make her breathe easier. Melissa was scared when we were taken into the treatment room. The doctor's assistant told her that this doctor did not like to give children needles.

The doctor explained the four signs of asthma trouble to me while he was examining Melissa. He told me to watch for a change in her wheezing, retractions, prolonged expiration, and respiratory rate while she received treatment with a compressor driven nebulizer. Then he went out to see another patient while the nurse measured metaproterenol and saline into a plastic nebulizer unit. She turned on the air compressor and a mist came out of the mouthpiece. She asked Melissa to hold the mouthpiece between her teeth and to breathe in and out. I saw a big improvement in Missy's breathing about two minutes after she started breathing in the mist.

The entire treatment lasted about eight minutes. Half an hour later, the nurse watched as I gave Missy the next treatment. Her peak flow score had been 60 when we arrived. After two treatments it was 200. I borrowed the compressor driven nebulizer to use at home every four hours. The doctor also prescribed prednisolone (an oral steroid) for three days and said to continue the theophylline as before and to give metaproterenol and cromolyn by nebulizer.

That evening Melissa had two more treatments at home while watching television. Her breathing was peaceful that night. The doctor called to check on her at 8:00 P.M. and I felt more reassured than I ever have. I knew I could fall asleep and not worry. The next morning she continued taking four medications: metaproterenol and cromolyn by nebulizer, long-acting theophylline, and prednisolone. She did some arts and crafts, made pudding for herself and her brother, and balleted around the house. I received another call at 4:00 P.M. from the doctor's office to check on her progress. That follow-up meant a lot to me.

The next morning she took her medicine. Then we had breakfast and went out to walk the dog. Missy and her dog ran far ahead of me up the hill. I was out of breath, but Missy was not. I brought Missy to school with her nebulizer and arranged for a health aide to give her a treatment at noon. When I picked her up at the end of the day, she was feeling fine.

This episode was different. I learned a lot and I know I'm going to learn much more. But the big difference is that it only took twenty-four hours for Melissa to recover. Now I have a written plan and know what to do. When the next episode comes, I will be ready for it.

■

Ms. Pelak's story was written more than ten years ago. Several of the medicines that Missy's mom used to bring her asthma under control would no longer be recommended. Albuterol is now used instead of metaproterenol as a quick relief medicine to open the airways because it causes fewer adverse effects. Though theophylline is used by some patients today, it is usually taken as an add-on medicine. Inhaled steroids, cromolyn, or nedocromil are the safest and most effective antiinflammatory medicines used to prevent asthma episodes.

■

Russ, age 18
Gail Wall

It was on Russell's sixth birthday when I knew he had a breathing problem that was not going to go away. We had the family and other guests at the house to celebrate his birthday. It was March, cold and windy. He came into the house, sat on my lap and said, "I can't breathe again." I held him, talked to him and stroked his cheek until he said, "I'm OK now."

When Russ had a cold our family doctor treated him with antibiotics. After that doctor died, we started going to a pediatrician. I told the new doctor Russell's history as best as I could. From then on Russ's colds were treated with a shot of epinephrine as well as antibiotics.

Russell joined a hockey league when he was 10 years old. It became evident at this point that sitting on Mom's lap and being treated with antibiotics and a shot of epinephrine was not going to help him breathe well enough to play hockey. But he stuck it out. Sometimes he had to come off the ice after a few minutes.

We moved to a new town and went to another pediatrician. Believe it or not, he was the first doctor to use the word asthma! He prescribed theophylline for the episodes. Russell

had stomach upsets and could not sleep when he took his medicine. However, I felt that we were making progress.

This pediatrician left his practice when Russell was 14. Since then Russ and I have coped as best we could. His only treatment has been emergency room visits. When I telephone the pediatrician's office I may reach three different pediatricians in a twelve-hour period. Each one gives different instructions.

Now Russ is 18 years old. In April and in June his asthma flared up. We made three trips to the emergency room with each episode, and things were worse than ever. Russ was very sick from this last attack. He had a violent headache and severe vomiting from too much theophylline. One doctor said stop the theophylline, one said continue it, and the third said switch to terbutaline. At this point I said, "I've had it! There is a doctor out there who knows how to deal with this and I'm going to find him!" I did. I called for an appointment and now I am trying to put my son's asthma history down on paper.

Russ is intelligent, talented (he will be an architect), and athletic. Yes, he is good at soccer, hockey, and baseball, and he would be an excellent athlete if we could master his asthma. And he is dead set against drugs. Theophylline is a drug. Yesterday Russ had a severe headache. I called and talked to one doctor who told me to continue the theophylline, add a strong pain killer for the headache, and to come in. We saw another doctor. He said he wasn't sure what to do. Maybe Russ should start taking cromolyn. Russ said, "I'm sick of filling my body with this junk. I can't eat. I can't sleep. I can't work. I don't want a painkiller and a new medication. I want to reach my potential. And these drugs I'm filling my body with aren't helping. I want my body clean."

We went home and he took two puffs of his inhaler. A few hours later, more inhaler. He was up coughing all night. At 6:00 A.M., after two puffs of the inhaler, I took him to work. He is a dishwasher at Howard Johnson's. He got out of the car and said, "Oh, God. I'll call you when I'm through with work." He took a deep breath. Another day to cope.

Russ is a muscular, six-foot-two-inch young man. He is too big to sit on my lap.

Help.

■

Russ and his mother came in to see me, and together we worked out an asthma treatment plan for Russ to take to college. One year later, he wrote me a letter describing how the changes we had made had affected his asthma and his life.

I have suffered from asthma for most of my 19 years. Many a cold winter night I have spent hour upon hour gasping for air in a hospital emergency room. I have battled with many bouts of "pneumonia" that left me underweight and demoralized. Every head cold I caught would immediately invade my lungs and spark breathing difficulty. On top of that, I suffer from side effects of the drug theophylline. Headaches added more discomfort. I had to choose, either breathe easier and accept the side effects or skip the drug and wind up in the emergency room. Some choice. I would always choose to accept the breathing difficulty. It seemed like the safest route.

I oppose any kind of drug-taking and feel that drugs and sports just don't mix. Though I knew I could breathe easier if I took drugs I chose to play without them. Recently I have learned that the theophylline was all right, the doctors were just giving me too much of it.

In 1985, four months before I was to leave for Arizona State University, I had one of the worst asthma attacks ever. I required emergency room treatment three times in one week. This was not good. I was going to be on my own soon and felt a need to get my asthma under control.

I visited a new doctor (you) and started reading about asthma and the medications used to treat it. I was amazed at the number of ways that asthma can be defeated. After some experimenting we figured out that if I reduced my theophylline dose I could get relief without getting headache, nausea, or sleeplessness. I would use albuterol to prevent or treat episodes caused by exercise. A short burst of prednisone could be used if my symptoms didn't clear quickly. You assured me that this plan would hold up, but if it didn't, you were confident we could work out another.

You also introduced me to the peak flow meter. What a device! For the first time I could actually "see" how well I was breathing. At first I thought of it as just another pain in the butt, another waste of time. One of my college roommates saw the peak flow meter and wanted to try it. When others came in to measure their peak flow I started a competition. The person with the highest score would win a prize (usually a hamburger or pizza). Over a period of months, I began equaling and then surpassing kids who didn't have asthma. What a thrill it was to actually see my progress. Due to the peak flow meter, I could see myself getting better and I was elated.

The peak flow meter also allows me to stay off medication because on days when I "see" that I'm breathing well, I simply don't take medication. One day after a couple of sets of tennis, I checked my peak flow and found it was a little under par. I immediately started taking medication, and two days later I was back up to my usual mark.

Today I sit here in sunny Arizona and my horrible memories of asthma seem to disappear. I feel stronger and healthier now than at any time in my life. When you get right down to it, asthma is just another opponent. As in any sport, you can defeat asthma with knowledge and practice.

■

Josh, age 5
Harriet Goodwin

"How long has this baby been wheezing?" asked the pediatrician in Peterborough, New Hampshire. We had all been praying for this doctor's arrival as the few general practitioners were so overworked. He didn't ask this question politely. There was a nasty, guilt-producing edge to the question. Like, "Lady, how long have you been so dumb?"

In truth, I had brought 18-month-old Josh in because he had had this odd, sharp cough all morning. There didn't seem to be any cold symptoms. I was torn between ignoring it and taking him in, thereby running the risk of being laughed at as an over-anxious mother.

"What wheezing?" I asked. And that was how I learned that my second and until now perfectly normal (well, almost), healthy baby had asthma. What a curse! Everyone knew asthma was a psychosomatic disease caused, of course, by mother! Oh God, Sigmund Freud has my number. This is it. I thought I had been doing such a good job of faking parenting.

Then came the shot of epinephrine. Then the twenty-minute wait in the waiting room while Josh turned ghastly pale white. Then the slightly congratulatory welcome back to the second shot — well, good, epinephrine will work on him. And then the prescription for a combination medicine (asthma syrup), to be administered every few hours for the next few days and then,

after that, as needed. There was probably a follow-up visit. It's hard to remember.

Josh was born in 1970 and now is almost 12. When Josh was 3 years old we determined that he was allergic to peanuts. We moved to Amherst shortly after and our new pediatrician advised us to see an allergist to define this problem and get advice on the care of Josh's frequent wheezing. The allergist said that Josh was allergic to peanuts and prescribed an epinephrine kit.

The years between Josh at age 3, with "occasional" asthma, and Josh at 7, when our "awakening" to the true nature of his condition occurred, are something of a blur to me. I don't remember using the asthma syrup very often. When Josh went to kindergarten at age 5, the teacher called and told me that he seemed more comfortable with the "four's" and seemed to belong there. That was fine with me, as I could tell that he was nowhere near being ready to deal with even the pre-reading. He was quite small for his age as well. His constant runny nose as well as his small, skinny size, made him seem a bit sickly, I guess.

Josh's first grade teacher said he often appeared tired and would nap under her desk during the afternoon. The next year his second grade teacher recommended a full evaluation of Josh's social, psychological, and educational status. The school psychiatric consultant diagnosed Josh as being chronically depressed.

On our first visit to the psychiatrist, he commented that Josh seemed very unwell. We agreed and said that perhaps April was a poor month for Josh allergy-wise.

That night, Josh had his first really severe asthma flare in a long time. We brought him to the office to see the new pediatrician who had recently taken over the practice. In between the first shot of epinephrine and the second one, he grilled us. What were we doing for this child's wheezing? Again I felt that pang of guilt that I had experienced in Peterborough.

The doctor seemed astounded and appalled when I told him that I gave Josh medication only if I heard him wheeze. "You've got to continue medication for at least two days after wheezing stops," he said. Patiently, he explained that he was reluctant to prescribe medicine unless necessary, but most people don't treat an episode long enough.

My little boy had asthma. It was as if I had never heard the words before. Deep shock set in. I had a very close friend who suffered terribly from asthma. This friend used to tell me that Josh was wheezing. I would bring Josh to swim at his lake cottage and he would say, "Harriet, Josh is wheezing." "Oh, it's nothing," I would say. At this time Josh was 4 or 5 years old. Not my Josh, he didn't have asthma. Not like that. When my friend dropped over and saw Josh, he said warningly, "He's wheeeeeezing." Why hadn't I taken it more seriously? I will never know. Perhaps just ignorance. I do know that it wasn't just Josh who had to be treated. We — Josh's father, Mike, and I — now had to be educated right along with Josh.

The first revelation was about the asthma syrup. Combination medicines are no longer recommended by the experts, said Josh's pediatrician. They contain unnecessary ingredients that can lead to bad side effects. So it was out with the combo and in with the theophylline. We tried one phyllin, this phyllin, and that phyllin.

At last, we settled on a long-acting theophylline tablet and taught Josh to master the fine art of pill-swallowing. What a breakthrough that was! Liberation from pouring liquids into those plastic measuring spoons and dribbling them down the poor child's throat.

All the while, the pediatrician provided support for Mike and me as we learned about asthma. Josh was always quite calm about all these new medical developments as one episode followed another that April. As I remember it,

we went to the office for epinephrine shots at least four times or more in ten days.

When our pediatrician decided to run a class for parents of children with asthma, our names were high up on the list of candidates for this series of meetings. Even as he worked on evaluating Josh's medication, adding, changing, deleting, improving, listening to those lungs, and listening again, our worst fears were alleviated by these wonderful classes. After hearing what some of the other parents had been through and were going through, we realized that Josh was not as bad off as we had thought. I can't describe what a relief it was to finally, once and for all, understand that Josh would not die in the ten minute interval between our house and the doctor's office, no matter how bad he sounded.

We learned about all of the different kinds of asthma medicines, how they work, and why they are chosen for use. We began to face the probability that Josh would take medicine for years, and that he might not ever "out-grow" it, although no one could predict anything and I still, to this day, hope that he will. We learned how to judge the severity of a flare by looking at the retractions at his neck. We learned how to use the stethoscope and were instructed in its use as a diagnostic tool at home. And then came the endless (or so it seemed) months of keeping a record, listening three times a day, writing down, in a sort of code, a day-by-day description of his condition.

I began to feel that I was partly the doctor. There were many consultations (by phone and in the office) during this initial period of treatment, which stretched over a year or more. At last we arrived at an effective combination of long-acting theophylline, metaproterenol, and an antihistamine. During this time, our pediatrician seemed to be constantly attending seminars on this stubborn disease, and trying new ideas. He liberalized his attitude toward the inhaler, and taught us to use it right along with the other medications. I think that was the final refinement, and it serves us in good stead. Our rule is that Josh may use the inhaler three times a day, but after that the doctor wants to hear about it and, most likely, to see him. This has almost never occurred.

It came as a big surprise to me when, last year, I had to be reminded that it was time to bring Josh in for a checkup. He had gone to the doctor's so often in the past that it never occurred to me that three months might slip by without a visit.

Josh underwent another series of allergy tests, but no strategic information turned up. He had his serum theophylline level checked several times. We increased his dose to 400 mg twice a day, which I thought was a lot, but it seemed to be just right for treating our 70-pound boy.

This May, Josh had his first bad episode in over a year. I attribute much of this good track record to intelligent and discriminate use of theophylline and the inhaler. One of the most important things I remember learning from the Parents' Asthma Group is how an episode may leave the lungs in a susceptible condition for weeks after the symptoms have gone. This placed our treatment approach in context for me and helped me to accept it.

I finally rebelled against keeping records after Josh had been quite well for a long time. I put away my stethoscope several years ago (although it is always there if I need it). I have learned to get all the lung information I need by pressing my ear right up to a bare chest. Josh is now almost completely in control of his own medication.

Once in a while there are complications. Just two days ago, he forgot he had taken his evening medicine and took it again. He was up a good part of the night vomiting and enduring stomach pain. Josh leaves me a note when it's time to refill the prescription. He had dropped his three

o'clock metaproterenol and allergy pill for several months over the summer. Just yesterday, I saw a big note that he left for himself on the kitchen counter near his pills:

JOSH TAKE YOUR THREE O'CLOCK PILLS

Josh is now in the fifth grade, reading on an early sixth grade level. He repeated a year, and thanks to the superb special education teachers and the proper medication routine, he is now back in a regular classroom. He is a happy and highly motivated boy. His depression in the second grade was probably related to his inadequately treated asthma. At last I am an educated parent with an educated child who knows about his asthma. I wouldn't have it any other way.

■

In 1987 Josh's mom reported on his condition.

Josh is now in tenth grade. Among his main interests at the moment is karate, which he has been studying for the past three years. He has held a blue belt for a while now and is hoping to achieve a black belt before he graduates from high school. Skateboarding has pushed breakdancing out of the picture recently, and Josh has just bought himself a motor scooter with some of the money he has earned working with his father. He shows a certain disdain for his tenspeed, but he's keeping his dirt bike.

Asthma? Oh yes, that's still a part of Josh's life. But it is no longer the way in which he identifies himself to others.

About five years ago Josh was hospitalized and we both learned a great deal from that experience. By living through it I lost my terror of "going to the hospital" as a worst-case scenario. Now I look at the hospital as a non-threatening place where they have all the same medicines that we do at home, but they also have a few more, some extra gadgets to dispense them with, and nurses who can make hour to hour observations. Although we have conquered our fear of hospitalization, it does increase my leverage with Josh when he gets careless with his medication routine. Just one reminder of that event convinces him to take his medicine.

Josh does take his medication on his own, except at times of severe distress. Sometimes he has trouble because he has been "careless" about his medication. I tell him what the doctor repeatedly tells me: it's his body, and if he doesn't take care of himself, he will get sick, not me. He has the responsibility to take the medication and limit his physical activities at these rare times. I have to face the fact that I can't yank him off his skateboard — he's going too fast, already out of sight and downtown anyway! Of course, it is hard for a parent to stay on the sidelines. By and large, I do, and for the most part, Josh manages quite well.

Josh has not taken theophylline in the past year. His headaches have decreased dramatically and evening nausea and vomiting are things of the past. He is stabilized on a routine of using the cromolyn inhaler 3 double puffs a day and the albuterol inhaler 3 to 5 times a day. He uses the albuterol before sports and sometimes at night. When he ceases to get relief from this routine, Josh uses a short burst of prednisone. This happens two or three times a year. We see the doctor every four months to review asthma care rather than to treat a flare.

Just recently, Josh had a brief but major crisis. The triggering complications were flu and an ear infection. Suddenly Josh went from just being sick and feverish to having great difficulty with his breathing. He begged me to take him to the doctor — an unheard-of request from Josh. His peak flow score was down and Josh had retractions. His breathing out took longer than breathing in. I was scared and out of practice. I was unsure about how to handle this episode. I started him on prednisone, and I managed to track down our doctor for guidance by phone. Over a few hours' time Josh seemed to turn a corner. The next morning he was much better.

Why is it always at night, never during office hours? This time I found out the answer — asthma always gets worse during the night. It's a steady twenty-four hour cycle, for everyone, better in the day, worse at night.

As a result of this crisis, we paid a visit to the office. As usual, we learned something new. Our doctor introduced us to the concept of dividing peak flow readings into the green, yellow, and red zones. We used these zones to formulate a written treatment plan. Now that we've established these guides for action, I feel like a general with a strategic battle plan that's almost guaranteed to work.

At this stage of my lengthy experience as an asthma parent, the hardest part for me is helping Josh decide what to do and when to do it during a crisis. The burden of that responsibility seems light when I look back to the pain, guilt, fear, and sadness I experienced when I first began to realize that I was the parent of a person who has asthma.

■

When I spoke with Josh in 1998, his asthma control was excellent. In the previous six years he had taken no oral steroids, had no emergency room visits or hospitalizations, and had not missed work. Asthma was rarely interfering with his physical activities or sleep. Josh wasn't taking any controller medicines, although he occasionally needed albuterol (a quick relief medicine) for symptoms during the winter. For the previous three years, he was using yoga to relax his airways. When he was hearing a mild wheeze or feeling a tight chest and was not carrying his albuterol inhaler, he focused on his breathing and was often able to relieve his symptoms.

■

Nathan, age 1
Marilyn Sansouci

Our fourth son, Nathan, was born in April 1981. He weighed 8 pounds, 10 ounces and was a very handsome little fellow. We were very pleased with him. He was healthy and fine until one day in November when he caught a cold. We treated it with aspirin and a decongestant. This didn't seem to help him at all.

By the third day he became worse. He began to cough quite frequently and he was breathing rapidly. By the time evening came, our baby was struggling to breathe. We immediately called an ambulance which took us to the hospital. He was put in an oxygen tent for several days. After taking chest X rays, the doctor said that our son had pneumonia. He gave him an antibiotic and after a week's stay in the hospital, Nathan was sent home. He did fine for three weeks but when he caught another cold, it turned into a nightmare.

Late one night I awoke from a sound sleep with a feeling that I should look in on the baby. I check on all the boys every night (a mother's routine) before I go to bed, but this time it was different. When I went into Nathan's room I heard him wheezing and coughing and gasping for air. I ran and woke my husband. We rushed our baby to the hospital and on the way total fear gripped me. I feared that this time we were going to lose our son. By the time we got to the hospital, Nathan's lips began to turn blue from lack of oxygen. He was put into an oxygen tent again, and all we could do was pray to God that our baby would be all right. I believe it was a miracle, an answer to prayer, that Nathan did survive. They took more chest X rays and did a test for cystic fibrosis, which was negative, and we were very thankful for that.

I remember feeling distressed and wondering how long this would continue before we would find out what was causing our little boy to get so sick so often. Approximately one week later, when I was to bring Nathan home from the hospital, I called his doctor to ask if he had made a diagnosis yet. He told me there was still no diagnosis and encouraged me just to be happy he was better. Well, by this time I had had my fill of finding out nothing concerning my baby. Certainly we were happy that he was better, but for how long? We knew something was terribly wrong but we just didn't know what. We decided it was time to change doctors. At this time we were referred to another pediatrician by a friend. The first time we visited this new doctor and I told him of Nathan's trauma, he diagnosed him as having asthma and began treatment with theophylline three times a day. Despite this treatment, Nathan was still hospitalized for asthma twice more before his first birthday.

In March of 1982 we joined a health maintenance organization. The next time Nathan had an asthma episode, he was examined by our new family doctor, who then phoned for a pediatric consultation. After he got off the phone he ordered three shots for Nathan. I believe the shots were epinephrine twice, followed by a long-acting epinephrine preparation. Nathan responded and was able to go home within an hour. He continued treatment with theophylline capsules and prednisone three times a day for a short period of time. This was the first time that he had an asthma episode and was not admitted to the hospital. We were so thrilled to be able to take our baby home the same night. It was beautiful not to have to go home to an empty crib. This was the beginning of learning about our son's asthma.

Nathan was fine for about a month and then he had another episode. This time our family doctor increased the theophylline dose but

Nathan couldn't tolerate the full amount. He got hyperactive and wouldn't sleep at night. He did calm down after it was reduced. The consulting pediatrician prescribed metaproterenol followed by cromolyn, both delivered by a compressor driven nebulizer three times a day. This amounts to a regular program of treatment and prevention at the same time.

Not long ago, my family doctor recommended that my husband and I attend the Parents' Asthma Group that was held in Amherst. We attended two two-hour sessions and are we glad we did. We learned a lot about asthma and how to detect episodes early and how to monitor these episodes. We also learned about various medicines used to treat asthma, their good effects and also their undesirable effects. It was good to share experiences with other parents: to hear what they were going through and how it affected them. It helps to know that we are not the only parents going through these problems.

In the beginning of Nathan's sickness, we feared for his life. At the Parents' Asthma Group we learned that it was rare for a child to die of asthma. Only one of every twenty-five thousand children with asthma die of it each year. If parents have adequate knowledge and see that their children get proper treatment, this tiny number will become smaller still.

Nathan is now 3 years old and doing much better. In the two years he has been on this new treatment plan, he hasn't needed to be admitted to the hospital once. He takes theophylline capsules twice a day except when he begins a cold, then I add another capsule at night. He takes metaproterenol and cromolyn by nebulizer three times a day. Since we've learned more about how to deal with Nathan's condition and he's been on this medication, he has gone as long as three months without an episode. Before he

was having them at least once a month. What an improvement!

■

Nathan's mom wrote this update in 1987, when Nathan was six years old.

In the past two years Nathan has had a tremendous improvement in his health. I am grateful for the knowledge I gained on how to deal with asthma and for the parents who shared their experiences on how to cope with asthma. It is nice to know that others have dealt with this problem. My husband David gives me a lot of support and help.

Nathan now has asthma episodes twice a year. He has one in the spring and one in the late fall. That is a real improvement from having an episode every other month. Nathan still takes a long-acting theophylline preparation three times a day. Recently he had an attack and we started giving metaproterenol by nebulizer four to six times a day. He also took prednisone twice a day for a week. After a couple days of treatment Nathan was fine and as playful and active as ever.

Nathan loves to ride his bike and play baseball with his three older brothers. He is excited about starting kindergarten this fall. I'm so happy with Nathan's progress. It is a relief not to be frantic and upset with worry if he does have an asthma episode. I believe the key to overcoming the problem of asthma is to detect it early and to give the child proper treatment.

Each child has different symptoms. In Nathan's case he will get itchy, usually behind his ears and on his chest, and he might be cranky for a couple of days. Then he will start symptoms of a cold and he'll start wheezing. Now that Nathan is getting older he knows when he starts to have trouble and he will come to me and ask for a nebulizer treatment.

Asthma is a problem, but as long as we know enough to treat it properly, we can go on and live normal happy lives. I am going to have my fifth baby this September. People have asked me, "Well, aren't you worried about your new baby having asthma?" Of course I hope and pray that this new baby will not have asthma. But I am not too worried, because my husband and I know how to deal with it.

■

I spoke with Nathan's mom in 1998, more than ten years after I last saw Nathan. He is now 17 and has excellent control over his asthma. During the past decade, he has not needed oral steroids or any urgent visits to a doctor or to be hospitalized for asthma. For the last five years, Nathan has taken no controller medicines. He plays on the high school basketball team and treats asthma symptoms with albuterol one or two games per year.

STORIES FROM THE 1990s

■

Karen Warren, age 22

The earliest memory that I have of asthma is the deafening sound of my own wheezing on the way to the doctor's office when I was ten years old. My chest ached and I wasn't getting any satisfaction from my attempts to gulp for air — it just wasn't there. Instead I took short, shallow breaths, which were equally unsatisfying. The next memory is the "green room" (my pediatrician had a "green room," a "yellow room" . . . etc.) where I cried as I received my first shot of adrenaline, and minutes later violently puked.

Following this first attack, I started taking theophylline (with applesauce). I still won't eat applesauce to this day. I took theophylline as directed for two weeks, and I was in the emergency room using a nebulizer four days after I stopped. The machine was terrifying and no one explained anything about what was going on. I think my parents aged more than I did that night.

Upon returning home from the emergency room I had a host of medicines to choose from: albuterol, cromolyn, theophylline . . . only we were never taught what each of the medications did, how much to take, when to take them. The cromolyn Spinhaler was not only a complete nuisance, but in addition, I hadn't been taught how to use it properly; half of the powder remained stuck in the tube, while the rest was choked out as I coughed upon inhaling.

Finally my parents thought it would be wise for me to see an allergist. One of my brothers had severe allergies, so perhaps, we thought, this was the missing link. After dozens of scratch tests and little blue-and-yellow bruises up and down my arms, they found that I was allergic to pollen, dust and mold spores. There went the carpet and my plants.

I was in junior high, and the albuterol seemed to be doing the job, with an occasional dosage of theophylline (although this left me nauseous and shaky). This regimen continued through high school, as I participated in soccer and had a rigorous, outdoor practice every afternoon. I recall taking the theophylline pills in the locker room; as long as I took them, I was all right, except when we did sprints. They sent me hacking and choking off the field.

During high school, I was in the emergency room again twice. Although the nebulizer was more familiar, I still didn't know how it was working to make me feel better.

My first semester at college was a nightmare. I visited the health services over half a dozen times that winter (in the middle of the night, of course) and became friends with the nebulizer. As far as the physicians were concerned, I was doing the right thing by coming in, but they had no advice for me on a long-term basis.

Consequently, I taught myself how to slow down an episode as I felt it coming on by taking small breaths and ceasing all activity. In addition, I learned to avoid situations, namely, any strenuous exercise, that would trigger my asthma. I felt frustrated and cheated by having to restrict my activity, and I often exceeded my limits. This stubborn behavior always resulted in moderate to severe attacks.

Now as I prepare to graduate, it seems I am back where I started. Since the flu last semester I have wheezed upon waking every morning. If I take an afternoon nap — I wheeze. And more recently, I have been unable to sleep through the night.

I drive to classes that are far away instead of having to deal with wheezing on the walk home. I have an inhaler at home, in my dorm, in my car . . . and I miss soccer and bike riding and the little things, like being able to take a really deep breath and feel satisfaction.

■

Karen came in for her first consultation in April 1993. She expressed these goals for her visit: "I would like to learn how to use the various pieces of asthma equipment properly — so I can best benefit from their use. In addition, I would like to feel that there can be an end to this restless-night, achy-chest, twelve-year pain in the butt."

I told Karen I expected her to achieve excellent control of her asthma, to have symptoms only rarely, and to be able to play any sport she wanted. We reviewed asthma in general and discussed asthma devices (holding chamber, peak flow meter, and peak flow diary), medicines, and environmental measures. I prescribed a seven-day burst of an oral steroid to be taken simultaneously with cromolyn and albuterol.

One week later, Karen reported she was sleeping through the night for the first time in three weeks. She woke without wheezing or coughing for the first time in six months and could laugh without coughing for the first time in a year. Karen stopped driving to her distant classes because she could now walk there without trouble.

In May 1993, one month after her initial visit, Karen came in for a follow-up visit. It had taken her seven days to recover from welding fumes in metal art class. She had a cold at the same time. I substituted an inhaled steroid for cromolyn as her controller medicine, and she improved steadily. She felt fine six days later.

In 1998, Karen told me that her asthma control is excellent. She has not taken oral steroids, nor has she visited an emergency room or an asthma doctor. She has missed no work due to asthma in the four years since her last visit. She stopped taking an inhaled steroid in 1996, and her only symptom at present is a slight wheeze when she has a cold. She is in excellent health, works out five days a week, and pretreats with albuterol prior to strenuous exercise.

■

Luke, age 7 months
Wendy Fulginiti

My son Luke is seven months old. Since his birth in August 1992, my husband and I have been telling the doctors that Luke coughs, sneezes and sounds very raspy, and occasionally spits up mucus. We were told this was normal for newborn infants.

At age 2 months, Luke developed a virus with a slight fever. After Luke was sick for three weeks, the doctor decided to run some X rays and lab work; all results were negative. At this time his coughing and spitting up mucus became much more pronounced. One afternoon when my mother was watching Luke, he was lying in his crib when my mom heard a violent cry from the other room. When she reached Luke, he was spitting up mucus and gasping for air. I called the doctor, who once again told me there was nothing wrong with Luke and that this was very normal for infants.

In early November 1992, we went back to the doctor, for a routine checkup. We discussed our concerns that Luke was still very raspy and coughing every few minutes throughout the day and night. I also voiced my concern that his eyes were awfully tearful. We were basically told that everything sounded clear and we should try not to worry about either of these concerns, because Luke was growing and appeared healthy. The doctor said, "If the coughing and sneezing continue when Luke is about a year old, we will run some tests on him." At this point I became so frustrated that I asked, "Could this be asthma or allergies?" I received no response other than, again, "I do not hear a wheeze. He really is too young to detect allergies." I decided to call the Second Opinion Clinic at Boston Children's Hospital. The doctor there agreed that the symptoms might be either asthma or allergies, but at Luke's age it was really difficult to determine. The doctor gave us some soybean formula to try.

At this point, we did not know where to continue in this battle, but we kept searching for the answers. During Thanksgiving, we discussed that we needed to find another pediatrician, one who would listen to our concerns and not make us feel like paranoid parents. Right after Christmas, my parents left for three weeks on vacation. When they returned in January 1993, my mother commented, "I can't believe Luke is still coughing and he sounds worse!" I agreed. I knew at this point that I had to find some answers to this grim situation.

Luke woke up the next Saturday much more congested. He was coughing non-stop (he could not catch his breath between coughs) and he was sneezing every few minutes. So we decided to take him to Boston Children's emergency room.

This visit became an eye opener. The doctor told us that Luke was coughing at an abnormal rate but that he did not know why. When the doctor listened to Luke's chest, everything sounded fine. However, when he timed Luke's breaths on his watch he felt that Luke was breathing slightly quicker than normal. The doctor recommended we contact an allergist and a lung specialist, and in the meantime gave him an antihistaminic to see if it would calm the cough. At this point, Luke was waking up on and off all night.

Two days later, I called the doctor's office and requested to see another pediatrician. Tuesday morning we went to see a new doctor. The doctor listened to our concerns. During the examination, she detected a slight wheeze and agreed that Luke was breathing slightly quicker than normal. The doctor explained to us that she wanted to try giving albuterol by nebulizer. We administered this to Luke and after 20 minutes, she came back to recheck him. The wheeze was gone and Luke's breathing had returned to normal. The doctor gave us referrals to see a lung specialist and an allergist. She prescribed cromoyln to be administered by compressor driven nebulizer. This was approximately three weeks ago. The lung specialist advised us to continue on this treatment and to return in two months for a follow-up appointment.

The allergist ran some allergy and lab tests and told us that if the test results proved positive, she would contact us for further consultation. Neither specialist would commit themselves that Luke may have asthma. At this point, my sister recommended that I read *Children With Asthma: A Manual for Parents* because she went through a similar experience with her daughter who has asthma.

After reading the book, I became even more frustrated, because I realized that Luke had very similar situations to some of the children in the book. Plus, I discovered that the nurse told us a very different way of using the compressor driven nebulizer than how the book explained to use it. We feel very frustrated over this whole situation. All we would like for our son is to determine what is wrong . . . and what we can do to help him. My husband and I feel so helpless. Presently, Luke is still coughing and sneezing throughout the day and night.

Luke has spent numerous hours with many different doctors, all of whom did not significantly help him. We were told nothing was wrong with our son, even though he coughed all day and night. Before our first appointment with you, we read *Children With Asthma,* which talks about asthma children like Luke, and we started filling out an Asthma Signs Diary, which helped us monitor Luke's condition.

■

When Wendy brought Luke in for his first visit in March 1993, she came with these written goals:

I would like to learn how to prevent my son from coughing and sneezing, without being a nervous mother. I would like to know if my son has asthma and if so learn everything I need to know to help him. I would like to see my son not coughing and not so stressed when I give him his medicine.

■

Wendy later wrote an account of that first visit, and the changes that she and her husband made in Luke's care after our discussion.

At the time of our first consultation, when Luke was 8 months old, my husband and I were unclear about asthma in general, and we were very frustrated over the chain of events we were experiencing with our other doctors.

At the first visit, we reviewed Luke's Asthma Signs Diary for the previous two weeks. He had had a cough every day. His total signs score usually ranged between two and five. You asked my husband and me to show how we administered Luke's cromolyn using the nebulizer. As we watched Luke we realized immediately that he was not getting much of the medicine. It was escaping from the top and sides of the mask. At that point we decided to use a mouthpiece with the nebulizer instead of a mask. We doubled his dose of cromolyn, added albuterol to the solution, and gave him prednisolone (an oral steroid) for seven days.

You recommended that we purchase several items to reduce dust within the household. We encased Luke's crib mattress in an allergy-type encasing, we bought a HEPA air filter for the bedroom, and we began keeping the dog out of the bedroom. All of these changes have improved our son's well being. We now have the knowledge, confidence and skills to keep our son from having major asthma problems. When Luke gets very excited, or if the weather is nasty, he still coughs. However, my husband and I have learned not to panic. If Luke continues to cough, we increase his dose of albuterol and try to eliminate the triggers. Luke is a very happy child. When he becomes cranky, his asthma usually needs attention.

■

Two weeks later, Luke came in for a second visit. He was doing extremely well taking daily cromolyn and albuterol. His parents had kept an Asthma Signs Diary each day, which showed that his sign scores had greatly improved (decreased). His parents had purchased a HEPA filter which seemed to be soaking up the cigarette smoke from the downstairs neighbors. They started using the Pari-Jet nebulizer and found that it has cut the total amount of time it takes to give four ampules of cromolyn each day from sixty to thirty minutes.

At Luke's appointment three months later, Wendy wrote, "We have gained vast amounts of knowledge on asthma. Our son is one hundred percent better than he was in February." At age 2, Luke stopped taking cromolyn by compressor driven nebulizer and started taking an inhaled steroid by holding chamber with mask.

At age 5, Luke takes an inhaled steroid daily and albuterol as needed for symptoms. His dad reports that Luke's asthma control has been good for the preceding year. He made two urgent visits to the doctor and needed two short treatments with an oral steroid. He has not had any major problems since the summer and has been able to play outside in the winter for long periods of time.

■

Erin Freed, age 34

I have had asthma for as long as I can remember. Both my parents dealt with it mostly as something I was probably exaggerating, because my sister Kerry obviously had it much worse. Kerry actually did get diagnosed by a doctor and got treatment. My parents didn't consider treatment for me . . . except the treatment of trying to get me to give up the act.

I only had asthma problems at a certain time of the year. I grew up believing that it was hay fever more than asthma. My father was allergic to ragweed, so I figured it was something like that. I believed that if I could only stay away from whatever it was out there that I was allergic to, I'd feel great. I never thought that it might be our household entourage of hairy mammals — we always had one dog and two cats — that were causing these problems.

One incident sticks in my mind. When I was about 9 or 10, I was wheezing so badly I couldn't practice my French horn. I felt under pressure because my father was the premier horn teacher in town, and he didn't believe I really had asthma. My mom called me into the living room to set up my chair and music stand so that my father could tell whether or not I was actually wheezing. After many doubtful glares, he gave me permission to forego practice that day.

For treatment, my father suggested playing the horn as much as I could when I was breathing well, so as to build strength in my lungs. Thus I developed a "no treatment, just tough it out" approach to my asthma. I remember during the height of my asthma and allergy season in August, I stayed at home wheezing and drinking mint tea. I was convinced that there was nothing I could do to help it. It would go away.

During my college years, I remember having attack after attack of asthma. Usually they were associated with exercise or exposure to cold air, dust, mold, cats, dogs, or horses. I remember bike trips when I could not keep up with my friends because I'd have to stop for ten minutes every so often to catch my breath. I remember allergy seasons beginning mid-August and lasting clear through September when I would stay inside as much as possible and try to open my lungs with herb tea. I remember climbing a mountain one day with some friends, wheezing heavily and using every bit of my strength to make it to the top. When I finally got there, I was amazed that so many other people were up there too, merrily bouncing around as if it had been no ordeal at all for them to have climbed up. Duh. You would have thought I would have gone to the doctor to find out what was wrong with me, but still I didn't.

It wasn't until I started having babies that my bouts with wheezing and sneezing turned into annual four-month battles with "bronchitis" and "pneumonia." The only treatment prescribed by my doctor was theophylline. The trouble would begin with hay fever in August, develop into a constant sinus drip during September, and then, wham, with the first cold of the season, I'd be flat on my back for three weeks with full-fledged bronchitis, green sputum and everything. If I recovered by Thanksgiving, I would still have one or two more episodes before the winter was out. Since I am the main breadwinner in my family, this created a serious problem. I began to fear using sick time for anything but real, bona fide mega-illness. It never occurred to me that there might be effective treatment out there beyond chicken soup and heavy doses of theophylline for an attack. I'm still very allergic to dogs and cats, and especially to houses in which dust and animal dander are allowed to build up. I also get symptoms with exercise and cold air.

■

At the time of Erin's first consultation, she was having ten episodes per year, the worst ones from August through November. Her physical examination was normal except that her peak flow score increased 10 percent after taking

two puffs of albuterol. I prescribed prednisone for seven days, an inhaled steroid, and albuterol. Two weeks later she no longer was waking at night nor did she have a cough. She wrote the rest of her narrative after beginning her new treatment.

■

What broke the cycle of illness in my life was a combination of events: I started using an inhaled steroid and a bronchodilator (albuterol) on a regular basis. I started taking vitamin C, learned about asthma, and began identifying the things that trigger my attacks and my periods of poor health. I also began exercising, usually running two miles a day.

I still have to deal with the attitude lock that my parents have been in since the beginning. They continue to believe that I exaggerate my symptoms when I visit them (their house is perennially covered with a soft layer of golden retriever hair). They get offended when my husband (he has asthma, too) and I bring our air cleaner with us when we visit.

■

In March 1998, five years after Erin's previous visit, she came in for a review of her status. Her asthma control is good and only interferes with activity two times a month or less. She is moderately satisfied with her ability to control asthma. She currently takes an inhaled steroid daily and albuterol as needed. She has a full-time job as a quality-systems supervisor and with her husband shares the responsibilities for their three children and the household.

Cynthia Miller, age 65

I lived in New York City until I was 5 years old. The summer I turned 4, I spent my birthday in bed with a cough. During the winters of '37, '38, and '39, I was often bedridden with bronchitis. My health must have been "fragile" as I had to rest a lot.

Ages 11, 12, and 13, I spent summers in Long Island, with lots of bike riding, swimming and tennis. Riding horseback, I always liked to ride up front to avoid the dust. On damp, muggy, still days, I always had trouble breathing. I had all sorts of tests, including allergy tests, which were positive for dust and mold. I was given no specific medicine or shots for allergies and was advised to sleep on a foam pillow.

I remember always needing my nap in the afternoon in May and early June. Muggy nights in May and June found me kneeling by the window with my nose pressed against the screen trying to get "more air." I was always very athletic, playing hockey, soccer, tennis, basketball, swimming competitively, and riding a horse and a bike. Only muggy air slowed me down. I have had sinusitis two or more times a year since childhood and rhinitis which I have treated with inhaled steroids for the past six years.

Between the ages of 20 and 60, I was married to a man who smoked four packs of cigarettes a day. The smell of cigarette smoke brings on sneezing and choking along with coughing. I don't wheeze very often.

At present, I have great trouble sleeping in an airless room, or exercising in humidity or heat. I keep the heat low in winter, since air blowing on me bothers me. When we changed from oil/hot air heat to gas/baseboard heat, I started sleeping better and choked less.

My coughing spasms can often come on unexpectedly. In one case I had just visited a huge indoor flower market. The next day I was in the hospital because of breathing trouble.

For the past six months, I have been aware of every breath. Last summer, I noticed I could not ride my bike in the heat. I could not breathe properly. The day I came down with this "bronchitis," I noticed a restriction in my lungs at the end of a deep breath in while I was biking uphill. The next day I was out of breath and could not walk uphill without gasping for air. This lasted for a week.

I want to learn whatever is necessary, including changes in my lifestyle, to ward off attacks. I want to familiarize myself with "clues" indicating an approaching problem, and if an attack starts, know how to immediately start remedying the situation. As a result of new knowledge and skills, I hope to gain confidence in dealing with my asthma problems.

■

Cynthia had a history of breathing problems for sixty years. She had been diagnosed with bronchitis three or four times a year and was hospitalized once for pneumonia in 1986. She was first diagnosed with asthma two weeks before her first visit with me and was treated with inhaled albuterol, an antibiotic, and a cough medicine.

A physical examination showed that Cynthia had signs of both asthma and sinusitis. I assessed her to have mild to moderate persistent asthma since childhood. I suggested that she read further about asthma, reduce triggers in her environment, and monitor peak flow. I instructed her in the use of a peak flow meter, holding chamber, and the technique of nasal irrigation (for her sinusitis). I also prescribed an oral steroid, an inhaled steroid, and albuterol, and I treated her for rhinitis and sinusitis.

Three weeks after her initial appointment, she said the improvement in her condition was "fantastic." She had kicked the dog and the cat out of the bedroom and had gotten rid of the carpeting to reduce allergens. She started using a mask for allergenic or dusty environments, purchased a HEPA air filter and vacuum cleaner, bought a filter for the furnace, and watched the asthma video I loaned her. Her cough had disappeared in four days, her mild wheeze had disappeared in five days, and her activity had returned to normal in about seven days. During the first week of treatment, she had occasional difficulty with sleep (probably due to the oral steroid). She found the nasal washes helpful. She felt like her old energetic self for the first time in many years.

Three months after her initial consultation, Cynthia wrote this update.

Having had pneumonia twice and severe "bronchitis" many times, I believe I had an unconscious fear of doing "top performance" — whether riding my bike as fast as I could go or hiking hills at a faster pace. Now the unconscious fear in my breathing is put at rest. My last asthma attack awoke me in a rage of coughing and choking. It was scary but I knew what to do. I finally have a handle on my own management, something I never had before.

My mind and body have been freed from a fear that I have had since I was a young child. Knowledge of asthma has given me the confidence to exercise more fully. Now that I know what to expect, my inner self no longer constantly asks me "what could happen if . . . ?" All this frees up a lot more energy and as I enjoy doing so many things, I find I have been able to move "smoothly" and joyously from one to an-

other. There are no more daily interruptions by breathing problems.

The knowledge and skills I have gained in the past four months enable me to feel free and secure in any place I go. I can now hike three miles without getting out of breath. I feel like the "little engine that could." I went up to the barn yesterday and did not bring my mask, as I did not realize how horribly dusty everything was. My breathing worsened immediately. My problem is I feel so good that I forget I have asthma and forget to carry my mask always with me. I must remind myself!

■

When we spoke in 1998, Cynthia reported that her asthma control continues to be excellent with the treatment plan we had worked out.

■

Daniel Rodriguez, age 45

My asthma was first diagnosed after I moved to Amherst, Massachusetts from New York City in 1973. Prior to that time, I did not have any respiratory problems. Over the years, the occasional episode has become a chronic condition.

For a long time I have been aware that my asthma appears to be very inconsistent. Sometimes when I am with cats I sneeze and have a tightness in the chest, other times there is no reaction. I can be under great stress and my asthma is fine, other times when I feel little stress I have asthma symptoms. It has been very hard to figure out how to improve the asthma because the asthma has seemed too unpredictable.

I know that there are certain triggers for me: when I am physically tired, emotionally upset, have a cold, or am in dusty areas. Pollutants, cold air, exercise, and allergens also trigger my asthma. I have tried to remain healthy and have, except for symptoms of diabetes that my doctor feels are directly related to my oral steroid use (prednisone, 5 to 30 mg daily for the past three years). I maintain a physically active lifestyle, have major professional responsibilities, and engage in social and sports activities.

I have, however, been unable to get off the prednisone except for a month or two in the past three years. The asthma almost always is a difficulty late in the day and during sleep. I wake up coughing almost every night. I use the prednisone in the evening generally before going to sleep.

In the 1980s I was hospitalized between twelve and fifteen times for asthma. My last hospitalization was in 1990 for pneumonia. I had one emergency visit in the past twelve months. I take prednisone, theophylline, and cromolyn every day. I also use metaproterenol by compressor driven nebulizer four times a day and albuterol by metered dose inhaler. I play tennis and swim, but about twice a month I have to lie down to rest because I don't have enough strength to walk. I wake up coughing almost every night. My peak flows before medicines were 100 to 160 in the three days before this visit. I have never used a holding chamber.

In 1988 I was seen by an allergist, who said my asthma was intractable. My pulmonary function test results were between 30 and 40 percent of normal in spite of my being treated very aggressively with prednisone. I had an enormous exposure to cat, dog, and horse dander as well as to dust and molds. I did not want to limit my exposure to my animals. For the next few years I administered epinephrine to myself by injection about twice a day.

The asthma attacks themselves are less severe than they used to be — fewer emergency room visits — but I have not been successful at reducing the drugs. Three times I have tried allergy shots and once I was put on methotrexate but stopped it because I noticed no effect.

My goal for this consultation is to reduce or eliminate my need for prednisone and to improve my asthma control. I have symptoms four to six times per day, and I have missed six to eight work days in the past year.

■

During the first consultation, Daniel blew a peak flow score of 320 after inhaling albuterol, a very low score for a man his height. My physical exam showed that he wheezed both when breathing in and breathing out. I observed Daniel using his inhaler and realized that he had a unique and completely ineffective technique for taking medicine: he put the metered dose inhaler mouthpiece in his mouth, then actuated three puffs of medicine in a row while taking a single breath, breathing in further with each puff. After this three-second maneuver, he held his breath for three seconds.

I explained and demonstrated proper use of an MDI: position the inhaler two inches away from the mouth, start to breathe in, and then release *one* puff of medicine; continue breathing in for five seconds, then hold your breath for ten seconds. Following this instruction, Daniel inhaled one puff of albuterol correctly. At that point he remarked "I really feel it. My breathing is better."

I taught him how to use a peak flow meter, the Asthma Peak Flow Diary, and a holding chamber; I also advised him to spend more time breathing in than breathing out when using his compressor driven nebulizer.

Given his asthma history and the physical exam, I assessed Daniel to have severe persistent asthma. I prescribed a high dose of prednisone (an oral steroid), an inhaled steroid, and substituted albuterol for the metaproterenol, which he was taking by compressor driven nebulizer. I did not change his cromolyn or theophylline dose. I suggested that he encase his mattress and pillows, keep the humidity between 25 and 50 percent, and buy dust-trapping bags for his vacuum cleaner.

Two weeks later, Daniel was able to blow a peak flow score of 640, twice the score he achieved at his first visit. I reduced his albuterol dose and switched him to an alternate-day schedule for taking the oral steroid to reduce the adverse effects. He started exercising for an hour a day, including thirty minutes of swimming. He felt no wheeze, observed no cough, and was sleeping through the night without symptoms.

Since I do not provide continuing care for patients with severe asthma, I referred Daniel to an allergist. I last talked to Daniel in 1998. He recounted that he had been hospitalized for one night in 1993 and three nights in 1996, and he had one urgent visit for asthma in the past five years. Two years after seeing me he had gradually gone off of prednisone, and he had needed that medicine for a total of only eight days in the preceding year.

The addition of a new asthma medicine (salmeterol) to Daniel's medicine routine in 1994 greatly reduced his symptoms. He now takes an inhaled steroid, salmeterol, and occasionally albuterol. Daniel often goes hiking and riding, but no longer loads hay or brushes his horses. His asthma does wake him up at night about three times a month, but it rarely interferes with his physical activity.

■

Shoshana, age 20 months
Tamara Barbasch

Shoshana has had troubles resulting from "allergies" since her birth in October 1992. Although these problems always fell within the "mild" range, they were troublesome to us because they were chronic: no matter what we did, they always returned. I began to notice her eczema when she was approximately one month old, and her skin was dry, rough, and prone to patches of redness or small, reddish bumps. Although she was completely breast-fed until she was 5 months old, she would "break out," especially on her cheeks, shortly after nursing — so I realized that she was reacting to the foods that I had eaten prior to her nursing.

In February of 1994, when Shoshana was 16 months old, she developed a cold with typical symptoms of nasal congestion and postnasal drip. On the fourth or fifth day, she became unusually irritable, demanding, clingy, and inconsolable. She cried repeatedly throughout the day in response to tiny problems which would otherwise never bother her (something dropped on the floor). This constellation of behaviors remains, to this day, as the most significant clue that an asthma episode is developing. At the time, however, I was unaware of its significance.

Later that day, Shoshana began to breathe rapidly and laboriously. I thought that she was simply congested and having difficulty breathing because of her stuffed-up nose. Shortly, the labored breathing developed into an audible wheeze. By this time, Shoshana was crying continuously, had developed a fever, and had vomited her dinner. At the pediatrician's office, we were told that Shoshana was probably having an asthma attack (she responded with some improvement to an updraft treatment of albuterol) and that she would have to be hospitalized that night. We spent two days at the hospital, learning about asthma (reading *Children With Asthma* over and over), and learning how to use a compressor driven nebulizer machine. Shoshana was given albuterol and prednisolone and was kept inside an oxygen tent. Her condition had improved within twenty-four hours. We continued the medicines, tapering as directed, for one week.

After this episode, we watched very carefully. I fantasized that the incident requiring hospitalization (which was extremely difficult for all of us) was a "fluke" and that Shoshana did not really have asthma at all. In fact, in mid-March Shoshana developed cold symptoms again without any asthma symptoms, so I was almost convinced that it would not happen again.

On April 25, 1994, during Shoshana's 18-month well visit to the pediatrician, her doctor detected mild bronchospasm and prescribed albuterol updraft treatments two to three times per day for several days. Although she had been exhibiting cold symptoms, Shoshana had given no indication that she was experiencing any difficulty breathing. I was still not convinced.

In early May, however, Shoshana began to exhibit a "cold" that lasted for five weeks or so. We now believe that this was allergic rhinitis in response to the pollination of trees in our area at that time. On May 13, the nasal congestion and nasal drip symptoms led to mild wheezing and coughing, which we treated with albuterol by compressor driven nebulizer. She then developed an upper respiratory infection, with a fever of 104 degrees, and more asthma symptoms. On May 25, Shoshana had moderate asthma symptoms and was prescribed prednisolone in addition to albuterol. Her pediatrician recommended and prescribed cromolyn to be taken daily, but I was hesitant because I was still not quite convinced that she needed daily medicine. She was having asthma symptoms less than once a week.

If she developed asthma only when she had nasal congestion and a nasal drip, I reasoned, then we should treat the symptoms as they appeared.

Shoshana's most recent experience with asthma, developing on June 20, has somehow led me to alter my thoughts regarding her treatment. Again, during this most recent episode, she had developed cold symptoms, otitis media in both ears (requiring antibiotic treatment), and asthma symptoms. The wheezing was particularly "stubborn" this time. We gave her albuterol by nebulizer thirteen times in twenty-four hours, yet she showed little improvement. The next day, we began administering prednisolone again.

I have finally realized that Shoshana's asthma is not going to simply "disappear," although, of course, I wish that it would! It is painful to see her suffer each time, and watch our child become "a different person" as she regresses to a crying, clinging, inconsolable "mess." The frequent albuterol treatments and prednisolone administrations have become much more difficult as Shoshana enters into a developmental period typical of toddlers, wherein she refuses to comply with absolutely anything we wish to have her do.

You made an excellent point during our telephone conversation when you said that parents must believe that their child needs to take a medicine that tastes terrible or causes discomfort. If they are not convinced, the child will sense their ambivalence and often refuse to take it. With Shoshana, I believe that part of the problem does have to do with exactly this fact: I have never felt entirely comfortable with what we have been doing.

The second part of the problem, however, is a result of her extreme mood and behavior changes during an acute asthma episode, which contribute further to her "negativism" in complying with any treatments. I find this part of the entire situation the most frustrating. When I am trying to help my child and she is spitting pred-nisolone all over me or vigorously struggling against me as I am trying to force the nebulizer mouthpiece to her lips, I feel hopeless, dejected, angry, frustrated, and depressed.

I have had enough of "reactive" treatment methods: I wish to treat my daughter's asthma "proactively" and prevent any further episodes, if possible. If cromolyn, the asthma "wonder drug," will work to do that, then I am ready to use it! My husband and I are both highly educated, highly motivated individuals who are interested in learning the details of how to make a treat-ment plan work properly. So I am appealing to you for some assistance in helping us to learn exactly what to do, how to do it, and why we are doing it — in order to make it work!

■

At the first consultation, I told Shoshana's par-ents that if they need to give more than six treatments of albuterol by compressor driven nebulizer in twenty-four hours during Shoshana's episode, that is a sign that the asthma is worsening or that their technique for giving medicine is ineffective. I showed them how to use a compressor driven nebulizer and watched Shoshana take a treatment. Even with the mouthpiece properly placed, mist contin-ued to come out of the top of the nebulizer cup both during inspiration and expiration. Usually, mist comes out only during expiration. When a child is inhaling and breathing the medicine mist into her lungs, you should not see mist es-cape. Clearly, Shoshana was not inhaling the medicine. What was wrong? We realized that Shoshana was breathing through her nose and no medicine was entering her mouth. So, I rec-ommended using the compressor driven nebu-lizer with a mask instead of a mouthpiece.

After recording Shoshana's asthma signs in a diary each day, her parents realized that she needed to take a controller medicine and started to give cromolyn by compressor driven nebulizer. Three months later they wrote this letter to me.

In the three months after her initial visit, Shoshana had two episodes of asthma. We found that delivering albuterol by nebulizer with mask was much more effective than using a mouth-piece. At this point, our pediatrician recom-mended a holding chamber with mask to give medicine. We were impressed with the small amount of time necessary for administration (which is extremely important when working with a toddler!) and the speed of the outcome. Within minutes after we administered albuterol, a wheeze would entirely disappear. Shoshana herself (23 months old) claimed that it made her "feel better," and she would ask for the inhaler herself when she began to feel uncomfortable. She very rarely, if ever, resisted using the holding chamber, in contrast to the nebulizer machine, which sometimes had elicited huge screaming fits. We were also happy with the holding cham-ber's portability and its effects on our mobility during Shoshana's asthma episodes.

After a four-week trial of giving cromolyn by compressor driven nebulizer, we switched over to an inhaled steroid, at her pediatrician's sug-gestion. Since then we have not had to use any prednisolone syrup and have not had any sleep-less nights filled with Shoshana's crying and mis-ery. She truly does seem to have asthma that falls into the mild range, and we are so glad to have determined that only a minimal amount of medicine is necessary.

I spoke with Shoshana's mother on the phone in 1998. She said that Shoshana's asthma control has been excellent for the past year. Now 6 years old, she has taken no oral steroids, has had no urgent visits to the doctor, emergency room, or the hospital, nor has she missed school. She continues to take a very low daily dose of an inhaled steroid by holding chamber with mask.

■

Jeffrey Wolfman, age 38

I was born in Oakland, California. At approximately 18 months, I was diagnosed with asthma. Both of my parents smoked and continued smoking until the mid 1960s. To the best of my recollection, I did not take any medications until elementary school. I was taken to the local hospital emergency room on numerous occasions for treatment whenever an asthma attack occurred.

I was an active, athletic child, always able to keep up with others in school sports. I played varsity basketball, soccer, and was on the ski team in high school. I attended college in Colorado, where I was involved in intramural sports. I placed 15th out of 70 in a bicycle race from Colorado Springs to Aspen in 1973. I took a combination medicine containing theophylline, ephedrine, and an antihistamine for my asthma from the time I was in elementary school until age 30.

I have always had difficulties with allergies and eczema. I was treated for my allergies through injection therapy during elementary school in California and then most recently for five years (1988–1992) in Boston.

At age 30 (1984), my doctor changed my medicine to theophylline. Seven years later, my doctor changed my brands of theophylline and quick relief medicine and added an antihistamine. This year I started taking a different antihistamine and started using an inhaled steroid.

In November of 1992, I was asked to participate in an experiment at Beth Israel Hospital,

testing the effect of cold air on asthmatic lungs and the relative recovery time to restore normal breathing after using various inhaled medicines. The study required that the subjects take no medicine of any type for twenty-four hours prior to the test. After fifteen hours without medicine, my bronchial passages became severely constricted, and my lung capacity did not even register on the peak flow meter. Normal breathing was restored after administering albuterol.

I have a number of allergies to certain foods, trees and grasses, and dust and animal dander. To deal with a drastic emergencies, I carry an EpiPen with me at all times. Over the last two years, I have begun to have noticeable difficulty breathing and have felt that my respiratory capacity has diminished significantly. I have become very sensitive to smoke, perfume, soaps, and a variety of environmental substances, pollen and dust in particular. Any minor physical activity, even climbing a flight of stairs, leaves me winded and feeling the need for asthma medicine.

During my consultation, I hope that I may be able to better understand the problems I have been experiencing and the changes in my asthma, and to develop a treatment plan using appropriate medicines that will allow me to resume some of my normal activities. I would like to have greater endurance with the least amount of medicine possible.

■

At Jeffrey's first asthma consultation, we discussed additional details of his asthma history. He had taken prednisone only once, in 1989, for nine days, and had no emergency room visits or hospitalizations for respiratory problems in the past twelve months. His family had a history of eczema, asthma, and hay fever. Jeffrey did not use a holding chamber to take his medicines. During the month prior to his first appointment, his peak flow score never exceeded

375 before taking a quick relief medicine, a low score for a man his age and height.

After some coaching during the physical examination, Jeffrey was able to blow a peak flow score of 550 before inhaling albuterol. His chest was clear. He demonstrated how he took his inhaler: he held the MDI at his mouth, began to breathe in, and simultaneously released one puff of medicine. He took two seconds to breathe in, then held his breath for six seconds. Both his inhalation and breath hold were too short for him to get the full benefit from his medicine. He also took his inhaled steroid before his beta$_2$-agonist (quick relief medicine), another error.

I assessed Jeffrey to have moderate persistent asthma that had required daily medicine since elementary school. Over the past two years, he had found that his tolerance to exercise and pollutants had decreased. He was taking an inhaled steroid, theophylline, pirbuterol (a quick relief medicine), and an antihistamine daily. He had not been properly instructed in use of the metered dose inhaler, holding chamber, asthma diary, or a peak flow meter, nor did he know which inhaler to use first. He did not know how long it took for his medicines to work or how long their effects lasted.

At the first visit, I recommended that Jeffrey add an oral steroid to his current medicines for the next seven days. This additional treatment would help clear his airways, reduce symptoms, and let him establish his personal best peak flow. I showed him the proper technique for using his inhaler and demonstrated use of the holding chamber with MDI.

Nine days later, Jeffrey came in for a second visit. He reported that he had taken his medicine as directed and started feeling better in two days. He felt more physically able than at any time in the past four years. Prior to his visit, he could not push his 10-month-old uphill in a carriage, nor he could roughhouse with his 3-year-old son. Most of his activities with his 3-year-old were "housebound" like reading and coloring. But at the time of his second visit, he was running with his family and was able to climb three flights of stairs at work or walk a mile and a half across a college campus without being tired. He had not used a quick relief medicine at night since starting the oral steroid burst. His 10-month-old, not his asthma, was waking him three times a night.

At a four-month follow-up visit, Jeffrey said he had no symptoms and that his asthma control was excellent. His personal best peak flow score was 650. Four years later, in 1998, his asthma control continued to be excellent. He was taking a low dose of an inhaled steroid and using albuterol daily. He was walking a mile a day and swimming regularly with his kids.

Chapter Two

The Basics of Asthma

You must work closely with a competent doctor to control your asthma safely and effectively. The information in this chapter can give you the asthma knowledge you need to communicate well with your doctor.

Asthma treatment has improved for almost everyone. If you live with asthma, the best you can feel today is much better than the best you could have felt five or ten years ago. But to achieve these results, you will have to learn what provokes your asthma and how these triggers work together to make you sick. You will need to learn how asthma works in your body and how to judge whether you have it under control.

Our understanding of asthma has changed greatly in the past ten years, as have the medicines and tools for treating it, raising our expectations for the results of asthma care. We now consider the primary problem in asthma to be inflammation of the airways. Inflammation causes the airway lining to swell inward, reducing the space left for air to flow. Bronchoconstriction, the tightening of the muscles around

the airways, plays an important but secondary role in asthma.

There are two types of asthma severity: overall severity and the severity of an episode. "Overall severity" classifies your asthma situation based on symptoms you have had over a period of weeks while your asthma was not being treated. This classification guides your long-term treatment plan. The severity of a given episode is determined by the degree to which your airflow is reduced and how intense your symptoms are during that episode. You adjust immediate treatment based on the severity of each episode. A person with mild asthma can have episodes that are mild, moderate, or severe. The same is true for people with moderate or severe asthma.

Many factors can trigger, or start, an asthma episode. A trigger may be a substance, a weather condition, or an activity. Allergens (specific substances that cause an allergic reaction) are the most important group of triggers for people with asthma. You can reduce your asthma symptoms by eliminating or reducing the presence of allergens and other triggers in your environment. Exercise is also an important trigger, but one you should not avoid. It usually causes trouble only if you are not following an adequate treatment plan.

Understanding asthma and learning to control it is not a casual task. You need to understand many pieces of the asthma puzzle before you can effectively and safely put them together. Common sense may not give you the right answer if your reasoning is based on incomplete knowledge. I suggest that my patients listen to advice only from experienced health professionals or from people who have read this book or the *Practical Guidelines for the Diagnosis and Management of Asthma.*

What Is Asthma?

If you have asthma, your airways narrow in response to various triggers, such as respiratory infections, allergens, and pollutants. We now know that inflammation is the primary culprit in this reaction. It narrows the airways by causing swelling, predisposes the airways to bronchoconstriction (the tightening of the smooth muscles that surround the airways), and increases the production of mucus.

If you have asthma, your airways are inflamed much of the time. Because your airways react to pollutants and other triggers more quickly and more easily than normal ones, we say that they are hyperresponsive. Your level of inflammation may change with the season, the environment, or with your medical condition or medicines you are taking. Even when you have no symptoms, the inflammation may be present in your airways, making you vulnerable to asthma triggers. We now know that long-term, untreated inflammation can also cause permanent changes in the structure and function of the lungs.

Expectations

You can control your asthma. You can eliminate all or almost all of your asthma symptoms. But in order to reach that point, you will have to know what it feels like to breathe normally. Until you know this, you will be unable to set your goal. That is why I say that low expectations (both by doctors and by patients) are the major cause of inadequately controlled asthma.

Almost everyone who lives with asthma can reduce their symptoms dramatically within two weeks after starting an effective treatment program. If you have mild or moderate asthma, you should be able to achieve excellent control of your asthma symptoms in one to three months. If you have severe asthma, your symptoms should decrease noticeably within two weeks. It may take two to six months of treatment, often trying combinations of several medicines, before you achieve the best control possible.

What were you conditioned to expect from your asthma? If you have been hospitalized ten times in the past fifteen years, you probably expect to be hospitalized again. If you have experienced a cough and wheeze for the past few years when you climb a single flight of stairs, you probably think that you have no choice but to tolerate this handicapped state. If your brother and sister had serious asthma problems in childhood, you may expect the same for your child who was just diagnosed with asthma. But the treatment of asthma has improved greatly. If you believe you can eliminate symptoms, you can do what it takes to accomplish this task. If you resign yourself to frequent symptoms, you will make no progress.

Many doctors provide good asthma care and many do not. A doctor who received specific training in asthma treatment and who cares for many patients with asthma will usually have a greater understanding of asthma and higher expectations for control of asthma. He should be able to estimate how long it will take for you to achieve excellent long-term asthma control. Your doctor's expectations are extremely important to your well being. Doctors, like patients, need to know what to expect from asthma and its treatment: what results are possible with intensive medical and environmental treatment, how long it should take for symptoms to clear, when to look for complications, when to review treatment techniques, and when to refer for a second opinion.

If you do not show a significant improvement within the expected time, you should discuss it with your doctor or seek a second opinion from an asthma specialist. Of course, no doctor can help you unless you do your share of the job: making environmental changes, taking medicine using good technique, and tracking your progress on a well-designed diary.

Short-term expectations are also important. Ask your doctor to estimate the time it will take for your medicines to start to work and how long it should take you to recover from an asthma episode. For example, if you are having difficulty breathing, you should know that your inhaled beta$_2$-agonist medicine usually works in five minutes. If it doesn't, don't wait half an hour for improvement. Instead, increase the intensity of your treatment according to your written plan or call your doctor. Proper expectations enable you to change treatment promptly and prevent an episode from worsening. If you are having an acute episode and start treatment right away, symptoms usually will start to improve within hours and should disappear within seven days. Call your doctor if this improvement does not occur.

Most doctors have taken care of many people with asthma. They have treated hundreds or thousands of asthma episodes. Almost every primary care physician (pediatrician, family care practitioner or internist) has had the experience of rescuing a patient who is frightened, wheezing, and breathing with great difficulty. Within minutes after the doctor gives inhaled medicine to dilate the airways, the patient's distress is relieved. The patient is grateful and praises the physician's good work. The physician is pleased that the patient improved so rapidly.

I tell doctors that it's all right to accept a patient's praise for clearing a serious asthma episode. But if an episode occurs a second time, it means the doctor and patient have not worked out a treatment plan that enables the patient to prevent episodes or to treat them earlier.

If your doctor believes that almost everyone with asthma can achieve excellent control over it, he will not rest until that has been accomplished or has been proved impossible. A good asthma doctor will keep up with the principles and techniques of treatment and carefully analyze your response to treatment. No patient with asthma symptoms should settle for less than excellent control until all of the current treatment methods have been tried.

Excellent Asthma Control

When you achieve excellent control of your asthma, you:

- have symptoms two or fewer times per week.
- can prevent almost all asthma episodes.
- rarely require urgent treatment for asthma from a doctor or emergency room staff.

- rarely miss school or work because of asthma.
- can exercise as hard and as long as you want.

In the 1980s, less than half of people with asthma could achieve this level of control. Now, almost everyone can. And the first step to achieving excellent control is to have proper expectations of how good you can feel and how active you can be.

When I talk about "asthma control" in this book, I am referring to the excellent control described here. (I discuss it further on page 218 in Chapter 8, "Working With Your Doctors.")

Basic Facts

I believe you can stay out of the emergency room and out of the hospital if you learn the basic facts about asthma and the medicines used to treat it. These facts will help you learn how to make sense of the many pieces of the asthma puzzle. When you understand these facts, you are well on your way to avoiding most asthma episodes and treating those which do occur at home.

HOW DO THE LUNGS WORK?

To understand the asthma condition and what happens during an asthma episode, you must start by learning what happens during the normal process of breathing. Breathing provides a continuous supply of oxygen to the body; you need oxygen to release energy from the food that you eat and to enable the body's cells to do the many jobs that keep you alive. About twenty percent of the air that enters your lungs is oxygen, a gas that is absorbed into the bloodstream deep inside the lungs. The blood carries oxygen to the billions of cells in

your body. As the body' cells function, they use up oxygen and produce another gas, carbon dioxide, which you eliminate when you exhale.

ANATOMY OF THE RESPIRATORY SYSTEM

As you breathe in, air flows through the nose or mouth, down the throat (pharynx), through the voice box (larynx), and continues down the windpipe (trachea) [see Figure 1]. The air then flows through tubes that branch as they extend into the lungs. The first three branches are known as the large airways or bronchi. From there, the air flows into progressively smaller passageways called small airways or bronchioles. The air continues to flow through these bronchioles as they branch ten to twenty-five times before reaching the air sacs (alveoli) where air exchange takes place (see Figure 2). Your lungs contain approximately eight million bronchioles and three hundred million tiny air sacs.

Oxygen leaves the air sacs and enters the surrounding tiny, thin blood vessels (capillaries). The blood carries oxygen away from the lungs to the body's tissues, including the brain and the heart. At the same time that oxygen enters the capillaries, carbon dioxide leaves and enters the air sacs. This waste product of chemical reactions in the body is eliminated when you breathe out.

The Muscles of Breathing

The main breathing muscle is the diaphragm, a large, dome-shaped muscle located between the chest cavity (which holds your heart and lungs) and the abdominal cavity (which holds your stomach, liver, and intestines) [see Figure 3]. In normal breathing, you contract and flatten your diaphragm when you breathe in. This enlarges the chest cavity

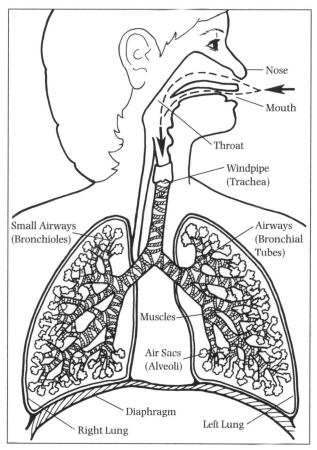

Figure 1. Normal Lungs

and creates a partial vacuum that draws air into the lungs. When the diaphragm relaxes into a dome shape again, the chest cavity becomes smaller and the vacuum disappears. Elastic fibers in the lungs, chest wall, and abdomen — which were stretched by breathing in — spring back and force air out of the lungs. In heavy or rapid breathing, you contract your abdominal muscles (abs) to force air out more effectively. The muscles between your ribs (intercostals) raise your rib cage to enlarge the chest cavity for breathing in. They lower your rib cage and compress the chest cavity to help with breathing out.

The Nose

The nose is a very effective air conditioner. Hairs at the openings of the nose (nostrils) trap large particles of dust. Mucus, a special fluid produced by glands in the nose, traps the smaller particles. Hairlike structures, called cilia, move the dirty mucus out of the nose. At the same time that air is being cleaned, it is being warmed to a temperature of about 95 degrees Fahrenheit. The air is humidified as it moves past the turbinates, bones that protrude into the nasal cavity (see Figure 4). By the time it reaches the trachea, the air you breathe in has a humidity of about 97 percent. Clean,

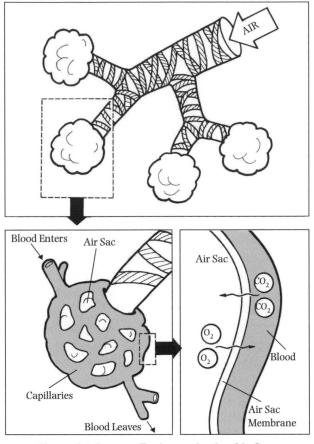

Figure 2. Oxygen Exchange in the Air Sacs

warm, humid air is less likely to trigger asthma symptoms than air that is dirty, cold, and dry.

The Lungs

The lining of the airways to the lungs is similar to the lining of the nasal passage. The humidifying, warming and cleaning process continues as air flows through the large airways (bronchi) and small airways (bronchioles). Mucus-producing glands and goblet cells manufacture a thin film of sticky fluid which traps foreign particles. Cilia on the ends of the cells lining the small airways gently sweep the particle-laden mucus to the throat (see Figure 5). From there, the mucus is either swallowed or coughed out.

THE ASTHMA REACTION

Asthma is an inflammatory condition. Once the process has started, inflammation is much like a ball rolling down a hill; it usually picks up speed unless something is done to block it. Early in inflammation, mast cells in the airways release chemicals called mediators (histamines, leukotrienes, and others). These mediators produce swelling of the airway lining and narrow

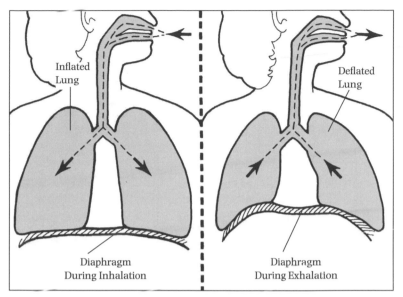

Figure 3. Main Breathing Muscle: Diaphragm

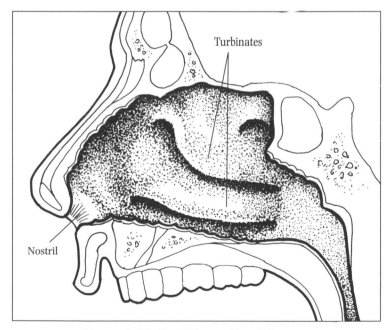

Figure 4. Air Conditioner: Nasal Passage

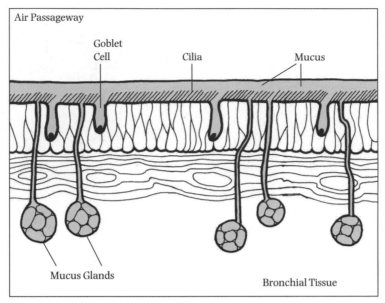

Figure 5. Air Cleaner: Cilia and Mucus-Producing Glands in the Lungs

the air passages. They also cause an increase in the secretion of mucus which clogs the airways and triggers more inflammatory cells to react. As the episode continues, white blood cells (eosinophils) accumulate and release more chemicals that exacerbate the inflammation. As the airways become increasingly inflamed, they are even more hyperresponsive to triggers. As these changes occur, you may have a wheeze, a cough, chest tightness, or breathing difficulty. You are having an asthma episode.

An asthma episode is any period of time when you have asthma symptoms that change your breathing or compel you to take additional medicine. This event almost always involves airway inflammation and can be set off by any one of many triggers.

The airways narrow three different ways during an asthma episode (see Figure 7). First, fluid and cells enter the lining of the airway as it becomes more inflamed. This causes the lin-

ing to swell inward and narrows the air passage. Second, the muscles encircling the airway tighten, which also narrows the air passage. Third, mucus glands in the lining of the airway secrete more mucus than usual. This mucus may narrow air passages even more and block some of them completely.

An asthma episode can also be called an exacerbation, problem, flare, flareup or attack. I seldom use the term attack because it implies a sudden, dramatic, and unpredictable onset. If your asthma is well-controlled, an episode will usually develop slowly and give you plenty of warning to change your treatment.

For some people, a single trigger can set off an asthma episode. For others, several triggers add up to cause symptoms. Common triggers include:

- Viral respiratory infections (such as colds and infectious bronchitis)
- Sinus infections

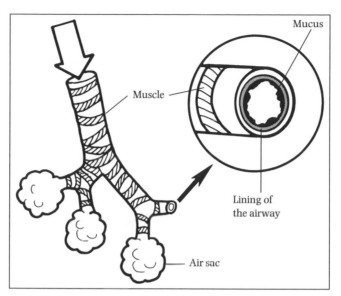

Figure 6. Normal Small Airway. Exterior view shows muscle encircling airway. Cross-section shows normal thickness of muscle, airway lining, and mucus.

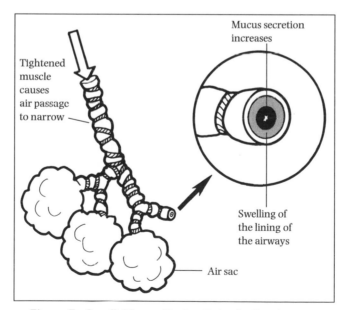

Figure 7. Small Airway During Episode. Exterior view shows narrowed airways and overinflated alveoli. Cross-section shows narrowed airway almost blocked by swollen lining and increased mucus.

- Exercise, especially in cold air
- Allergens (such as house dust mites, pollens, molds, animal dander, cockroaches, and some foods)
- Irritants (such as cigarette smoke, perfume, dust, and chemicals)
- Physical events like yelling, crying, or laughing.

SIGNS AND SYMPTOMS OF ASTHMA

A symptom is any indication of the asthma process that you can feel. Common symptoms include tight chest, shortness of breath, wheeze, increased breathing rate, cough, and a change in the sensation of breathing which you may experience leading up to and during an asthma episode. Some symptoms can be difficult to identify and quantify because each person feels and describes them differently. Some people may not notice symptoms at all if they have become accustomed to them.

I ask my patients to learn the four signs of asthma: wheeze, cough, increased breathing rate, and retractions (sucking in the chest skin). A sign is a symptom that can be observed by another person. Some of the symptoms listed above are also asthma signs. By observing these signs in young children, parents can determine what treatment their child needs.

Symptoms and signs can start within minutes after you are exposed to a trigger. In response to the trigger, mast cells in your airways release mediators that can cause inflammation, bronchoconstriction and secretion of mucus. Usually, symptoms continue to worsen once they have begun. In some cases, your symptoms may diminish and disappear within 30 to 90 minutes without treatment. However, these symptoms may return in a few hours.

DOES EVERY EPISODE NEED TREATMENT?

It is a good idea to treat every episode, since its severity is not predictable at the outset. Since early treatment leads to the best result it is usually wise not to delay. Treatment should be based on a home treatment plan that you have decided on in advance with your doctor.

Naming and Diagnosing Asthma

You may not hear your doctor use the word "asthma." Some doctors recognize the symptoms of asthma and treat it with asthma medicines but do not call it "asthma" to avoid worrying a patient. Instead, they may describe the situation as bronchitis, a chest cold, or a wheezing problem or diagnose you with RAD (reactive airway disease). Yet typically, if you have been sick with "bronchitis" five times in two years, you will be happy to hear the word "asthma." You will be relieved to have a diagnosis that can be treated effectively. If you are not told that you have asthma, you are being deprived of the opportunity to learn about it. Information you read about viral bronchitis does not fully describe the bronchitis that accompanies asthma. You won't be able to find a book in the library on RAD or "wheezing problems." You won't know to discuss the problem with friends who have asthma. On the other hand, if you do know you have asthma, then you can begin learning about it and working with your doctor to develop a treatment plan that brings your asthma under control.

DIAGNOSING BY HISTORY

In most cases, a doctor who pays close attention to your story will begin to suspect asthma. Asthma stories, like the ones in the first chapter, often include episodes of coughing, wheezing, shortness of breath or a tight chest, or previous episodes of bronchitis or pneumonia. Asthma should be considered in anyone who has been diagnosed with bronchitis or pneumonia more than once in a year. Perhaps your story includes hospitalization for a respiratory problem or medicines taken for breathing trouble. Often, you will be able to identify certain conditions when symptoms occur, such as during pollen season, after exercise, during exposure to tobacco smoke, or after laughing or crying hard. All of these are clues to you and your doctor that you may have asthma. You may have asthma even if you have never wheezed and don't have allergies.

DIAGNOSING BY PHYSICAL EXAM

If you are having an asthma episode at the time of your visit to the doctor, the physical examination may show one or more of the four major signs of asthma trouble: coughing, wheezing, breathing faster than usual, and retractions, which means "sucking in" of the chest skin between your ribs (children) or at the front of your neck (adults). If these signs improve one to ten minutes after you inhale a quick relief medicine (albuterol), the diagnosis of asthma becomes almost certain.

TESTING LUNG FUNCTION

To confirm a diagnosis of asthma, your doctor will measure your airflow before and after treatment with albuterol (or another quick relief medicine). In the office, some doctors may use a spirometer, a machine that measures how much air you can blow out in one second (forced expiratory volume: FEV_1). Spirometry also measures flow rates at several points in the breathing cycle and the usable volume of air in the lung. If you have untreated asthma, your FEV_1 will improve at least twelve percent after

inhaling albuterol, unless your airways are significantly blocked by inflammation (swelling). Some doctors use a peak flow meter to measure how much air you breathe out in a fast blast. If your doctor uses a peak flow meter, an increase in airflow of fifteen percent or more will confirm a diagnosis of asthma.

You could have a history consistent with asthma but show little or no improvement in airflow after inhaling albuterol. This could be due to significant ongoing inflammation in your airways.

Natural Course of Asthma

Most people who develop asthma symptoms have a genetic tendency or predisposition to do so. This means that the likelihood of developing asthma is usually present at birth. If one parent has asthma or allergies (atopy), each child has a twenty-five percent chance of developing asthma. If both parents have asthma or atopy, the chances are roughly fifty percent. The likelihood of a child developing asthma if neither parent has it is somewhere between five and fifteen percent.

Several factors increase the risk of developing asthma:

- Asthma occurs about twice as frequently in infants who live with a mother who smokes. Smoking by either parent increases the risk for infants to develop allergies.
- A premature baby is four times more likely to develop asthma than a term-birth baby.
- Eighty percent of children who develop asthma have allergies (are atopic).
- Some people develop asthma symptoms after they experience a viral respiratory infection. This is particularly true of infants

and young children who have been infected with the respiratory syncytial virus.

Half of all children with asthma develop their first symptoms by age four, but symptoms can start at any age. One quarter of all people who develop asthma do so after age forty.

The tendency to have hyperresponsive airways lasts a lifetime. However, many young children will stop having symptoms during elementary school. These symptoms may return for no apparent reason many years later. If your asthma symptoms started in your teen years, they are less likely to disappear.

The severity of episodes or presence of symptoms often decreases as children grow older. There are several possible reasons for this. The size of their small airways increases greatly in the first few years of life. As a result, inflammation and bronchoconstriction can no longer block airflow as completely. Certain viruses damage the airways more easily in very young children, which can increase the severity of an episode. In addition, respiratory infections (which often trigger asthma symptoms) are less frequent in older children and adults than they are in preschoolers.

Each person has an individual pattern of asthma episodes. Episodes may be seasonal or intermittent because of specific triggers, such as spring allergens or cold air. Symptoms vary in how fast they come on and how intense they are, depending on the trigger and the amount of underlying inflammation in the airways.

Do not assume that you have a serious asthma problem if you have been hospitalized for asthma. Most hospitalizations could have been avoided. Perhaps you did not receive an effective treatment plan or were not told how important it is to reduce the triggers in your environment. A good preventive program, which includes avoiding triggers and taking medicine to control inflammation, will prevent most hospitalizations.

CAN ASTHMA CAUSE PERMANENT LUNG DAMAGE?

Recent studies show that if airway inflammation remains untreated for several years, permanent changes in lung structure can occur. Effective treatment of asthma, especially long-term control of inflammation, can prevent this damage in many cases. People with asthma who smoke or live in an area with high air pollution suffer lung damage more frequently than people without asthma.

DO PEOPLE DIE FROM ASTHMA?

Death from asthma is unusual. The total number of deaths from asthma each year is a little over 5,000, one-tenth the annual number of deaths from motor vehicle accidents. One of every 22,000 children with asthma and one of every 2,000 adults with asthma will die from it this year. Asthma experts agree that most of these asthma deaths could be prevented by proper diagnosis and treatment. They also agree that the main cause of asthma death is the failure of the doctor or the patient to recognize the severity of the problem in time to start effective treatment.

Monitoring Peak Flow Scores and Asthma Signs

Asthma causes more emergency room visits and more hospital admissions than any other chronic illness of childhood, and is also a major cause of emergency visits and hospital admissions by adults. You can avoid these traumatic events if you know how to blow a peak flow and have the skill to accurately observe the four signs of asthma trouble.

PEAK FLOW

Your peak flow score is the fastest speed at which you can blow air out of your lungs. Peak flow is a sensitive measure of how your airways are doing. Measuring your peak flow score allows you to identify an asthma episode early and begin treatment promptly. It measures how much air you can "blast" out of your lungs in a fraction of a second. Peak flow is measured with a simple, inexpensive device called a peak flow meter. This device can be used easily and accurately by almost every person five years of age or older.

The peak flow score depends mainly on the status of your large airways. It will be highest (your personal best) when these airways are absolutely clear, without any narrowing due to inflammation, bronchoconstriction, or mucus. Doctors use the personal best score as the basis for guiding both your daily treatment and assessing your response to asthma episodes.

ASTHMA SIGNS

Children under five often cannot describe their symptoms and usually cannot blow an accurate peak flow. For this reason, you observe the four signs of asthma trouble and score them as accurately as possible to assess your child's status. Each sign is scored based on its frequency or intensity. The total score for all four signs tells you how severe an episode is and guides you to follow the appropriate treatment. Classifying the severity of asthma episodes is discussed more fully later in this chapter.

The four signs of asthma trouble are:

- Coughing
- Wheezing
- Breathing faster
- Sucking in the chest or neck skin (retractions)

Coughing is the most common sign of asthma. Asthma-related coughing is often described as dry and nonproductive, but it may be coarse and bring up mucus. Coughing occurs more often when your airways are hyperresponsive. It also occurs when your body attempts to clear the mucus from the airway. The severity of coughing is scored by how often you cough in one minute.

You may easily overlook your coughing, especially when your asthma has been poorly controlled for a long period of time. In this case, you may unconsciously ignore the cough because you have become accustomed to it.

Wheezing is the high-pitched, whistling sound that occurs when air flows through narrowed airways. It is scored with the naked ear (no stethoscope). A wheeze is mild if it occurs only at the end of breathing out (expiration). As the episode worsens, the wheezing becomes louder and may be heard throughout expiration and then during inspiration as well. If many of your airways become totally blocked, too little air will move through them to produce a wheeze at all. A severe episode is signaled by the absence of wheezing, along with severe retractions or prolonged expiration. As you improve with treatment and some of your airways start to open, your wheezing will disappear.

Most people *breathe faster* than usual when they are having an asthma episode. To check your normal breathing rate, either count your breaths for a full minute or count for half a minute and multiply by two (see Table 1). Fast breathing is often the first sign of an asthma episode in an infant. In young children, it is often easier to watch the belly move in and out rather than to notice the chest move.

If your airways are significantly blocked, you may have difficulty breathing out, so expirations are prolonged. This effect slows down

Table 1. Range of Normal Daytime Breathing Rates

	Per Minute
0–2 years	25–50
2–5 years	20–30
6–14 years	15–25
Adults	10–20

the overall breathing rate. In this case, a slow breathing rate along with severe retractions signals a severe episode. After treatment has begun to clear some of your airways, your breathing rate will increase.

Your breathing rate usually slows down during sleep. An increase in the nighttime rate should be scored the same way as an increase in daytime rate.

Sucking in the chest skin (retraction) occurs when your child cannot draw air into her lungs fast enough. As the chest cavity expands, a vac-uum is created inside the chest and the soft tissues of the chest wall are pulled inward. You will notice that the tissue between the ribs, above the breastbone and above the collarbone may be sucked in (see Figure 8). This sign is much more obvious in a slim child than in a chubby one. Some slim children suck in their chest skin a little bit when they are breathing normally. Learn your child's usual breathing pattern so that you can detect a change. In an infant, retractions may be an early sign of an asthma episode. In adults, retractions are more notice-able in the front of the neck than in the chest wall. Neck muscles will begin to stick out as the person strains to increase the volume of the chest.

If you are the parent of a young child with asthma, you can learn the four signs of asthma trouble by watching your child during an asthma episode and by paying close attention to the signs. You can learn the signs in your doctor's office while your child is being treated

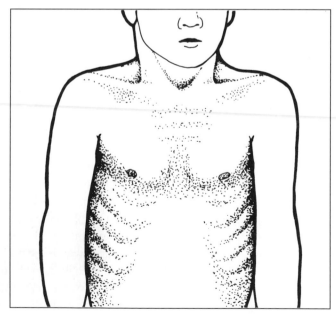

Figure 8. Sucking in the Chest Skin: Retractions

for an episode. With practice, you will be able to notice whether each sign is improving or worsening as the episode continues. Once you can judge the severity of your child's signs, you can judge her progress.

If you are a teenager or an adult with asthma, you can benefit from learning to observe the four signs of asthma in yourself. There is space to record cough and wheeze in the Asthma Peak Flow Diary (see Chapter 6, "Using an Asthma Diary"). Scoring peak flow and asthma signs together will help you learn how your asthma responds to triggers and medicines. While you are learning the asthma signs, it helps to have an observer assist you. As you become more sensitive to your signs, you should be able to perceive earlier on your own that an asthma episode is beginning.

EARLY CLUES

Some people experience very individual symptoms or signs which indicate that an asthma episode is "brewing." You may be able to identify a particular clue several hours or a day before an asthma episode starts. These clues are unique for each person and should not be confused with the four signs of asthma (which can be observed, scored, and used as a basis for treatment for almost any person with asthma). The clues my patients have described most often are an itch on the neck, a yawn, or "the look" in their child.

■

The Look
Pat Esposito

Monday night, two-year-old Mark was wide awake and restless. He didn't fall asleep for another two hours. Mark awoke in the morning with bags under his eyes and "the look." This should have rung an alarm in my head, but I guess I was tired and just not tuned in.

Tuesday, Mark looked a little wiped out, but played happily all day. He went to bed at 7:30 P.M. and fell asleep immediately. At close to 1:00 A.M., I was awakened by Mark's coughing and rushed to his room. He had a full expiratory wheeze and was anxious. I had missed starting the medicine on time and Mark had a rough night. Next time I'll start his medicine when I see "the look."

■

A clue that regularly precedes an asthma episode can serve as a signal to start treatment. Early clues are particularly helpful in children who are too young to express their complaints. Some teenage and adult patients have identified their own clues and know to pay attention to them. Early clues can be grouped as changes in mood, changes in facial appearance, changes in breathing, verbal complaints and others.

Mood changes: watch for anything different from normal behavior. You may become aggressive or quiet; overactive, grouchy, mopey, grumpy, or tired; or easily upset, nervous, or sad.

Facial appearance: Your face may change, becoming either red or pale, or look swollen. Other facial clues include dark circles under the eyes or increased perspiration.

Breathing changes: You may cough, breathe through your mouth, feel short of breath, yawn, or sigh.

Other clues: You may have an itchy chin or neck. Some young children stroke their necks in response to this itchy feeling. A child might say that her neck "feels funny" or maybe that she just doesn't feel well. Some people complain of a hurting chest, a feeling that the chest is filling up, shortness of breath, fatigue, headache, or a dry mouth. You may notice that some other mannerism, not mentioned here, also foretells your asthma episodes.

EARLY WARNING SIGNS

Some asthma educational materials list the following as "early warning signs" of an asthma episode: incessant cough, difficulty breathing, chest starting to get tight or hurting, breathing faster than normal, and getting out of breath easily. These are not *early* warning signs. They are the real thing — actual signs and symptoms of an asthma episode under way. It is time to act. If you wait for these signs to worsen before you do anything, you will be late in treating. And when treatment starts late, you are likely to have a more serious and prolonged asthma episode.

EMERGENCY SIGNS

If you have any of the following signs, it is an asthma emergency:

- breathing hunched over
- bluish fingernails or lips
- difficulty walking or talking
- severe retractions
- a slow breathing rate

Appearance of any of these signs means you must go the emergency room or call 911 immediately. If your asthma is well controlled, it is extremely unlikely that you will ever have these emergency signs.

Asthma Severity

CLASSIFYING OVERALL SEVERITY

Your asthma exists even when you are not having an asthma episode. The 1997 NHLBI *Expert Panel 2: Guidelines for the Diagnosis and Management of Asthma* identifies four levels of asthma severity: mild intermittent, mild persistent, moderate persistent, and severe persistent. The intensity of treatment needed is different at each level. Asthma experts estimate that about thirty percent of people with asthma have a problem that is mild intermittent, thirty percent have mild persistent asthma, and thirty percent have moderate persistent asthma. Ten percent have persistent asthma that is severe.

The *Guidelines* assess each level of severity based on the history of a person's symptoms when they were taking no asthma medicine. Any person with asthma symptoms that occurred more than twice a week (on average) before beginning treatment has persistent asthma. If this applies to you, your doctor can determine whether your persistent asthma is mild, moderate or severe by looking at three factors: the frequency of daytime symptoms, the frequency of nighttime symptoms, and your peak flow score (see Table 2). In children under 5, who cannot blow a peak flow score, overall asthma severity can be assessed by noting the frequency of daytime and nighttime signs and symptoms.

Your doctor will classify your asthma at the most severe level at which you have any one of the indicators. For example, if you have nighttime symptoms twice a week, you have moderate persistent asthma (even if your peak flow and daytime symptoms are in the mild persistent category.) If your physical activity is usually limited, you have severe persistent asthma.

Once your doctor has assessed your overall asthma severity, he can help you work out a

Table 2. Classifying the Overall Severity of Asthma — Based on Status Before Treatment

Mild intermittent asthma
- Peak flow score 80% or more of personal best*
- Daytime symptoms twice or less per week
- Nighttime symptoms twice or less per month

Mild persistent asthma
- Peak flow score 80% or more of personal best*
- Daytime symptoms more than twice a week, but less than once per day
- Nighttime symptoms more than twice per month

Moderate persistent asthma
- Peak flow score between 60% and 80% of personal best*
- Daytime symptoms every day
- Nighttime symptoms more than once per week

Severe persistent asthma
- Peak flow score 60% or less of personal best*
- Daytime symptoms continual
- Nighttime symptoms frequent

*The personal best peak flow is established when the airways are completely clear of inflammation and bronchoconstriction.
Adapted from the NHLBI *Expert Panel Report 2: Guidelines for the Diagnosis and Management of Asthma,* 1997.

medicine routine that controls airway inflammation and prevents symptoms. People who have persistent asthma require daily controller medicines even if their symptoms are mild. Quick relief medicines like albuterol are taken in response to asthma episodes as needed. Table 3 outlines the general guidelines for treatment. (See Chapter 3, "Asthma Medicine," and Chapter 7, "Asthma Treatment," for more complete discussions of asthma treatment.)

CLASSIFYING THE SEVERITY OF ASTHMA EPISODES

The term "asthma episode" refers to a period when you have any asthma symptoms or take additional medicine. The severity of an episode is assessed by the events that occur during that single episode. If you have mild inter-

mittent asthma, you might have a mild episode one month and a severe episode several months later, even though you have few symptoms between episodes. To treat an episode effectively, it is important to assess each one individually.

The severity of an episode should be classified within one of the asthma treatment zones which are based on your personal best peak flow score or the total score of asthma signs (see Figure 9). The treatment zones correspond to the colors of a traffic light — green, yellow, and red — with each color representing a different severity. Green mean "Go," yellow means "Caution," and red means, "Stop! Danger!"

In the green zone, your breathing is normal. The yellow zone indicates an episode of mild or moderate severity. To distinguish between mild and moderate, I divide the yellow

Table 3. Long-Term Asthma Treatment Based on Severity

Mild intermittent asthma
- No daily medicines needed to control airway inflammation
- Quick relief medicine taken as needed for symptoms

Mild persistent asthma
- Low dose of daily medicine to control airway inflammation
- Quick relief medicine taken as needed for symptoms

Moderate persistent asthma
- Medium dose of daily medicine or combination of daily medicines to control airway inflammation
- Quick relief medicine taken as needed for symptoms

Severe persistent asthma
- High dose of daily medicine or a combination of medicines to control airway inflammation
- Quick relief medicine taken as needed for symptoms

zone into two parts: the high yellow zone (mild episode) and the low yellow zone (moderate episode). The red zone identifies a severe episode. The zones provide the basis for using a written treatment plan at home to manage your asthma.

Adults

The fastest and most accurate way to judge the severity of an asthma episode at home is to measure the airflow from your lungs with a peak flow meter. The treatment zones for people over age 5 are based on the personal best peak flow score. A score of eighty percent of the personal best or higher falls within the green zone. A score from 65 to 80 percent is in the high yellow zone, while a score of 50 to 65 percent is in the low yellow zone. If your score is less than 50 percent of your personal best peak flow score, it falls into the red zone (see Table 4). Assign a score that falls on the boundary between two zones to the higher zone.

Children

For children under age 5, parents can use the four asthma signs to assess an episode. Each of the four signs is scored separately (see Table 5), and the total score defines the asthma treatment zone. I recommend scoring cough and respiratory rate on a scale of zero to three, and wheeze and "sucking in the chest skin" on a scale of zero to five. Absence of a sign earns a score of zero.

The *total score* for all four signs determines the severity of the episode and the type of treatment (see Table 6). A total score of zero means that there is no episode. If your child scores from 1 to 4, she is having a mild episode. A total score of 5 to 8 indicates an episode of mod-

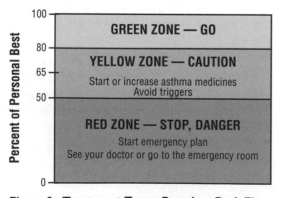

Figure 9. Treatment Zones Based on Peak Flow

Table 4. Judging Episode Severity By Peak Flow Score

Asthma Treatment Zone	Peak Flow Score*	Episode Severity
green	80% or more	no episode
high yellow	65% to 80%	mild episode
low yellow	50% to 65%	moderate episode
red	less than 50%	severe episode

*Asthma treatment zones are calculated based on the personal best peak flow score.

Table 5. Scoring the Four Signs of Asthma

Cough		Breathing Faster	
None	0	None	0
Less than 1 per minute	1	Up to 50% increase	1
1–4 per minute	2	50–100% increase (double)	2
More than 4 per minute	3	More than 100% increase	3
Wheeze		Sucking in the Chest Skin	
None	0	None	0
Exhale only	1	Barely noticeable	1
Throughout entire exhale	3	Obvious	3
Both inhale and exhale	5	Severe	5

erate severity, while a total of 9 or more signals a severe episode and the need for emergency measures.

- *Cough* is scored by its frequency each minute over a period of five minutes. Less than one cough per minute is scored as 1, one to four coughs per minute is 2, and more than four coughs per minute is 3.
- *Wheeze* is scored by its position in the breathing cycle. A wheeze at the end of exhale is 1, a wheeze throughout exhale is 3, and a wheeze on both inhale and exhale is 5. During a severe asthma episode, a wheeze may disappear temporarily. When this happens, it should be scored as a five.
- *Breathing faster* is often the earliest sign of an asthma problem. An increase of up to 50 percent higher than the usual breathing rate scores a 1, 50 to 100 percent (double) of the usual rate scores a 2, and more than double the usual rate scores a 3. If a child's normal breathing rate is 24 breaths per minute, she would score a 1 with a rate between 24 and 36. A rate of 37 to 48 would score a 2. A rate over 48 would score a 3.
- *Sucking in the chest skin* (retractions) between the ribs (in children) or at the front of the neck (in adults) scores 1 if barely noticeable, 3 if obvious, 5 if severe.

Once parents can assess the severity of these four signs, they can use the total score to identify their child's treatment zone and start to treat accordingly.

Table 6. Judging Episode Severity by Total Score of Asthma Signs

Asthma Treatment Zone	Total Signs Score	Episode Severity
green	0	no episode
high yellow	1–4	mild episode
low yellow	5–8	moderate episode
red	9 or more	severe episode

Asthma Triggers

A trigger is an object, act, or event that makes asthma worse. Triggers can be allergenic substances, irritants, viruses, physical events, activities, chemicals, medical conditions, or medicines. Allergens are a special type of environmental trigger for any person with asthma who also has allergies; they are discussed in a separate section of this chapter. Many triggers, including allergens, can be avoided once you identify them. Avoidance can greatly reduce your symptoms and need for medicine; it may eliminate the need for emergency visits to the doctor or hospitalizations.

To avoid your triggers, you first must acquire a good understanding of possible triggers and learn how to identify them. By keeping an asthma diary, you will be able to analyze your exposure to potential triggers and see how you react to them. Once you understand your triggers, you can reduce or eliminate them. In some cases, this can be done easily. In other cases, it may require a change in habits and take time before an effect is noticeable. Many people are willing to tackle the job once they realize that avoiding triggers can reduce the frequency and severity of their symptoms and also their need for medicines.

Sensitivity to triggers varies greatly from person to person and even in the same person at different times, depending on how much in-flammation exists in the airways. Some people develop symptoms of asthma after contact with a single trigger. Others may not have any trouble with a particular trigger unless they have underlying inflammation produced by a previous trigger (see Figure 10).

A person with hyperresponsive airways may have an asthma episode with any one of the triggers mentioned previously. Other people have an asthma episode only when two or more triggers (such as exercise, cold air or a viral respiratory infection) occur simultaneously. Some triggers may cause the airways to be inflamed for as long as eight weeks. Contact with a cat can cause such long-standing inflammation. Weeks after the cat exposure, contact with a trigger that usually doesn't cause symptoms may result in another episode.

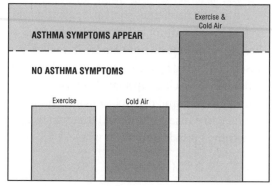

Figure 10. Asthma Triggers. Triggers often add up to cause symptoms.

VIRAL INFECTIONS

Viral respiratory infections, including bronchitis and pneumonia, are very common triggers of asthma episodes in people of all ages. These viruses can invade any part of the respiratory system including the upper airway (the nose, throat, or sinuses) or the lower airway (trachea, bronchi, or bronchioles), as well as the lung tissue itself. Viruses cause the air passages to narrow and increase airway hyperactivity by causing inflammation. A viral infection may also reduce the ability of your airways to respond to a quick relief medicine that usually helps open the airways. Since viral infections are a major trigger, it is very common to have a viral infection just before or at the same time as an asthma episode.

You can reduce your exposure to viruses, but it is a major undertaking. I do not recommend that people stay at home to prevent exposure to viruses. However, it would make sense to keep a child who gets severe asthma episodes away from playmates who are sick with a viral respiratory infection. I do recommend an influenza vaccine in the fall as a preventive measure for all people who take asthma medicine daily or for those who have severe asthma episodes several times a year.

Antibiotic medicines such as penicillin and erythromycin cannot kill viruses. Therefore, these medications do not help treat an asthma episode triggered by a viral infection. However, antibiotics help clear up some bacterial infections (sinusitis) and mycoplasma infections (which can cause pneumonia) that can trigger an asthma episode or make it worse.

ENVIRONMENT

Environmental factors frequently trigger asthma episodes. The effect of environmental triggers may not show up right away but may cause problems later if not addressed. Fortunately, most people do not have to tear their homes apart to provide a healthy living situation for themselves or their children with asthma. The vigor of environmental control should match the severity of your asthma problem. If you have mild intermittent asthma, you should prohibit smoking in the house. If your asthma is well controlled, it may not be necessary to make further changes. If you take medicine daily to prevent or treat your asthma, I encourage you to actively reduce the triggers in your environment.

If you smoke a cigarette, a cigar, or a pipe in the house, you are hurting yourself or your child with asthma. If you have asthma and are a smoker, I doubt that you can achieve excellent control of your symptoms, even if you take more than the usual amount of medicine. If someone else in your household smokes anywhere in the house, he or she is making your asthma worse.

It makes little sense for you to take medicine for asthma if someone in your household continues to smoke — that's like trying to put out a fire while someone else is fanning the flames. I cannot demand that family members who smoke quite smoking, but I do strongly suggest that they not smoke anywhere in the house or in an enclosed space, such as the car. In addition to the smoke itself, the odor of tobacco may trigger asthma symptoms.

Some additional common irritants are dust, deodorants, perfume, paint, and air that is too wet or too dry. Irritants are substances that affect everyone's ability to breathe, but people with asthma usually have a more severe reaction to them. For example, one of my patients develops asthma symptoms whenever she walks down the soap aisle in the supermarket.

Fumes from car exhaust and smoke from factory chimneys or burning leaves can also trigger an episode. These irritants trigger asthma by acting directly on the tiny cells of the airway.

House dust can be both an irritant and an allergen. Invisible particles of house dust come from the disintegration of rugs, mattresses, stuffed toys, the skin of pets, and the bodies and feces of house mites and cockroaches. They float in the air and fall all around. If you have asthma symptoms more than twice a week, you should make an effort to decrease the dust in your environment. Since you spend more time in the bedroom than in any other room, concentrate your effort there. The allergenic components of dust are discussed further in the "Allergies and Asthma" section of this chapter. A table listing the time and cost involved in carrying out avoidance measures is included in that section as well.

If your home is heated by a forced-air system, you can replace the standard filters in the system with an electrostatic air precipitator, which reduces the dust in the air. Central electrostatic air precipitators are available from air conditioning distributors or heating contractors for about $100. Various freestanding filter systems are available for use in a single room of a house or office. One of the most effective systems is the high-energy particulate air (HEPA) filter. Freestanding room units cost from $110 to $500. They can be purchased from allergy catalogues, stores that sell respiratory therapy equipment, drug stores and many local department stores.

Any airborne chemical that causes odor or fumes may cause symptoms. You should avoid hair sprays, perfumes, paints, and scented soaps if they have caused any breathing difficulty in the past. Sometimes cooking odors and smoke cause an asthma episode. An exhaust fan in the kitchen can reduce this possibility.

> ### ▶ TO REDUCE BEDROOM DUST
>
> - Keep books, toys, knickknacks, stuffed animals, and other dust-collecting objets to a minimum.
> - Vacuum carpets weekly and shampoo them occasionally. Use a vacuum cleaner with a double-thickness vacuum bag that does not leak dust.
> - Use a mask when vacuuming, or ask another family member to do the vacuuming.
> - Wipe woodwork, closets, and drawers daily with a damp rag.
> - Launder curtains frequently. Avoid heavy floor-to-ceiling drapes. Use short curtains or blinds instead.
> - Store only this season's clothes in the closet. Keep the closet door closed.
> - Seal hot-air vents in the home with tape, or cover them with five or six layers of cheesecloth or a filter made for that purpose.
> - Purchase high-efficiency mechanical filters and replace or clean furnace filters each month during the winter.
> - Encase pillow, mattress, and box spring in mite-proof, airtight covers.
> - Wash bedding in hot water (130 degrees Fahrenheit) every two weeks.
> - If your or your child's condition does not improve with these simple measures, consider removing carpets and curtains, cleaning heating ducts, and using a HEPA air filter in the bedroom.

Room air should be a comfortable temperature. Cold air may trigger an asthma episode. Hot air may dry the mucus produced in the airways and interfere with the normal cleansing process of the lungs.

The ideal humidity is between 25 and 50 percent. This allows enough moisture for the cilia in your nose and lungs to perform their cleaning activities. Air with a higher moisture content may act as an irritant and may also promote the growth of molds and dust mites. Lower humidity can cause discomfort because it dries out the lining of the nose, mouth, and throat. You can check the humidity in various parts of your house with a humidity gauge which can be purchased at a hardware store for $10 to $15. If the humidity is higher than fifty percent, you should reduce it by using a dehumidifier, improving ventilation, and reducing obvious sources of water. You can install an exhaust fan in the bathroom and insulate basement walls (including a vapor barrier) to decrease condensation of moisture on them (sweating).

Wood stoves create a special problem for people with asthma because of the smoke these stoves draw into the house. As hot air, filled with smoke, rises up the chimney, cold air is drawn from the rest of the house into the stove. This indoor air is replaced by air from the outside containing the smoke that has just left the chimney. Thus, even a wood stove that does not leak draws sooty air into the home. To solve this problem, burn your stove hot to ensure more complete burning and less smoke; less smoke outside the house means less smoke will be drawn back into it. Attach a catalytic converter to cut smoke pollution further. Newer wood stoves generally come with good pollution control devices. Smoke from a neighbor's house may also cause symptoms.

THE WORK ENVIRONMENT AND ASTHMA

Exposure to certain substances in the workplace can trigger asthma episodes and increase asthma severity over time. A person with a predisposition to asthma may start to have trouble for the first time in an unhealthy workplace. In fact, it is estimated that occupational asthma may account for two to fifteen percent of new asthma cases. The longer a person is exposed before leaving the area or before the problem is resolved, the longer asthma trouble will persist. Early transfer of the worker may prevent permanent disability. Severe symptoms caused by the workplace may last for years after the exposure has ended.

Some occupations present greater potential risk to a person with asthma or a person who has a predisposition to developing asthma. However, almost any work situation can be made safer by proper ventilation, safe procedures and equipment, and attention to health and safety concerns. Asthma is most often triggered by airborne substances, which may be inhaled as small particles or gases. However, substances can also be absorbed through the skin or mucous membranes.

It is often difficult to link symptoms that occur in the workplace directly to an environmental cause. In addition, when only a few people are affected, an employer may devote insufficient energy to tackling the problem. However, under the Occupational Safety and Health Act of 1970, every working person in the United States is entitled to safe and healthful working conditions. This law is enforced by the Occupational Safety and Health Administration (OSHA). Its sister organization, the National Institute for Occupational Safety and Health (NIOSH), carries out research on health and safety in the workplace. Both of these organizations and the U.S. Environmental Protection Agency (EPA) can provide information if you have concerns about your health in the workplace (see p. 296).

A SELECTED LIST OF OCCUPATIONS THAT CAN CAUSE ASTHMA

- **veterinarian:** dog or cat dander
- **painter:** varnish
- **grain handlers:** grain dust
- **bakers, millers:** allergy to flour
- **woodworkers, carpenters, sawmill operators:** dust, especially from specific woods (e.g., western red cedar)
- **metal work (refining, plating, tanning):** metal dust
- **pharmaceutical:** medicines, chemicals
- **photography (darkroom):** chemicals
- **hospital staff, health professionals:** latex, sterilizing chemicals
- **fur dyers:** chemicals

EMOTIONS

Emotions do not cause asthma. For many years it was said that asthma was due to a defective mother-child relationship or some other psychological problem. I don't know where these ideas came from, but I do know that they are wrong. Asthma is an inflammatory disease, resulting from a complex series of chemical interactions. It is now well known that asthma is caused by genetic, physical, and environmental factors. For some people, emotional factors may add to the intensity of an asthma episode.

Although emotions don't cause asthma, they can indirectly trigger an asthma episode. Laughing, yelling, or crying may cause coughing or wheezing since these actions stimulate the vagus nerve that extends into the lungs. Impulses traveling along the nerve activate certain cells in the airways to release the chemicals that cause an asthma reaction. In this way,

the emotions produce a reflex or trigger of asthma.

Consider this scenario. A 10-year-old boy gets into an argument with his parents about doing the dishes. They scold him, and he runs out of the house yelling. A few minutes later he is wheezing. Did the emotions cause this asthma episode? Indirectly they did, since an emotional event generated two triggers: yelling and running. Yet, if this boy were acting in a school play and had to yell and run, he would also start to wheeze even though no emotions were involved. Proper preventive treatment for his asthma would make these symptoms unlikely in either scenario.

Emotions can aggravate an episode that is already in progress. For example, when people are upset or anxious, they often breathe faster (hyperventilate). Faster breathing, in turn, can cause the airways to narrow further.

If your asthma is well controlled, as it can be for almost all people, asthma should have little or no impact on your emotional well-being. I have found that children whose parents learned how to treat asthma early and effectively at home rarely were frightened by an episode.

If asthma is not well controlled, the effects on your emotions may be serious indeed. It may take weeks to recover psychologically from a single visit to the emergency room. A hospital stay may have even worse effects. Some children entered my practice after having been subjected to years of poorly controlled asthma, requiring numerous trips to the emergency room and hospital admissions. Often they and their parents appeared as dependent, helpless individuals who were terrified of, or resigned to, the next asthma episode. They had little or no understanding of asthma as a process, nor could they imagine what they should do about it. After a year of education and support, most of these children and their parents learned how to manage asthma episodes competently. As a result, they became more outgoing and confident.

Stress and Asthma

Asthma experts believe that stress plays a role in exacerbating asthma and triggering asthma episodes, but the nature of that role is not well understood. Having asthma can create additional stress in your life; you can reduce that stress by gaining knowledge, skills, and confidence about managing asthma episodes. When an episode is under way, anxiety may cause you to breathe faster, which, in turn, worsens your symptoms. If you have a plan for treating your asthma and you concentrate on carrying it out, you are less likely to become anxious. If you have learned a relaxation technique, you may be able to decrease your breathing rate and slow the progression of your symptoms.

Conditioned Response to Triggers

When a person has an asthma reaction without the physical presence of the trigger, it may be due to a conditioned response developed from previous experience. For example, suppose that for several years a woman developed asthma symptoms every time she smelled roses. Then her doctor presents her with an odorless silk rose and she develops the same symptoms as before. Is she faking the symptoms? No, her experience with real roses has led her to a conditioned response. Her symptoms were triggered by the sight of the rose. The smell was no longer necessary.

In the past, patients whose asthma was hard to control were referred for mental health treatment by doctors who believed that psychological problems were a major cause of asthma episodes. This is no longer the case. Now we have a much better understanding of the med-ical causes of asthma, and have developed treatment that is effective for almost all people with asthma. Only special circumstances call for psychological counselling.

EXERCISE

Exercise is a trigger for 80 to 90 percent of people with asthma — but it is the one asthma trigger that you should *not* avoid. If your asthma is poorly controlled, you probably will feel a tight chest, or have a cough, wheeze, or discomfort in breathing after you run up two flights of stairs. During longer exertion (like distance running) you may feel these symptoms while you are exercising, after you have finished, or both. Symptoms produced by exercise are similar to symptoms produced by other triggers, except that they don't last as long and a tight chest is very common. If your asthma is well controlled and you take simple preventive measures before exercise, you should be able to exercise vigorously without symptoms. Exercise will help you keep your heart and breathing muscles strong and efficient. As a result, they will have to do less work and require less energy during an episode.

By following a recommended warm-up routine and taking asthma medicines *before* you begin to exercise, you can prevent symptoms from coming on. Most people with asthma can prevent symptoms by taking one or two puffs of albuterol five to thirty minutes before they exercise. Albuterol and other quick relief beta$_2$-agonist medicines provide protection for three to four hours. You can continue to take albuterol every three to four hours as needed. A long-acting beta$_2$-agonist medicine (salmeterol) can prevent symptoms related to exercise for up to twelve hours and should be taken thirty to sixty minutes before exercise. (If you are already taking salmeterol as a daily medicine, you should not take additional doses before ex-

Table 7. Pharmacotherapy for Exercise-Induced Asthma*

Medication	Dose	Time Taken Before Exercise	Duration of Effect	Potential Side Effects
short-acting beta$_2$-agonists	2–4 puffs by MDI	15–30 minutes	2 hr	tremor, palpitations
salmeterol	2 puffs by MDI (not to exceed 2 puffs every 12 hr; not to be used as rescue)	30–60 minutes	12 hr	tremor, palpitations
cromolyn or nedocromil	2–4 puffs by MDI	10–20 minutes	2 hr	none
inhaled corticosteroids	8–16 puffs/day**	weeks†	weeks†	dose-related
ipratropium bromide	2–4 puffs by MDI	1 hr	2–3 hr	none
oral theophylline	5–10 mg/kg/day in divided doses	days†	hours†	nausea, tremor

MDI = metered dose inhaler

*For lists of allowed, banned, and restricted substances and methods, refer to the rules and regulations of the sponsoring or governing organization for the relevant sport or contest.

†Ongoing therapy.

**Dr. Plaut's note: This inhaled steroid dose provides daily therapy for persistent asthma and reduces the hyperresponsiveness of your airways. The dose will be lower for some preparations.

Taken from: Storms, WW, Joyner, DM. "Update on Exercise-Induced Asthma: A Report of the Olympic Exercise Asthma Summit Conference." *The Physician and Sportsmedicine* 1997;25(3). Reprinted with permission of McGraw-Hill, Inc.

ercise.) General recommendations for medicines, doses, frequencies and duration of effect are summarized in Table 7. Follow your doctor's specific recommendations.

Outdoor exercise often takes place in cold air, a common asthma trigger. Although you can warm the air by trying to breathe through your nose, this strategy is usually not practical in competition. Use a mask to help warm the air before you inhale it. The mask can also reduce your exposure to pollens and pollutants.

If you have mild or moderate asthma and are receiving proper treatment, asthma should not cause you to limit your activity. A toddler can run around outside. A grade-schooler can participate fully in all gym class and recess activities. High school students can play any sports they choose. Adults, too, can exercise without restriction and engage in every sport. Obviously, if you are in the middle of an asthma episode, your ability to exercise will be limited. If you have severe asthma, discuss the level of your activity with your asthma specialist. In this case, he may recommend less strenuous exercise, more medicine, or both.

Sometimes parents may not realize that a child with asthma is limiting activity. The father of one of my patients was surprised to hear his soccer-playing son Jim tell me that he plays goalie because he gets a tight chest or starts to wheeze after playing a few minutes in a more active position. Once Jim started doing his warm-ups and pretreating with albuterol, he could play any position without experiencing symptoms. The mother of a basketball player told me that her daughter was able to play the whole game now that she pretreated with two puffs of albuterol. Previously, she had often been pulled out in the second quarter to take her inhaler.

Athletes and Asthma

People with asthma can exert themselves at a competitive level without discomfort if they follow an effective warm-up and treatment plan. My patients compete in hockey, soccer, cross-country running, basketball, swimming, tennis and track at a varsity level in high school and college. You should be able to play any sport, even if it is a demanding endurance sport.

Many competitive athletes who have persistent asthma take inhaled steroids daily to prevent airway inflammation and asthma symptoms. These steroids act to fight inflammation in the body. They are *not* the same steroids banned by the NCAA and USOC, which some athletes take to build muscle mass and enhance performance. It is extremely important that coaches, athletes and teammates understand that the inhaled steroids taken by people with asthma are safe and accepted. To learn which medicines are banned or permitted by the NCAA and USOC, consult the *Athletic Drug Reference.*

To train rigorously, you need to get a full supply of oxygen from your lungs. To do so, your airways must be completely clear of inflammation and bronchoconstriction. Once your airways are clear, your lungs and heart will be able to work optimally. Only then will you be able to give your arms and legs an adequate workout and train to your full potential.

Dr. Peyton Eggleston, an expert on exercise-induced asthma, recommends an intensive warm-up routine that can protect you from asthma symptoms for 30 to 90 minutes. It includes 10 to 15 minutes of stretching, a slow jog for 5 to 10 minutes and then ten 30-second sprints at two-minute intervals. The initial sprinting exercise lowers your airway responsiveness so your subsequent reaction to exercise is milder. Pretreatment with quick relief medicine and warm-up allow an athlete with asthma to train and perform at peak intensity. You can work out an individualized warm-up plan with your doctor. If you develop symptoms during exercise, your treatment plan probably needs adjustment.

My 18-year-old patient Sarah is a competitive athlete who achieved excellent control of her asthma and became an outstanding runner.

■

Achieving Excellent Control
Sarah Riley
First visit in the 1990s

I have had asthma since childhood, but had no problems between the ages of 12 and 17. My asthma problem started again during the beginning of my senior year in high school. I was running cross country, as I had been for the past five to six years, and was expected to do quite well, as I had won the California state championship the year before. At the beginning of the season, I began to have problems breathing. The first time it really hit me was at the Stanford Invitational. It was extremely hot that day and very dry and we were running on the golf course near the horse stables. I had some trouble during the race and was very stuffed up and sneezing quite a bit. Since I knew I was allergic to horses, I attributed my symptoms to them.

I didn't have much competition during the middle part of the season, so it was hard to judge if I was doing well or not, but I had a feeling that things were not going as well as they had in the past. One meet we had in Hayward, California really showed me that there was something wrong. I ran a terrible race. Then I went down to the state meet and expected to contend for another title. I just remember trying to hard to stay up with the leaders, but not being able to get enough air in my lungs, feeling weak and getting passed by people I had always beaten before. It was the single most frustrating experience of my life.

I had visited several doctors and each of them had given me different types of asthma medications: cromolyn, theophylline, a nasal steroid and an antihistamine, but nothing helped. I felt that because my asthma was not life threatening, the doctors didn't feel it was really all that serious or important. But to me it was important. It was getting in the way of the things I wanted to do, the goals I wanted to achieve.

It was then that I went to a pulmonary clinic, where I was told that I had exercise induced asthma and allergic rhinitis and was told to increase my dose of cromolyn and albuterol. I took those drugs for the remainder of the cross-country season and through my spring track season, but my running did not improve all that much. I found that I had the most problems when it was very dry and hot, and when it hadn't rained for a long period of time. At our state qualifying meet (for track) in Berkeley, California, for example, it was very dry and the air quality was terrible. At that meet I had a very hard time breathing. I stopped all my asthma medicines after that meet because they didn't seem to be helping.

The next year I attended Notre Dame and ran cross country in the fall. When I started having problems again, the university doctor put me on theophylline and for a week I was on prednisone. My season was sub-par. I was able to keep up with everyone on the team during practices, and I could stay with everyone for the first mile to mile-and-a-half in a race, but from that point on I felt as though I could not make my legs move. It's not as though I was hyperventilating or wheezing during that last half of a race; I just felt like I was in oxygen debt. My arms and legs felt heavy and tired.

It was extremely frustrating because I didn't feel that I had asthma, especially exercise induced asthma, because I was not wheezing or anything. I just couldn't get enough oxygen to my muscles. I used my inhalers before every race that year and I didn't feel that they helped at all, so before my last race I did not take them and I performed about the same as I had been all year. I also took myself off the theophylline and started not taking any medication at all, because I didn't think the medicine was doing anything for me.

Finally, in December of 1991, I went to an asthma specialist. I felt that for the first time someone understood my situation and we worked together to find medicines that would work. The specialist taught me how to use a holding chamber and prescribed an inhaled steroid to be taken daily. I also took cromolyn prior to exercise. He also taught me how to use a peak flow meter. Keeping track of my peak flow really helped me to understand what was happening when I had an asthma attack and I could see that the medicine was working. Now I can use the peak flow meter to determine when I need to take my albuterol. I also started using the holding chamber, which helped the medicine to be more effective. Two weeks after the consultation I had no tight chest, no cough, no trouble getting my breath. While running, I finally felt like I was getting oxygen to my muscles.

After I learned what medicine to take and how to take it, my times began to drop and running became easier. During the spring track season, I surpassed all of my previous personal records. I began my sophomore cross-country season with confidence and had an extremely successful season, including wins at the National Catholic Meet and Indiana Intercollegiates. I finished sixteenth at the NCAA regional meet (the year before I had not even finished in the top 100).

I am so glad that I finally learned the right way to take my medicines. My asthma never forced me to seek emergency help, but it was a serious handicap to my running, which had been and still is a big part of my life.

■

The following year, Sarah won All-American honors in cross country and broke Notre Dame's school record for the 5,000-meter event. Seven years later, she works as a personal trainer and an assistant track coach at the University of Chicago. She is a frontrunner in 10-kilometer road races.

What Sport Should You Play?

Pick the sport you like and get good at it. If you and your doctor have worked out a good treatment plan, you can pursue almost any sport, with the possible exception of scuba diving. Swimming is the competitive sport which doctors recommend most frequently to people with asthma: it takes place at the proper temperature and humidity, and events don't last very long, so it is less likely to trigger an asthma episode.

Swim if you want to swim, but you have many other choices. Because almost all patients with well-controlled asthma can partici-

pate in any sport, I want them to play the sport they enjoy the most. After all, Bill Koch has asthma and he won an Olympic silver medal in cross-country skiing. He used proper asthma medicine to protect himself against the double triggers of strenuous exercise and cold air.

Exercise Induced Asthma (EIA)

You may have heard the term "exercise induced asthma" (EIA) before, perhaps in reference to your own situation. It may or may not be an accurate label for your asthma. Sarah was told she had EIA, but she really had regular asthma with exercise as a major trigger of her symptoms. The term EIA applies to people who have asthma symptoms and reduced airflow *only* after exercising vigorously for three minutes or more. They have symptoms at no other time. By "vigorously," I mean running or biking at nearly full capacity, not walking a few blocks or bringing in the groceries. If someone complains of a tight chest, wheezing, breathlessness, or cough when they run up a few flights of stairs, they have uncontrolled asthma, which gets worse with exercise, and they need daily treatment. People with exercise induced asthma need to take albuterol and go through a warm-up routine before exercise to prevent symptoms.

Some of my teenage and adult patients came to their first office visit complaining that they simply could not get in shape. No matter how hard they trained, they didn't seem to be getting more fit. They developed a tight chest or felt out-of-breath during training and assumed that everyone must feel the same way. This is common for people with asthma. They can't reduce those symptoms by training more, because it is the exercise that is causing the problem. The symptoms prevent them from improving their fitness. My 12-year-old patient Adrianne Hall thought she was running well.

Then she realized that if she pretreated with albuterol before working out, she could train to her full potential. Here is her story.

■

The Trophy
Adrianne Hall
First visit in the 1980s

I first learned that I had asthma when I was on the swim team in the fifth grade. I was always having to slow down in practice and breathe every stroke. My friends were able to swim the length of the pool in just one breath, leaving me far behind. At the time I believed that I was merely out of shape, but my pediatrician suspected otherwise. He heard some wheezes in my chest and said I had mild asthma. My sister and father both have asthma, so I was not freaked out. My doctor prescribed theophylline to be taken for a week. It caused headache and vomiting. The next time I had trouble with a tight chest he prescribed an adrenergic (beta$_2$-agonist) inhaler. I mastered the inhaler technique, and began seeing results. I thought that was the end of my asthma, but it was not to be the case.

I lost interest in swimming after sixth grade and joined the track team the next year. I have never been much of a sprinter and was in relatively good shape, so I figured that my best bet was to run a long distance event. I would practice long and hard, but when it came to running in meets, my time seemed to be stuck at three minutes or above in the 880-yard run, and I was never able to place.

It was still the middle of track season when my doctor came by our house to visit with my mother. He asked me how things were going, and I mentioned that I was running the half-mile.

Then he asked whether I used the inhaler before practice. I told him that I didn't need to, my breathing was fine.

He quizzed me some more, "How do you feel at the end of the half mile?"

"Just like everybody else," I replied. "They are breathing hard and I am too."

"Actually," he said, "you can't know that you feel like everybody else. You might try using your inhaler before practice the next couple of days."

I didn't answer him, but the next day I did use it and really felt the difference. Over the next week I cut twenty seconds off my time. As a result, I was picked to run in the individuals competition in our region of the state. Most importantly, though, I was awarded a huge trophy by the team when they named me the Most Improved Player.

Allergies and Asthma

An allergy is a condition in which the body's immune system overreacts to a foreign substance that has been breathed in, swallowed, touched or injected. The job of the immune system is to recognize and fight harmful substances that invade the body. In an allergic reaction, the body identifies a normally harmless object as an invader, and reacts. This response causes inflammation which can affect cells and tissues in many parts of the body, including the respiratory tract, skin, eyes or gastrointestinal tract.

You can develop allergies only if you are genetically predisposed to do so. If you are susceptible, your immune system responds the first time you encounter an allergen. Your body makes antibody immunoglobulin E (IgE) specific to the allergen. The antibodies attach themselves to mast cells in your lungs. Then, when you encounter the same allergen a second time, the antibodies are waiting. When the allergen connects with the antibodies on the mast cell, chemicals are released (including histamine and leukotrienes) that cause inflammation. This inflammation is the beginning of the asthma reaction and it occurs every time you are exposed to a sufficient dose of the allergen.

But developing an allergy requires more than a genetic predisposition. You also need to be exposed to the allergen and become sensitized to it. The likelihood of sensitization depends on how much allergen you are exposed to and for how long. Common allergens include animal dander, house dust mites, mold spores, cockroaches, and pollens from trees, grasses, or weeds. Adults who work with wood, chemicals, animals, agriculture, or food production may have allergy problems related to occupational exposure. Allergists estimate that about 75 percent of children younger than 16 years of age with asthma have allergies. About 50 percent of people who develop asthma as adults have allergies.

ALLERGY TESTING

Anyone who takes asthma medicine daily, misses school or work because of asthma, has been seen in the emergency room more than once, or has been hospitalized for asthma should be tested for allergies. In addition, allergy testing is recommended for any person who has hay fever or eczema (a reddish, itchy skin condition), a history that suggests a reaction to a specific allergen, or a strong family history of allergies.

If your history and skin tests are positive to a specific allergen, you can often avoid the allergen or reduce your contact with it. The same approach can be taken with any other trigger of asthma. In addition, some people who are allergic to a substance may benefit from allergy shots (immunotherapy). If your skin test to a pet or pollen is negative, you do not need to avoid it, as long as it does not cause you to have symptoms.

If you are allergic, a blood test may reveal an increased number of eosinophils, white blood cells often associated with allergies. An elevated level of IgE antibodies also suggests allergies. Skin testing involves pricking, scratching or injecting small amounts of suspected allergens into the skin. A positive reaction is judged by the amount of swelling produced in response to the allergen. A RAST (radioimmunosorbent test) can be used to identify specific allergies in some cases. In general, it is less sensitive than a skin test, but can be used if the results to the skin test will be affected by a medicine or a rash, or if skin testing is not available.

AVOIDING ALLERGENS AND IRRITANTS

The most effective way to avoid asthma symptoms and stay out of the emergency room is to avoid your asthma triggers. Some aspects of allergy avoidance can be expensive but many are not, such as placing filters over open windows and heating vents and using light bulbs to dry out a damp closet area (see Table 8).

Many people are hesitant to do the work required to reduce triggers because they do not realize how much it will help them. In fact, reducing triggers in your environment usually reduces your need for asthma medicine. Once you learn how allergens trigger your asthma reaction and cause continuing symptoms, you may decide to tackle the task. Improving the environment for a person with asthma can help other family members feel better, too. Dan Joslyn's mother, Audrey Eldred, wrote this account.

■

Dan's Story
Audrey Eldred
First visit in the 1990s

After the tests showed Dan was allergic to cats and house dust, we made changes at home. First we found homes for all our cats. That was very sad, but very necessary. Second, we got a cleaning service that uses a vacuum cleaner with a HEPA filter and especially mild cleaning solutions. This is expensive, but it's rather nice coming home to a clean house. Also, we encased Dan's mattress, got rid of some upholstered furniture, and stripped down his room. To compensate for all we removed, we gave Dan free rein to cover his walls with sports pictures, all secured with tacks. No frames to collect dust. We wash all Dan's bedding in very hot water every two weeks. He uses a soft, folded baby blanket as a pillow, and that also gets laundered. Meanwhile, my husband's allergy symptoms have improved because of the general cleanup in the house.

■

In order to reduce or eliminate allergens, you first must know where to find them in your environment and then what measures for removing them are most helpful. Much of the next two sections is informed by the writing of Dr. Thomas Platts-Mills, an allergist and one of the nation's leading experts in allergy avoidance.

ALLERGENS IN THE HOUSE

Ordinary house dust, a mixture of harmless fibers, human skin scales, dirt and potent allergens, is a major source of allergens. The most important allergen it contains comes from the pulverized skeleton and feces of the house dust mite. Other components can come from cockroaches, cats, dogs, and some other mammals.

Pollens from trees, grasses, and ragweed — which enter the house through doors, windows, on clothing, and in dust — also contaminate the indoor environment.

Reducing dust, especially in the bedroom, will help reduce dust mite infestation. Dust mites eat dead, dry skin flakes (human dander), and they grow best in warm, moist environments. Bedding, carpeting, and upholstered furniture are ideal homes for mites. (Strategies for reducing dust were previously discussed in the "Environment" section of this chapter.) To help reduce humidity and moist conditions, consider the following changes:

- Keep humidity between 25 and 50 percent.
- Place an exhaust fan in the bathroom and vent the clothes dryer to the outside.
- Use an air conditioner to prevent the high heat and humidity which stimulate mite growth.
- Repair or treat basement leaks and condensation.
- Remove basement or ground floor carpeting that stays damp.

Time and cost involved in implementing these measures are estimated in Table 8.

Pets

Cats live in a third of all American households and cat dander is probably the most allergenic material known. Some people with asthma will have symptoms within 15 minutes of exposure to cats. Other people have a low-level reaction that does not cause obvious symptoms but makes them more vulnerable to other triggers. It is hard to get rid of cat allergen because it is small, floats in the air for hours, becomes embedded in carpets, and sticks to the walls. Removing carpets and using a HEPA filter will help.

Table 8. Time and Cost for Allergy Avoidance Measures

Allergy Avoidance Measure	Cost	Labor/week
Find new home for cat or dog, or keep outdoors	$0	*
Bathe cat or dog every other week	$0	varies
Wash stuffed animals in hot water	$0	10 minutes
Freeze stuffed animals	$0	5 minutes
Place 25 watt light bulb in closet; heat will reduce humidity and thus mold growth	$.40/week	*
Vent clothes drier to outside	$5–$20	*
Filter for air conditioners	$8	*
Six nonleaking vacuum cleaner bags	$8–$12	*
Wear mask during exercise in cold air or in pollen season	$9–$45	*
Humidity gauge	$10–$35	*
Filter for heating vents	$12–$40	
Ventilating hood over stove	$80–$250	*
HEPA air filter for room	$100–$270	*
High-quality vacuum cleaner	$195–$800**	*
Dehumidifier cuts mold growth	$200+	*
Air conditioner eliminates pollen	$270+	*
Central air purification system	$1,000	
Seal sweaty walls	varies	*
Fix leaking pipes	varies	*
Clean heating ducts	varies	*

*Takes no time after initial purchase or installation.
**Check *Consumer Reports*.

The most effective way to get rid of cat aller-gen is to give your pet away. This will greatly re-duce your need for oral and inhaled steroids. After you find a new home for your pet, it may take six months for the level of cat allergen to drop significantly. You can speed this process by steam cleaning or removing carpeting and cleaning all surfaces, including walls. If you cannot give your cat away, bathing it gener-ously with water every other week will reduce your exposure to cat dander.

Although dogs cause less asthma trouble than cats, allergen is also found in their dander, hair, and saliva. Some people are allergic only to certain breeds of dog. Rabbits, guinea pigs and gerbils can also cause allergies, as can bird feathers.

Cockroaches are the major allergen found in multiunit housing in urban areas. Extermina-tion rarely helps, since cockroaches move in from other units and some of the extermina-tion chemicals cause asthma symptoms.

In rural areas, mouse and rat urine becomes part of the house dust and may cause allergies when inhaled. Rodent control can help reduce these allergens.

Plant pollens are allergens for many people with asthma. Plant pollens are lightweight, so they stay in the air, unlike many animal products. Plants release pollen during a predictable time period of the spring, summer, or fall. If you know what pollens you are allergic to and when they are in the air, you can increase the dose of your controller medicine to reduce their effect. To reduce exposure during certain seasons, keep windows closed. If you want to keep the windows open, place a filter between the bottom of the window and the window frame.

Molds can cause inflammation in your airways year-round in temperate climates. To grow, molds need the moisture and dirt or dander that is often found in carpets. Vacuum carpets weekly using a cleaner with a double thickness bag or HEPA filter. Wash walls and air conditioner and refrigerator reservoirs with bleach to reduce mold. A dehumidifier will reduce moisture in the room but will not clear problems due to damp floors because organisms can still grow there. To reduce problems due to outdoor molds, identify and avoid areas of high exposure, such as decaying leaves, mown grass, and barns.

Other Allergens in the Home, School and Workplace

Ever since the oil crisis in the early 1970s, tight construction designed to reduce energy loss has resulted in poor ventilation and air exchange in buildings. Allergens, particulates, and gases build up instead of being exhausted. The humidity is also increased, a condition that can encourage the growth of mold. Some building materials emit pollutants such as formaldehyde. Filters in the heating, ventilating, and air conditioning systems are helpful in addressing these problems, but they must be properly maintained and changed regularly to be effective. Newer construction often includes air exchangers that continually bring in fresh air and warm it before it circulates through the building. This design achieves energy efficiency without sacrificing air quality.

Make a plan and get started. Do things that are easy and inexpensive, at least one new item each month. Tackle the big projects as you have the time and money. But get started. It will be a huge help to everyone in your family with asthma or allergies.

IMMUNOTHERAPY (ALLERGY SHOTS)

Immunotherapy (allergy shots) works by interfering with the allergy reaction. I recommend allergy shots for people who show significant asthma symptoms in response to allergens they cannot avoid, even though they have improved their environment and are taking standard medicines for asthma. For example, a veterinarian who is allergic to cats will benefit from allergy shots. In contrast, a person who owns a cat and keeps it indoors should give the cat away, wash it every other week, or let it live outdoors. People who are allergic to or intolerant of asthma medicines, or who are unable to learn how to take their medicine, may benefit from immunotherapy.

Immunotherapy can be very helpful in carefully selected patients. Patients who are highly sensitive, have rhinitis in addition to asthma, and are between the ages of 6 and 50 are most likely to benefit. It has been found useful for people with asthma who have allergies to dust mites, pollens and cats. People with allergies to food, medicines, and dander from animals other than cats usually do not respond well. Allergy shots help only against the allergens given in the injection. They do not help eliminate the problems a person has with non-allergic triggers.

If allergy shots are started, they should be continued for a minimum of one year before deciding whether or not they are helpful, unless the shots cause adverse effects. Since avoidance of allergens is the safest and most effective treatment, shots are not generally given for an allergen which can be avoided, such as a pet. The shots do not replace standard treatments for asthma, but are given in addition to them.

The most effective duration of immunotherapy has not yet been determined. Some physicians give allergy shots until symptoms have been gone or greatly reduced for one year, for three years, or for a maximum of five years. After completion of immunotherapy, one-third of patients will continue to have a significant reduction in symptoms, one-third will have some persisting benefit, and one-third will show little or no continued benefit. If the shots produce no improvement within one or two years, they should be discontinued.

Allergy shots can provoke an asthma episode. They should not be given when you have asthma symptoms. Rarely, a shot may cause a severe anaphylactic reaction, which can be life-threatening. For this reason, the shots should only be given in an office prepared to treat such an emergency.

Cautions to Consider Before Starting Immunotherapy

- If you are wheezing, you are much more likely to have a bad reaction to an allergy shot. Wait to start immunotherapy until your symptoms have cleared.
- Do not take allergy shots if you are using a beta-blocker medicine, because beta-blockers increase the risk that you will have a serious adverse reaction to the shots.
- Do not start immunotherapy during pregnancy, because of the rare possibility that the shots will cause a serious allergic reaction that could harm an unborn baby.

FOOD ALLERGIES

People with asthma tend to be allergic (atopic) to many substances, including foods. In the general population, true food allergy occurs in 1.5 percent of adults and 4 to 8 percent of infants and young children. Compared to inhaled allergens, food is an infrequent trigger of asthma.

Most reactions to food are due to food intolerance, rather than a food allergy. For example, lactose intolerance, which causes abdominal pain, bloating and diarrhea when a person drinks milk, is due to the lack of a certain enzyme (lactase) in the body, not an allergy.

A true allergic reaction to food can trigger an immune response very similar to the asthma reaction. Any food can cause an allergic reaction, but there are a small number of foods that most often cause trouble, even in tiny amounts. These include eggs, milk, peanuts, soy, tree nuts (walnuts, pecans, almonds, brazil nuts, pistachios, cashews, hazelnuts, pine nuts, hickory nuts), wheat, fish, and shellfish. If you know that you are allergic to any of these foods, check ingredient lists carefully.

In addition, some food additives and preservatives can cause adverse reactions. Sulfites, a food preservative, can trigger severe asthma episodes, particularly in people who have severe persistent asthma. Sulfites cause trouble for about 8 percent of people with severe persistent asthma. Sulfites are added to some wines and beers, dried fruit, some processed foods, shrimp, some frozen foods, and some over-the-counter and prescription drugs.

People with asthma who also have food allergies may be at greater risk for having a severe reaction to their allergenic food. A severe allergic reaction to food can be life-threatening if you are not prepared to treat it when symptoms first appear. Severe reactions, or anaphylaxis, involve a hypersensitive response throughout the whole body, not just the airways. Symptoms include an itchy rash, hives, shortness of breath, a tight chest, wheeze, a drop in blood pressure, and ultimately, loss of consciousness. If not treated promptly, anaphylaxis can lead to death. These severe reactions occur most often after eating peanuts, tree nuts or shellfish.

If you are at risk for having a severe allergic reaction, you and your doctor should work out an emergency plan. Your doctor will prescribe an epinephrine kit for you to carry with you at all times. When administered at the onset of severe symptoms, an epinephrine shot can stop symptoms from progressing. You should *always* seek medical attention right after you have an anaphylactic reaction, even if your symptoms improve after you administer an epinephrine shot. Symptoms may reappear and you may still be in danger.

The best way to treat food allergies is to avoid the foods that give you trouble, once you have identified them. Immunotherapy has not been very successful and is not recommended. For many foods, avoidance is feasible. People run into the most trouble with food prepared outside of their own homes. Careful consultation with a restaurant manager and chef about ingredients and cooking practices can improve your chances of eating out safely and enjoyably. When you go food shopping, check ingredient lists *every* time you shop, since manufacturers may change ingredients without a warning of "new" or "improved" on the front panel of the product.

The Food Allergy Network in Fairfax, Virginia specializes in providing up-to-date information on food allergies and recommending services. This group publishes an excellent newsletter on food allergies and sends food allergy alerts to all members when special incidents arise, such as a change in ingredients or a labeling error.

Special Considerations for Diagnosis and Treatment of Asthma

COUGHING AND ASTHMA

A cough is the most common sign of asthma in children and the second most common sign in adults. If you cough at night, cough with exercise, cough in polluted areas, and have other symptoms of asthma such as wheezing or a tight chest with exercise, your asthma is easy to diagnose. A person who has had a cough for more than two weeks may have asthma even though she has no other signs of it. For many people, a cough is the only sign of asthma. For others, it is often the first sign of an asthma episode.

Almost any kind of cough can be due to asthma. A typical asthma cough is short, high-pitched, and nonproductive (does not clear mucus from the lungs). But an asthma cough may also be low-pitched and productive. The cough may occur several times per minute and keep you from sleeping. If you cough at night or with exercise, that usually means that your asthma is not well controlled.

COUGH VARIANT ASTHMA

Some people who have had a cough for many weeks have entirely normal physical examinations, normal lung function tests and peak flow scores which do not improve significantly after inhaling a quick relief medicine (bronchodilator). For this reason, many experts recommend treatment with inhaled or oral steroids to eliminate the cough and confirm the diagnosis. After the diagnosis is made, treatment will depend on the frequency and intensity of symptoms.

■

Twenty Years of Coughing Asthma
Beth Gradone
First visit in the 1980s

Every time I got a cold, I coughed. Endlessly. But I never, ever wheezed. I thought every kid coughed for months after they had colds. Twenty years ago, when I was a 9-year-old living in the suburbs of Boston, no one knew that asthma could cause a chronic cough. Every winter of my childhood found the family vaporizer by my bed and all kinds of concoctions for suppressing coughs in the family medicine cabinet.

None of it ever worked. I'm told I coughed in my sleep, when I fell asleep at all. From November to April, I frequently slept sitting up all night to avoid a tight-chested cough. I remember taking codeine cough syrup in college. The combination of codeine and lack of sleep at night made it impossible for me to stay awake during the day. My roommate took notes for me when I slept through lectures.

In November 1983, my usual cold and cough started, then the cold subsided and the cough stayed on. This time the cough worsened until one night my chest was so tight I didn't know if I'd be able to keep breathing until the morning. The next day, I went to see the doctor.

Fortunately, though the doctor didn't hear a wheeze, she suggested a trial of metaproterenol mist. Within minutes I started to feel better and by the end of the treatment I felt normal. My diagnosis is mild asthma. I've figured out that my main trigger is an upper respiratory infection with post-nasal drip.

Thinking back, I remember having a hard time keeping up with my karate class in the winter. We met in a large but cold room. I coughed and was short of breath all the time. I had thought I was out of shape, but I wasn't. Since I started taking proper medicine for asthma, my breathing is normal, exercise doesn't slow me down, and coughing is not a problem.

MISDIAGNOSIS OF ASTHMA AS BRONCHITIS, BRONCHIOLITIS, OR PNEUMONIA

Approximately one hundred thousand children and one hundred thousand adults in the United States are hospitalized each year with a diagnosis of acute bronchitis, a viral infection of the large airways. Most of them actually have asthma. Bronchitis can be caused by any one of several viruses but does not usually require hospitalization. It is rarely caused by bacteria. Doctors may have difficulty distinguishing between bronchitis caused by a simple viral infection and bronchitis present in the asthma reaction because both illnesses have the same symptoms. However, if your symptoms persist for a long time, it is likely that a viral infection triggered your asthma. Bronchitis that recurs, especially during the same season every year, is usually due to asthma.

To determine whether asthma is a significant part of your problem, your doctor can treat you with an inhaled quick relief medicine. If your symptoms are due to asthma, the medicine may open your airways within minutes, increasing your airflow and decreasing your symptoms. If you have only a viral infection, the asthma medicine will be of little help. It is also possible that you can have symptoms of bronchitis more than once (asthma) but not improve with quick relief treatment. In this case, treatment with an oral steroid and albuterol for one week will often resolve your symptoms and confirm that asthma is your underlying problem.

Bronchiolitis is a viral infection of the smaller airways which occurs in children under two years old. It causes cough, wheeze, fast breathing, and retractions, all signs of asthma. It is uncommon to have a second episode and rare to have a third. Therefore, two episodes of bronchiolitis should raise the possibility that the diagnosis is asthma.

Infants who are coughing and breathing more rapidly than usual are often misdiagnosed with pneumonia. Frequently, the correct diagnosis is asthma, triggered by viral pneumonia. Ten years ago, doctors did not know that infants could have asthma. We now know that they can. The only way to find out whether asthma medicine will help an infant with breathing difficulties is to administer it. This can be done by treating an infant or a young child with inhaled albuterol by compressor driven nebulizer or by holding chamber with mask. If the child has asthma, the cough and rapid breathing will often improve or even disappear during the treatment.

If a child's symptoms have lasted for several weeks and inflammation is a significant factor, albuterol alone will not improve the child's symptoms. In this case, the doctor will need to treat the inflammation with an oral or inhaled steroid before the diagnosis of asthma can be made.

REACTIVE AIRWAYS DISEASE (RAD)

Reactive airways disease (RAD) is a term that doctors often use to name a respiratory illness with wheezing and coughing when they are not sure it is asthma. Wheezing or coughing episodes occur in almost half of children under the age of six at one time or another, especially during viral infections. Children with RAD who cough or wheeze more than two days a week for weeks at a time have asthma and will require daily treatment to control their asthma symptoms. On the other hand, when symptoms are occasional, episodic treatment is adequate.

The treatment of RAD is identical to that used to treat an asthma episode. But use of the term RAD often keeps parents from learning about asthma. Since books on RAD are not available, parents can't read or talk with their friends about it. Parents tell me they would have been able to take better care of their young child if they had realized that the term RAD had been used as a substitute name for asthma. Whenever I use asthma medicine to treat a child, I tell parents their child has symptoms of asthma and may actually have asthma. I do not use the term RAD. Parents can benefit from learning about asthma and its treatment even though their child's symptoms may disappear in a year or two.

UNDIAGNOSED ASTHMA

Most people know they have a breathing problem before they are diagnosed with asthma. They are aware of a cough, a wheeze, or some discomfort in their chest. But some people are completely unaware that they have a problem, or else they think they are just out of shape. Sally Kinder was one of these people.

Undiagnosed
Sally Kinder
Written in the 1990s

Finding out I have asthma was quite a surprise to me. It never occurred to me that I had difficulty breathing. Last Spring, I told you that

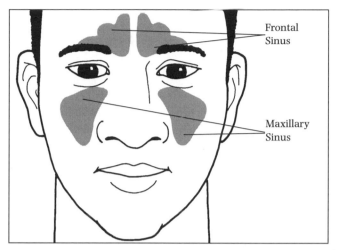

Figure 11. Frontal and Maxillary Sinuses. If you have sinusitis, pressing on your face over these sinuses may cause pain.

my son Andrew resisted taking albuterol with a holding chamber. He preferred the compressor driven nebulizer. You suggested that I take a puff of albuterol so that I could appreciate the bad taste. I immediately started to breathe more smoothly. I was stunned. Only then did I recall that when I ran in cold weather my chest hurt and that sometimes I have had a cough that lasted for weeks.

At your suggestion, I took albuterol and prednisone for a week to establish my personal best peak flow. I now treat my occasional asthma symptoms with albuterol. I was amazed that even with a cold I have almost normal energy and walking up the steps in our house is no longer fatiguing.

A few months ago, I had a persistent cough at night but I didn't have a cold. After taking two puffs of albuterol, the cough was alleviated and I was able to sleep comfortably. My asthma is not a big problem, but it sure feels nice to know how to clear my minor symptoms.

CHRONIC OBSTRUCTIVE PULMONARY DISEASE (COPD)

Sometimes chronic cough and wheezing do not mean that a person has asthma. Thirteen million Americans with these symptoms have chronic obstructive pulmonary disease, or COPD. Most of them are over 55 years of age and have a long history of smoking. COPD refers to two closely-related diseases of the respiratory system: chronic bronchitis and emphysema. Its long-term course can be halted but not reversed. Some of the symptoms can be reduced by the use of bronchodilator and anti-inflammatory medicines like those used in asthma treatment.

MEDICAL CONDITIONS THAT CAN MAKE ASTHMA WORSE

Sinusitis

Sinusitis is an inflammation of one or more of the sinuses that drain into the nose. The sinuses are hollow spaces in the skull that connect to the nose (see Figure 11). The cells lining the sinuses produce a thin layer of mucus that traps inhaled particles and bacteria. Tiny hairs, called cilia, clear mucus from the sinuses into the nose and then into the mouth or throat. When inflammation blocks the opening of a sinus, the mucus accumulates and bacteria multiply in it, causing an infection.

A sinus infection can trigger an asthma episode, and, for unknown reasons, keep asthma from responding to treatment. As a result, your symptoms will continue and you will be more sensitive to other triggers until the sinus infection is cleared.

Sinusitis is common in people with allergies. Chronic exposure to smoke, swimming or diving may prevent the cilia from functioning normally and thus increases the likelihood of sinusitis. Infection often occurs in the sinuses of the upper jaw (maxillary) or forehead (frontal).

Some symptoms of sinusitis are pain over a sinus (which may increase when you bend over), headache, toothache, nighttime cough or cough when getting out of bed, colored discharge from the nose, throat clearing, bad breath or bad taste, and puffiness and dark areas below the lower eyelids. When you visit the doctor with these complaints, he will ask you about your symptoms and your experience with allergies. He will also conduct a physical examination that includes applying direct pressure over the sinus areas.

Sinusitis lasting a few days or weeks is termed "acute" and improves when treated with antibiotics. Sinusitis that has lasted more than two months is considered to be "chronic" and requires more intensive treatment. Antibiotics, decongestants, inhaled steroid nasal sprays, and irrigation with salt solution (saline) can all be used to treat sinusitis (see Sidebar). Sometimes, allergies can be controlled by an antihistamine.

 NASAL WASHING TO PREVENT SINUSITIS

Washing the inside of your nose with a salt solution (saline) can help keep your sinus passages open and reduce the likelihood of inflammation and infection. It can be done daily if sinusitis is frequent, or less often if it occurs only during a respiratory infection (cold).

To make this solution, mix a level 1/2 teaspoon of table salt with 8 ounces of warm water. Pour 1 ounce of this solution into a saucer or your cupped palm. Inhale saline through one nostril while blocking the other nostril. Repeat this procedure on the other side.

Other methods include using a "neti" pot, a bulb syringe, a spray, or a specially fitted Water Pik.

Allergic Rhinitis

Allergic rhinitis is an inflammation of the tissue lining the inside of the nose. It is provoked by allergens and can be seasonal, due to pollens or grasses, weeds, and trees. Molds, dust mites, or animal danders can cause trouble year-round. If allergic rhinitis is not treated, it may prevent your asthma symptoms from clearing even if you are taking asthma medicine in doses that are usually effective. It may also increase your sensitivity to triggers. People with rhinitis complain of sneezing, a runny or itchy nose, or stuffiness of the nose or head. When you go to the doctor with these complaints, he will review what your symptoms are, when they occur and what exposure brings them on. A physical exam often finds swelling of the tissue lining the nose, a clear discharge, a line across the nose (due to rubbing upwards), and dark areas below the lower eyelids.

The most important treatment for rhinitis is to avoid the offending allergens. If you do this, you will need to use much less medicine. Other helpful treatments are nasal irrigation with saline, use of inhaled nasal steroids or cromolyn, oral antihistamines, and decongestants. Inhaled nasal steroids should be taken daily, starting a week before your allergy season begins or throughout the year depending on your symptoms. Oral antihistamines will stop the itching and swelling from occurring but will have no effect on the swelling already present. Inhaled decongestant sprays provide short-term relief but often cause increased symptoms if used for more than three days.

Gastroesophageal Reflux (GER)

Gastroesophageal reflux occurs when the contents of your stomach back up into your esophagus. Normally a sphincter valve between them prevents this from happening. When it does occur, the acid present in stomach material stimulates nerve endings in the esophagus. This commonly causes chronic cough in children and adults who may or may not have asthma. Other symptoms include heartburn and sour taste. These symptoms occur more often after a heavy meal, when lying down, and at night.

In addition to stimulating nerve endings, acidic materials from the esophagus may enter the airways and trigger the asthma reaction. Experts believe this is one of the causes of nocturnal asthma. Expert opinion varies widely on the importance of GER's role in causing asthma symptoms. If your asthma is not responding well to standard treatment, it is reasonable to consider GER as a possible cause.

Other Diagnoses

If asthma symptoms do not respond to standard treatment, a specialist should be consulted to review the treatment plan and techniques for taking medicine and to consider other diagnostic possibilities. In children these diagnoses include cystic fibrosis, an inhaled foreign body, habit cough, vocal cord dysfunction, malformation of the airways, and bronchopulmonary dysphasia. Possible diagnoses in adults include chronic obstructive pulmonary disease, congestive heart failure, pulmonary embolism, and laryngeal dysfunction.

PREGNANCY

Women who are pregnant may experience a change in asthma severity during their pregnancy. In about one-third of women asthma improves, in one-third it remains the same, and in one-third it becomes worse. If your asthma worsens, your doctor will suggest that you increase your medicine dose to bring the asthma under control. After it improves, a decrease in medicine is possible. Close monitoring of your asthma will help you and your doctor make the adjustments you need. Asthma severity usually returns to pre-pregnancy levels about three months after the baby is born.

You must maintain excellent asthma control during your pregnancy because your unborn baby needs a normal supply of oxygen for proper growth and development. A treatment plan that emphasizes reducing triggers (especially tobacco smoke), monitoring peak flow, controlling airway inflammation, and treating asthma episodes early will minimize the need for medicines.

Treatment is based on the level of your asthma severity during pregnancy, as well as the intensity and frequency of symptoms and episodes. If you have persistent asthma, you need to control airway inflammation with a daily controller medicine. Inhaled medicines are preferred because they are less likely to cause adverse effects. Cromolyn and inhaled steroids (specifically beclomethasone) have been widely used by pregnant women with asthma and are recommended by *The Pharmacotherapy of Asthma During Pregnancy: Current Recommendations and Future Research.* Oral steroids may be necessary for severe asthma that cannot be controlled with inhaled medicines.

Taking the medicines that the U.S. Food and Drug Administration (FDA) has approved to control asthma during pregnancy is much less likely to hurt your baby than living with asthma that is not under control. Discuss any medicines you are taking or plan to take with your doctor.

Medicines to Avoid During Pregnancy

- all alpha-adrenergic oral decongestants, except for pseudoephedrine
- epinephrine (adrenaline), except for treatment of anaphylaxis
- immunotherapy: may be continued but should not be started during pregnancy

Pregnancy may also exacerbate conditions such as rhinitis and sinusitis, which can then affect asthma. About one-third of women will have significant nasal symptoms during pregnancy; sinusitis is six times more prevalent in pregnant women. Reducing triggers and nasal washing with saline can help reduce nasal problems. If sinusitis occurs, intensive treatment is important so that asthma control can be maintained.

During labor and delivery, it is especially important to maintain good oxygen supply to the baby. Any regular asthma medicine routine should be continued during labor. If you have had oral steroid treatment during pregnancy — either daily, a recent one-week burst, or three separate bursts during the past year — supplementary corticosteroids during labor and delivery are recommended. Asthma episodes during labor are uncommon.

INFANTS WITH ASTHMA (CHILDREN UNDER 12 MONTHS OF AGE)

Because infants are more likely to get into asthma trouble quickly, they present some special challenges to parents and doctors. There are several reasons for this: the anatomy of an infant's lungs, their inability to talk or to blow a peak flow, the inexperience of new parents, and outdated medical knowledge.

Since the airways of children under one year of age are much smaller than the airways of older children, they can become blocked more easily and quickly. For this reason, an infant's condition may deteriorate much faster during an asthma episode. Also, infants are not able to tell their parents that they have a tight chest or a wheeze. Parents of an infant usually have not yet learned their child's moods or their normal behavior and deviations from it. And because these parents have had little experience with asthma, they often have not learned how to judge the severity of an episode. Parents can learn to assess asthma in their infant based on the four signs of asthma.

Until recently, doctors did not know that infants have enough muscle around their airways to cause bronchoconstriction, once presumed the main factor in an asthma episode. We now know that inflammation plays the key role in asthma. Infants are affected by inflammation and by bronchoconstriction, too.

Asthma has to be diagnosed before it can be treated properly. Infants who have fast breathing, cough and wheeze are frequently diagnosed as having bronchiolitis, bronchitis or pneumonia. Sometimes that is the right diagnosis. However, these illnesses don't usually occur more than once in infancy, whereas asthma episodes may occur repeatedly. If signs of respiratory illness occur more than once, the diagnosis of asthma should be considered.

MEDICINES THAT MAY MAKE ASTHMA WORSE

Beta-blocker Medicines

Beta-blocking medicines, or beta-blockers, are commonly used to treat high blood pressure, angina, migraine headaches, glaucoma, tremors, and hyperthyroidism. Some popular brands of beta-blockers include Lopressor, Corgard, Inderal, and Tenormin.

If you have asthma, a beta-blocker can make your symptoms worse. This may mean increased cough and wheezing, reduced peak flow scores and, rarely, a severe and sudden asthma episode (bronchospasm). Even one drop of a beta-blocker solution in your eye can cause bronchoconstriction within minutes. If you have hyperresponsive airways and have never experienced asthma symptoms before, a beta-blocker medicine may bring them on.

If a beta-blocker medicine is exacerbating your asthma, treatment with the usual quick relief medicine (a beta$_2$-agonist, like albuterol) will probably not clear up your symptoms. An alternative quick relief medicine is available (ipratropium bromide), but it does not act as quickly to relax constricted airway muscles. If you have a medical condition that is being treated with a beta-blocker, discuss possible alternative treatments with your doctor.

Sensitivity to Aspirin and Other Nonsteroidal Antiinflammatory Drugs

If you are sensitive to aspirin, it can cause severe reactions, including asthma episodes and massive swelling of nasal or sinus walls. An aspirin-sensitive person is probably also sensitive to medicines chemically related to aspirin, such as ibuprofen (Advil, Motrin, Nuprin), indomethacin, and others. All of these medicines are nonsteroidal antiinflammatory drugs (NSAIDs). They are widely used to treat pain, fever, inflammation, cardiovascular disorders, rheumatolgic problems (arthritis), and blood clotting disorders. Most NSAIDs are taken by mouth, but some are applied to the skin or eyes and can also cause an asthma reaction.

If you have asthma, there is about a 10 percent chance that you are sensitive to aspirin, as compared with less than 1 percent of people who do not have asthma. Children rarely have aspirin sensitivity. If you are an adult with asthma and also have nasal polyps, chronic rhinitis, and sinusitis, the likelihood that you are sensitive to NSAIDs increases to between 30 and 40 percent. If you fall into the high-risk category or have a history of reactions to aspirin or NSAIDs, your doctor will advise you to avoid these medicines.

Possible substitute medicines include acetaminophen (Tylenol), salsalate (Disalcid, MonoGesic, Salflex, Salsalate, Salsitab), choline magnesium trisalicylate (Trilisate), sodium salicylate, and methyl salicylate (Thera-Gesic, Panalgesic). Some of these substitutes are chemically similar to the NSAIDs, but have smaller quantities of the chemical that causes trouble. Discuss possible substitutes with your doctor.

Chapter Three

Asthma Medicines

The indications and dosages of all medicines in this book have been recommended in the medical literature and conform to the practice of asthma experts throughout the country. However, the information provided here is general and may not apply to your specific situation. Do not change your medication routine without discussing the change with your doctor.

Some medical problems are easy to treat. For example, for a case of strep throat you would take penicillin three times a day for ten days. You do not have to adjust the dose, decide how many days to take it, or whether to add other medicines.

 COMMON ABBREVIATIONS

CDN   Compressor driven nebulizer
DPI   Dry powder inhaler
MDI   Metered dose inhaler

Asthma treatment is different. The type and dose of medicines you need may change with the season, your location, or other factors, and will vary with triggers such as viral infections, allergens, pollution, cold air, and exercise. For most people with asthma, it takes between several weeks and several months to work out a treatment plan that leads to excellent asthma control.

Your doctor may take one of two approaches to help you control your asthma. She can prescribe intensive treatment until you achieve excellent control, and then reduce the number and dose of medicines to the lowest amount which maintains control. This is the "step-down" plan. With step-down treatment, you will often experience great improvement in a matter of days. You will soon learn what it feels like to breathe normally and will develop a positive outlook on your asthma condition and treatment.

The other approach is to start by prescribing a single medicine in a low dose and then increase the dose of medicine and add others until excellent control is achieved. This is the "step-up" plan. This method, which was used frequently in the past, often leads to prolonged symptoms, continued vulnerability to triggers, reduced activity, and discouragement. Therefore, I use the step-down method with all of my asthma patients.

All people with mild asthma can experience great improvement in their symptoms within two weeks of starting treatment. However, it may take months before an effective combination of learning, medicine and environmental changes can be established for a person with moderate or severe asthma (see Chapter 8, "Working With Your Doctors"). You can accomplish about half of the job using medicines alone, but the medication plan must be fine-tuned, taking peak flow scores, asthma signs and symptoms, and unwanted medicine effects into account. Fortunately, there are many effective medicines to treat asthma and many ways to control your environment to reduce or eliminate the triggers of asthma. People with moderate asthma can almost always work out a fully effective and convenient plan that causes minimal or no adverse effects. Most people with severe asthma can reduce their symptoms and increase their activity greatly after they establish an effective management plan with an asthma specialist.

You and your doctor are partners in developing, adjusting, and carrying out an effective asthma medication plan. This chapter will offer you the background, guidance, and tools you need to participate fully in this process. First, you will find a general overview of asthma medicines and discussion of the two major medicine categories: controllers and quick relief medicines. Then I provide detailed information about specific asthma medicines in each category. This chapter describes what each medicine is, when it should be used, how it works, how long it takes to work, and what adverse effects might occur.

The uses and dosages of all the medicines in this book have been recommended in the medical literature for home use. They conform to the practice of asthma experts throughout the country. However, the information provided here is general and may not apply to your specific situation. You will see the phrase "you should" frequently in this chapter. I intend the "you" in this phrase to include your doctor, who provides guidance, judgment, and prescriptions for your asthma treatment. Do not change your medicine routine without discussing the change with your doctor.

This book is designed to help you work together with your doctor, not alone. It will provide the foundation for you to be involved fully in your asthma treatment. With this foundation, you can learn to care for most asthma episodes at home, based on the treatment plan you have worked out with your doctor. If you do not agree with the treatment plan your doctor recommends, do not keep your disagreement to yourself. State your concerns. Your doctor should be aware of them. If you and your doctor still cannot agree, it may be time to request a second opinion or find a new doctor.

Understanding Your Medicines

You have the right and the responsibility to know what medicines are being prescribed for you. In order to take your medicines properly, you need clear instructions for each one. Asthma expert Dr. Thomas Creer has compiled a list of questions you should be able to answer before you leave the doctor's office:

- What is the name of this medicine, and what is it used for?
- How does it work?
- What are the possible adverse effects?
- Exactly when, and for how long, should you take it?

- How long does it take for the medicine to start to work, and when does it reach its peak effect?
- What should you do if it doesn't seem to be working?
- What should you do if you miss a dose by mistake?
- What should you do if you take an extra dose by mistake?
- Are there any medicines or foods that you should not use while taking this medicine?
- Are there any medical conditions that might affect the use of this medicine or be a reason not to take it?

If you don't understand your doctor's directions for taking your asthma medicines, either you don't know enough about asthma and the medicines used to treat it, or your doctor is not giving you a clear explanation. Either situation is unsatisfactory. There is no room for guesswork or miscommunication in asthma. A guess may cause serious problems. Never let the fear of asking a "stupid question" prevent you from clarifying an important point; there are no stupid questions when you are concerned about the medicines you are taking. After you have read this book closely, you should be able to understand any clear explanation given by a doctor.

For asthma medicine to work effectively, you need to take it in the amount and with the frequency prescribed by your doctor. If the routine suggested for you is not convenient, be sure to let your doctor know. She may be able to change the dosing schedule, prescribe a longer-acting form of the medicine, or prescribe a different but equally effective medicine.

MEDICINES USED TO TREAT ASTHMA

The two main kinds of medicines used to treat asthma are controller medicines (controllers) and quick relief medicines. Controllers are taken on a long-term basis to control symptoms. Quick relief medicines are taken in response to asthma episodes. You may hear quick relief medicines called "rescue medicines," because they are used to rescue a person having asthma symptoms.

Controller Medicines

Controller medicines are taken daily and work to prevent airway inflammation and reduce inflammation that may exist. Inhaled steroids are the most effective medicine in this group. Inhaled steroids both reduce existing inflammation and prevent future inflammation. Cromolyn and nedocromil, which also fit in the controller category, prevent future inflammation but do not reduce the inflammation you already have in your airways.

Other controller medicines are taken daily to reduce and prevent symptoms through different mechanisms, such as dilating the airways (bronchodilation) or affecting the way cells in the airways react to triggers. Long-acting beta$_2$-agonists, leukotriene modifiers, and theophylline fall into this category. They are almost always taken as an "add-on" to inhaled steroids.

Inhaled steroids, which are usually used as controllers, may be given in high doses to reduce inflammation during an asthma episode. In this case, they provide relief of symptoms.

Quick Relief Medicines

Quick relief medicines, also known as "rescue" or "backup" medicines, are used to treat asthma episodes. They include beta$_2$-agonists like albuterol, levalbuterol, pirbuterol, and terbutaline, which relax smooth muscles that have tightened around the airways. Because of this effect, these medicines are also called bronchodilators. Ipratropium, also a bronchodilator, takes slightly longer to begin working.

Oral Steroids

Oral steroids have two functions. They reduce inflammation effectively over several hours and therefore are used to relieve severe asthma episodes. When taken daily or every other day, they serve as long-term controller medicines for severe persistent asthma.

New Medicines

Our understanding of asthma and the medicines used to treat it continues to grow. The more an asthma medicine has been used, the better doctors and researchers understand who might benefit from using it, what benefits to expect, and what adverse effects might occur. A new medicine works in a unique way to treat asthma and may help people who were not able to achieve excellent asthma control with full doses of established medicines. If you can develop an effective asthma treatment plan using the established medicines, you do not need to risk using new ones. If you cannot, then your doctor will probably refer you to an asthma specialist to review your treatment options. Among those options may be a recommendation to try a new asthma medicine.

INFORMATION ABOUT ASTHMA MEDICINES

In this chapter, you will find the following information about each asthma medicine:

- Background information includes what the medicine is supposed to do, under what circumstances you should take it, and the mechanisms by which the medicine works.
- A selected medicine list provides generic and brand names. The same medicine manufactured by different companies may be sold by a single generic name and several brand names and may come in different forms and dosages. Brand names are included for identification, not as endorsement of one product over another.
- "Time factors" explains how long it takes for the medicine to begin working (onset of action), how long until it reaches maximum effect (peak effect), and how long the effect lasts (duration of action).
- "Possible adverse effects" describes reactions to medicine which you may experience and distinguishes between effects that are common, uncommon, or rare. Many adverse effects are more of a nuisance than a medical problem, and this section will help you tell the difference.
- Dosage information includes general recommendations about how much medicine is taken at once and how often it is taken. It also describes the mode of administration for each medicine, either by inhalation (metered dose inhaler, nebulizer, or dry powder inhaler) or by mouth (tablet, capsule, liquid). The doses given in this chapter are the usual amounts used at home, but they may vary with individual circumstances. Your doctor will prescribe the specific dose for your home use. (Higher doses are often used in a doctor's office, emergency room, or hospital.) Large doses are listed in milligrams (mg) and small doses in micrograms (mcg). One milligram contains one thousand times the dose as one microgram (1 mg = 1,000 mcg).
- "Comments" provides additional relevant information that does not fit into the above categories.

A Note on the Adverse Effects of Medicines

Most people who take asthma medicines do not have serious adverse reactions to them. Common reactions to medicine, such as shakiness after taking albuterol, are more of a nuisance than a medical concern. If you do notice a change in the way you feel that worries you, discuss it with your doctor. In my discussion of possible adverse effects, I will identify those that should prompt you to seek medical attention.

When it comes to possible adverse effects, all asthma medicines are not equal. My patients and I do not worry about some medicines, including cromolyn and nedocromil, inhaled quick relief beta$_2$-agonists (albuterol), and ipratropium. These medicines have been around for long enough to show that the most common adverse effects are mild and infrequent. Serious adverse effects from these medicines are rare.

Inhaled steroids are the most effective controller medicines for asthma. Their most common adverse effects are hoarseness and yeast infection in the mouth (moniliasis). Use of inhaled steroids over a period of months or years is associated with an increased risk of reduced linear growth (height) in children and an increased risk of the occurrence of cataracts, glaucoma, and osteoporosis in older patients. The risk of these adverse effects can be reduced by using a holding chamber and rinsing your mouth with water and spitting out after each dose. The benefits and risks of taking inhaled steroids are discussed in more detail in the "Inhaled Steroids" section of this chapter.

In general, an inhaled medicine is less likely to cause adverse effects than a medicine that is injected or taken orally because it can be taken effectively in small doses. However, because inhaled medicines are breathed into the lungs, they can cause cough and bronchospasm. This reaction can worsen your asthma symptoms temporarily. If taking an inhaled medicine causes your asthma signs, symptoms, or peak flow scores to become worse, consult your doctor before you take another dose of medicine.

You can reduce the likelihood of having an adverse reaction to some inhaled medicines by taking the medicine with a holding chamber, rinsing your mouth and spitting out after each puff, and minimizing the amount of medicine needed by avoiding your asthma triggers and treating episodes early. The bad taste of medicine can be reduced by using a holding chamber or sucking a mint either before or after inhalation.

Oral steroids are a wonder medicine for asthma, but can cause adverse effects when they are taken more than 14 days per year. However, this is rarely necessary, and many people don't need to take them at all. Some people with severe asthma, or whose asthma has been untreated for a long time, may require longer treatment with oral steroids to bring their asthma under control. Only an asthma specialist should prescribe oral steroids to be taken continuously for more than two weeks. The specialist will make sure that you are using the right combinations of controller medicines, are inhaling them properly, and have eliminated the most common asthma triggers from your environment. These steps will reduce your need for oral steroids to a minimum.

Coexisting Medical Conditions

Asthma medicines may affect some health problems or medical conditions. Under some circumstances, the medicine should not be used at all, while others require close monitoring. In the discussion of each medicine here, you will find the more common health problems listed. Even if your particular condition is not mentioned, you should discuss any health concerns or medical conditions you have with your doctor before taking a new medicine.

Interactions Between Medicines

Before you begin taking a new medicine, you should discuss with your doctor any medicines you are currently taking, over-the-counter as well as prescription. Some medicines interact, making one or both of them less effective. In other cases, two different medicines taken simultaneously may produce effects that are too strong or cause greater adverse effects. Finally, as mentioned earlier, a few medicines (such as beta-blockers) actually make asthma worse.

Pregnancy

Pregnancy may affect asthma and may require you to alter asthma treatment. A woman needs to have her asthma under excellent control to ensure that her unborn baby receives the oxygen it requires for growth and development. Many asthma medicines can be used safely during pregnancy. The need for medicines can be reduced by decreasing or eliminating exposure to asthma triggers. An unborn baby is at greater risk from poorly controlled asthma than from asthma medicine.

Controller Medicines

STEROIDS (CORTICOSTEROIDS)

The steroids used in the treatment of asthma are similar to the corticosteroids pro-

---

 SUMMARY OF ASTHMA MEDICINES

Controller Medicines are recommended for almost all people with persistent asthma to use daily. These medicines keep an asthma episode from starting by controlling inflammation.

- *Inhaled steroids* are the most powerful inhaled medicine for controlling inflammation and asthma symptoms. They are taken daily to treat persistent mild, moderate, or severe asthma.
- *Nedocromil* can often enable people with mild or moderate persistent asthma to achieve excellent asthma control.
- *Cromolyn,* when it is given by nebulizer, is often very effective for children under 4 with mild or moderate persistent asthma. Some adults with mild persistent asthma find the metered dose inhaler (MDI) preparation helpful.

Other controller medicines can be added to treatment by an inhaled steroid to improve control of symptoms at a lower dose.

- *Long-acting beta$_2$-agonists* are useful for people who do not achieve excellent control of symptoms by using an inhaled steroid alone.
- *Leukotriene modifiers* are useful for some people who continue to experience asthma symptoms while taking a moderate dose of an inhaled steroid. Sometimes these medicines are used alone to treat mild persistent asthma.
- *Theophylline* is a bronchodilator with some ability to reduce inflammation. The long-acting preparation can help reduce asthma symptoms at night.

Quick relief medicines are added to your medicine routine during asthma episodes.

- *Beta$_2$-agonists* are the primary medicines taken to open the airways during an asthma episode.
- *Ipratropium bromide* also opens the airways during an asthma episode, although not as completely or as rapidly as beta$_2$-agonists do. If you cannot take beta$_2$-agonists, your doctor may prescribe ipratropium as a substitute.

Table 9. Actions of Asthma Medicines

Controller Medicines	Action
cromolyn	Prevents inflammation Can be used to pretreat before exercise or contact with allergen
inhaled steroids	Prevent inflammation Reduce existing inflammation
leukotriene modifiers	Block the action or production of leukotrienes, which opens the airways and reduces inflammation
long-acting beta$_2$-agonists	Slowly open the airways Can be used to pretreat before exercise*
nedocromil	Prevents inflammation Can be used to pretreat before exercise
oral steroids	Prevent inflammation Rapidly reduce existing inflammation Reduce production of mucus Improve airway response to beta$_2$-agonists
theophylline, long-acting	Slowly opens the airways
Quick Relief Medicines	
beta$_2$-agonists	Rapidly opens the airways Short-acting Can be used to pretreat before exercise
ipratropium	Rapidly opens the airways† Short-acting

*Some long-acting beta$_2$-agonist medicines have been approved for use before exercise. Do not exceed the maximum daily dose.
†Ipratropium does not dilate the airways as rapidly as beta$_2$-agonists do.

duced naturally by your adrenal gland. Your body produces them to deal with inflammation and physical stress and to regulate metabolism. The steroids used to treat asthma differ from the hormones that have been used by athletes to increase their muscle mass (anabolic steroids). Corticosteroids are available for home use in two forms, inhaled and oral.

INHALED STEROIDS

Inhaled steroids were first used to treat asthma in the United States in 1976. Most people with persistent asthma take them daily for months or years to reduce and prevent airway inflammation and prevent asthma episodes. They can be used safely by almost every person with asthma.

Table 10. Available Forms of Asthma Medicines

Medicine Name	Form Available
inhaled steroids	MDI, DPI, CDN
cromolyn	MDI, CDN
nedocromil	MDI
oral steroids	Oral
theophylline	Oral
long-acting beta$_2$-agonist	MDI, DPI, Oral
leukotriene modifiers	Oral
beta$_2$-agonists	MDI, DPI, CDN, Oral
ipratropium	MDI, CDN

Inhaled steroids are recommended for the initial daily treatment of most people who have persistent asthma. Persistent means that you have a history of asthma symptoms more than two days per week (on average) when you are not being treated for asthma. Our current understanding and experience with inhaled steroids makes it clear that these are the most effective inhaled antiinflammatory medicines available. They provide the greatest benefit when treatment is started early after prompt diagnosis of persistent asthma. When treatment is delayed by two years or more, the airways may have already suffered permanent damage.

Through a variety of mechanisms, inhaled steroids control symptoms, reduce existing inflammation of the airways, and prevent future inflammation. They decrease swelling of the airway lining by blocking movement of cells to the inflamed area and reduce production of mucus by cells that line the airways. Inhaled steroids also prevent formation of substances called leukotrienes, which can cause bronchoconstriction. They decrease the hyperresponsiveness of the airways and help them respond better to beta$_2$-agonists (quick relief) medicines. To be fully effective, inhaled steroids must be taken every day in the proper dose, using proper technique. Taken in high doses for a short period of time, inhaled steroids can re-

Table 11. Inhaled Steroids

Generic Name	Brand Name	Form
beclomethasone	Vanceril, Beclovent, Qvar	MDI, DPI
budesonide	Pulmicort	DPI, CDN
flunisolide	Aerobid	MDI
fluticasone	Flovent	MDI, DPI
triamcinolone	Azmacort	MDI

duce the duration and severity of an asthma episode.

Time Factors

- In recommended doses, it may take less than one week for an inhaled steroid to start reducing and controlling inflammation in the airways. However, the medicine may not reach its full effect for four weeks. The length of time required depends on how much inflammation already exists in the airways, and on which medicine preparation and what dose is taken.
- When you stop taking an inhaled steroid, it may take several weeks for the medicine effect to disappear completely.

Possible Adverse Effects

- Yeast infections of the mouth and hoarseness are common. Most people normally have yeast cells growing in their mouths. Use of inhaled steroids reduces the local immune control, allowing yeast to multiply and cause symptoms.
- The risk of developing cataracts and of developing glaucoma is somewhat increased.
- Linear growth (increases in height) may be slowed in some children. In four studies, growth was slowed by 0.4 to 0.6 of an inch during a seven- to twelve-month period. The doctor will record your child's height regularly to watch for a slowing of growth. Some studies suggest that "catchup" growth occurs. Whether taking inhaled steroids has an effect on final adult height has not yet been determined.
- At very high doses, inhaled steroids may cause some of the same adverse effects as oral steroids. Occurrence of these effects is infrequent, but exact rates are not available.

- The risk of osteoporosis is increased in postmenopausal women. It may be reduced by taking a calcium supplement (1,000–1,500 mg per day), vitamin D (400 units per day), and an estrogen replacement.

Reducing the Risk of Adverse Effects from Inhaled Steroids

Inhaled steroids control inflammation in the airways better than any other asthma medicine. This control is essential for preventing asthma episodes and protecting the long-term health of the lungs. I prescribe inhaled steroids for almost all patients over the age of 4 who have persistent asthma, as well as for some who are younger. I always mention that slowed growth is a possible adverse effect in these children but that the benefit to be gained from taking inhaled steroids far exceeds this risk.

The risks associated with taking inhaled steroids are low, and they are related to how much you take. The lower the dose, the lower the risk. So, it makes sense to reduce your dose to the lowest amount that will prevent inflammation in your airways. After your asthma is brought under excellent control, your dose of inhaled steroids should be stepped down gradually. The step down can be done by reducing the dose 20 to 25 percent every two to three months until your symptoms recur or your peak flow scores drop. The steroid dose one step above that point is your lowest effective dose. You can monitor the process by recording your peak flow scores or your child's asthma signs in an asthma diary. If your doctor has not tried to establish your lowest effective dose, you may be taking a higher dose of inhaled steroids than you actually need. The goal of treatment is to achieve excellent control while taking the lowest possible amount of medicine. To do this, you will need to:

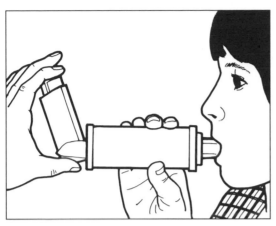

Figure 12. Holding Chamber. Using a holding chamber to take inhaled steroids increases the amount of medicine that reaches the airways and decreases the likelihood of adverse effects.

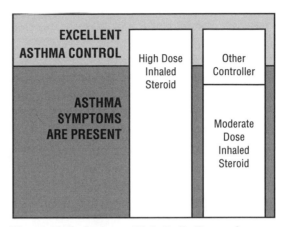

EXCELLENT ASTHMA CONTROL

High Dose Inhaled Steroid

Other Controller

ASTHMA SYMPTOMS ARE PRESENT

Moderate Dose Inhaled Steroid

Figure 13. Reducing a High Daily Dose of Inhaled Steroids. You can control moderate or severe persistent asthma with a high daily dose of an inhaled steroid or a moderate daily dose of an inhaled steroid along with another controller medicine.

- Reduce triggers in your environment.
- Use a holding chamber when taking an inhaled steroid by metered dose inhaler (see Figure 12).
- Rinse your mouth with water and spit out after taking a dose of an inhaled steroid to reduce the amount of medicine absorbed into your bloodstream.
- Continue to monitor your asthma status with an asthma diary.

Reducing a High Daily Dose of Inhaled Steroids

If you still need a high dose of inhaled steroids after your doctor has tried to reduce the dose, you may benefit from adding another controller medicine to your treatment routine (see Figure 13). Nedocromil, long-acting beta2-agonists, leukotriene modifiers, and theophylline can reduce the inhaled steroid dose needed to control asthma symptoms. After you begin taking one of these controller medicines, your doctor can reduce your inhaled steroid dose in a step-wise fashion, allowing a two- to three-month period of adjustment before making another change. Monitoring peak flow scores and asthma signs with an asthma diary will help you make these adjustments.

Dosage

Dose varies depending on which brand and preparation of inhaled steroid you take and on your age and asthma condition. Do not change your medication routine without consulting your doctor. The dose you need is directly related to your asthma severity, although it can often be reduced through environmental measures. Adding other controller medicines also may allow use of a lower dose of inhaled steroids. Tables 12 and 13 list the low, medium, and high doses of inhaled steroids recommended for daily use by adults and children. Notice that the number of puffs varies depending on which inhaled steroid preparation you use. The experience of one of my patients demonstrated how important it is to under-

Table 12. Adults: Estimated Comparative Daily Dosages for Inhaled Steroids

Generic Name	Brand Name	Form	Micrograms*	Low Dose†	Medium Dose†	High Dose†
beclomethasone	Beclovent	MDI	42	4–12	12–20	more than 20
	Vanceril	MDI	42	4–12	12–20	more than 20
	Vanceril	MDI	84	2–6	6–10	more than 10
budesonide	Pulmicort	DPI	200	1–2	2–3	more than 3
flunisolide	Aerobid	MDI	250	2–4	4–8	more than 8
fluticasone	Flovent	MDI	44	2–6		
		MDI	110	2	2–6	more than 6
		MDI	220	1	1–3	more than 3
		DPI	50	2–6		
		DPI	100		3–6	more than 6
		DPI	250		1–2	more than 2
triamcinolone	Azmacort	MDI	100	4–10	10–20	more than 20

*Micrograms (mcg) per puff by MDI or per inhalation by DPI.
†Number of puffs or inhalations.

Table 13. Children Ages 12 and Younger: Estimated Comparative Daily Dosages for Inhaled Steroids

Generic Name	Brand Name	Form	Micrograms*	Low Dose†	Medium Dose†	High Dose†
beclomethasone	Beclovent	MDI	42	2–8	8–16	more than 16
	Vanceril	MDI	42	2–8	8–16	more than 16
	Vanceril	MDI	84	1–4	4–8	more than 8
budesonide	Pulmicort	DPI	200		1–2	more than 2
flunisolide	Aerobid	MDI	250	2–3	4–5	more than 5
fluticasone	Flovent	MDI	44	2–4	4–10	more than 10
		MDI	110	1	2–4	more than 4
		MDI	220		1–2	more than 2
		DPI	50	2–4	4–8	
		DPI	100	1	2–4	more than 4
		DPI	250			more than 2
triamcinolone	Azmacort	MDI	100	4–8	8–12	more than 12

*Micrograms (mcg) per puff by MDI or per inhalation by DPI.
†Number of puffs or inhalations.

Dr. Tom Plaut's Asthma Guide for People of All Ages

82

stand the strength of different inhaled steroid preparations.

I received a letter from Michael, an adult patient who was having unexpected asthma trouble. For two years, Michael's asthma had been under control while he was taking a low-to-medium dose of an inhaled steroid: two puffs of Aerobid in the morning and two puffs in the evening. Then, Michael's HMO pharmacy changed his steroid brand to Azmacort. He continued to take two puffs in the morning and two puffs in the evening, because he was not instructed otherwise. After two months on this new routine, Michael wrote that he was now getting winded easily, his daily peak flow scores had dropped from 650 to between 500 and 550, and he needed to take albuterol, a quick relief medicine, much more often. Why was Michael having so much trouble all of a sudden? Had his asthma worsened?

The table of steroid doses gave us the answer. Michael wasn't taking enough puffs of his new brand of inhaled steroids to maintain excellent asthma control. Originally, Michael needed four puffs of Aerobid each day to control his asthma. Four puffs of Aerobid contains a medicine dose equivalent to ten puffs of Azmacort. The pharmacy had cut Michael's dose in half by changing brands. No wonder he was having asthma symptoms! A few weeks after I increased Michael's dose to ten puffs of Azmacort daily, his peak flow returned to normal and his symptoms disappeared.

It is important that you take the daily inhaled steroid dose you worked out with your doctor. You will not improve if you take a dose that is too low or do not inhale the medicine correctly. Once you have achieved excellent control, you and your doctor will work together to bring the dose to the lowest possible level while maintaining control (step-down treatment). Since you need to rinse and spit out after each dose to wash out excess steroid, it is most convenient to take a dose only once or twice a day.

Comments

- Early and continued treatment with inhaled steroids can prevent permanent lung damage.
- Controlling airway inflammation with daily inhaled steroids can reduce the likelihood of a severe episode requiring the use of oral steroids.

ORAL STEROIDS

Oral steroids are used as reliever medicines in the treatment of moderate or severe asthma episodes because they rapidly reduce inflammation, swelling, and production of mucus. They also may be used to control the inflammation in severe asthma when inhaled steroids are not effective.

Oral steroids, first used to treat illness in the United States more than forty years ago, were considered a miracle drug in the treatment of arthritis. In those early days, their side effects were not well known, and some people suffered serious problems, such as osteoporosis, adrenal insufficiency, or growth retardation. However, now we have much more complete knowledge of their use. We understand when to start using oral steroids and for how long.

When used with care, oral steroids are a safe and effective treatment for acute asthma episodes. Oral steroids can also be used every other day with other controller medicines for the long-term treatment of people with severe asthma.

SHORT-TERM USE OF ORAL STEROIDS

Oral steroids are extremely effective in the treatment of acute asthma episodes and can often keep you out of the emergency room or hospital. They rapidly reduce airway inflammation, causing the swelling of the airway lining and the production of mucus to decrease. This is why oral steroids are usually needed to treat a moderate or severe asthma episode. In addition, they make the smooth muscles around your airways more responsive to quick relief beta$_2$-agonist medicines.

Many people with asthma will require a short burst of oral steroids once or twice during a year. People who need more frequent bursts usually have asthma that is not well controlled and need an adjustment in their treatment plan.

Generic names of short-acting oral steroids include prednisone, prednisolone, and methylprednisolone. Of the available oral steroids, only short-acting preparations are recommended for treating asthma episodes, because they suppress the normal production of steroids by the adrenal gland (an adverse effect) for less time than medium- or long-acting preparations. Generic preparations of short-acting oral steroids are usually safe, effective, and inexpensive.

Possible Adverse Effects

Almost all adverse effects are related to the frequency, dose, and length of time an oral steroid is given.

The following mild effects may be seen after one or two days:

- Insomnia. This common adverse effect of oral steroids can be reduced by taking the full dose in the morning.
- Minor symptoms of increased appetite, a feeling of well-being or other mood changes, and weight gain due to fluid retention are common and may come on within a few days. The feeling of well-being may be followed by moodiness when the medicine is stopped.
- Acne.
- Stomach upset, which is sometimes caused by oral steroids, can be reduced by taking them with food.
- Muscles and joints may ache for a few days after discontinuing use.

See your doctor if:

- you develop hip pain, possibly a sign of a serious problem.
- you are exposed to chicken pox and are not immune. Oral steroids may allow the chicken pox virus to spread widely through your body.

Dosage

The usual dose of an oral steroid for short-term use is 0.5 mg to 1.0 mg of medicine per

---

Table 14. Selected Oral Steroids

Generic name	Brand Name	Form	Dose Available
prednisone	many	liquid	5 mg/5 cc
prednisolone	Prelone	liquid	15 mg/5 cc, 5 mg/5 cc
	Pediapred	liquid	5 mg/5 cc
prednisone	Deltasone	tablet	1, 2.5, 5, 10, 20, 25, 50 mg
prednisolone	none	tablet	5 mg
methylprednisolone	Medrol	tablet	2, 4, 8, 16, 24, 32 mg

pound of the patient's weight, up to a maximum of 40 to 60 mg per day (expert opinions vary), for short-term use. Oral steroids are often given in a "burst," one or two times a day for three to seven days, during an acute asthma episode.

Experts disagree on whether to stop an oral steroid burst abruptly or to taper the dose over several days. Before the peak flow meter was available, it was difficult to judge if a patient with a bad asthma episode had improved enough to stop taking oral steroids. Many doctors discontinued oral steroids gradually, to make sure symptoms would not reappear. However, tapering the daily dose after a burst increases the risk of adverse effects by prolonging your exposure.

Monitoring peak flow scores or asthma signs can give you a very good idea of how much your airways have improved. Most patients who have taken oral steroids for seven days or less can safely discontinue them abruptly after their peak flow scores have returned to the green zone and remained there for twenty-four hours. Symptoms return in only a small number of people, perhaps one out of ten, who follow this routine. This means that nine out of ten are spared the effects of a longer course of an oral steroid. If you have taken an oral steroid for more than two weeks, withdrawal should be gradual and closely monitored by your doctor.

After stopping an oral steroid, you should monitor your peak flow scores or the total score of your child's asthma signs to insure that the asthma condition remains stable. Any worsening calls for you to contact the doctor to change your treatment plan.

Most steroid bursts effectively eliminate symptoms and bring peak flow or asthma signs scores to normal within three to seven days. If an oral steroid is started early enough, it may be needed for only three or four days and rarely for more than two weeks. By starting an oral steroid promptly, you catch the inflammation process before it picks up speed, and the medicine can reach its maximum effect quickly.

If you use an oral steroid daily for more than fourteen days, a shift to an alternate-day (one day on, one day off) schedule is advisable. When prescribing such a schedule, your doctor may initially give you twice your previous daily dose as a single dose every other morning. This leaves the total dose unchanged, but suppression of the adrenal gland is decreased. Your doctor will then gradually reduce the dose.

If you have taken an oral steroid for a total of more than fourteen days in the past six months, your adrenal gland may not respond fully in the event of a major physical stress. You will require extra steroids in the case of a serious accident, burn, or surgical procedure. Supplemental oral steroids should be given the day of and the day following each of these events, as well as the day before surgery.

LONG-TERM USE OF ORAL STEROIDS (MORE THAN TWO WEEKS)

Oral steroids may be used for the long-term treatment of severe asthma. This treatment can enable a person with severe asthma to lead a normal life when other measures have failed. The duration of use may vary from two weeks to more than a year. Since serious adverse effects may occur with this kind of use, you should not take an oral steroid for more than two weeks without consulting an asthma specialist. Allergists and pulmonologists who care for patients with severe asthma problems agree that an oral steroid should be used long-term only when other intensive treatment programs — which include monitoring, medicines and environmental changes — have failed to enable a person to lead a fully active life. Experts estimate that about 5 percent of people with asthma fall into this category.

I have often found that patients who have come to me taking daily oral steroids did not really need them. After we had worked out an effective treatment plan of environmental changes, peak flow monitoring, and proper use of inhaled steroids, they were able to discontinue their long-term daily use of oral steroids.

Unlike short-term treatment, long-term treatment with oral steroids should be withdrawn gradually. This is because it takes time for your adrenal gland to return to normal levels of steroid production. A prudent taper that is closely monitored by your doctor should allow you to avoid the medical complications that can occur with abrupt withdrawal.

Possible Adverse Effects

From the following list of adverse effects, you can see that you ought to be under the care of an experienced specialist if you are taking oral steroids daily or every other day, on a long-term basis. You can discuss these possible effects in more detail with your specialist. The exact frequency of their occurrence is not known. Alternate-day treatment with less than 20 mg of oral steroids does not commonly cause significant adverse effects. Most changes come on gradually over a period of months, and some people may escape significant adverse effects completely. When taken for more than two weeks, oral steroids

- may cause acne, stretch marks on the skin, thinning of skin, increase in body hair, facial puffiness, swelling of the feet or lower legs, rapid weight gain, headache, or mood changes.
- may cause osteoporosis (loss of calcium from the bones), which may lead to frac-

tures, especially in postmenopausal women.
- may raise blood pressure, particularly in older patients
- may slow a child's normal rate of growth (in height). Your doctor should monitor your child's growth to check for this effect. Growth may be stunted to a greater degree by uncontrolled asthma.
- increases the risk of developing cataracts and glaucoma.
- may cause symptoms of diabetes but not diabetes itself.
- may cause potassium deficiency, which can cause symptoms of irregular heartbeat, muscle weakness or cramping, unusual tiredness, or weakness.
- may cause nausea, vomiting, cramps, menstrual irregularities, abdominal pain or burning, or dark stools.
- may cause reactivation of tuberculosis.
- may cause symptoms such as muscle aches or depression when you stop taking them or reduce your dose.

Dosage

The dosage for long-term oral steroid use is adjusted to your needs and is usually much lower than the standard short-term dose. Most people who require this treatment will do well on an alternate-day schedule, taking a single dose of between 5 and 20 mg every other morning. Recent research by Dr. Richard Martin at the National Jewish Medical and Research Center showed that taking an oral steroid once a day, between three o'clock and five o'clock in the afternoon, is equally or slightly more effective than taking it at other times. If an afternoon schedule is more convenient for you, discuss this possibility with your doctor.

CROMOLYN AND NEDOCROMIL

Both cromolyn and nedocromil are inhaled controller medicines: they prevent inflammation in the airways, but cannot clear inflammation that already exists. They are among the safest medicines used to treat asthma. If you have mild persistent asthma, you may be able to achieve excellent asthma control by taking one of these medicines daily. They are also used to prevent exercise-induced asthma. Although they are chemically distinct from each other, cromolyn and nedocromil exert their effects in a similar way, which is why I discuss them together here.

Cromolyn and nedocromil work to prevent the onset of asthma episodes by blocking the release of chemicals within the airways which cause bronchoconstriction, swelling and increased production of mucus. It may take from one to six weeks for cromolyn and three days for nedocromil to produce this antiinflammatory effect. Effective treatment will be marked by a decrease in the intensity and frequency of asthma episodes. When used as pretreatment before exercise or contact with an unavoidable asthma trigger, both cromolyn and nedocromil provide protection within minutes. They do not help in treating an asthma episode that has already started because they can neither reduce inflammation that already exists nor dilate the airways.

Delivered by nebulizer, cromolyn has been used safely by infants and young children. When delivered as 4 ampules per day with the usual nebulizer cup (or two ampules with a medicine-retaining nebulizer cup), cromolyn is an effective controller medicine for the majority of young children with mild persistent asthma. Some older children and adults use it by metered dose inhaler to prevent exercise induced asthma (EIA) and asthma episodes.

Nedocromil is recommended for the treatment of mild persistent asthma in people age 6 and older. For a person with more severe asthma, nedocromil can reduce the need for a high daily dose of an inhaled steroid while maintaining excellent asthma control.

For nedocromil or cromolyn to protect you most effectively against airway inflammation, the medicine needs to reach deep into your airways. This requires that your airways be open, not inflamed or constricted. Therefore, when you start taking one of these medicines, many doctors will simultaneously prescribe oral steroids for seven days or inhaled steroids for thirty days. For the first month, you should also take a quick relief medicine before inhaling cromolyn or nedocromil to dilate your airways further. Once excellent asthma control is established, you will no longer need to take the quick relief medicine before or with treatment. Whether nedocromil or cromolyn alone will produce excellent asthma control will depend on the severity of your asthma and how well you can improve environmental factors that trigger your asthma symptoms.

When used in the recommended dose, nedocromil acts faster and is generally more effective than cromolyn in reducing symptoms and preventing episodes. Nedocromil is also more effective than cromolyn in inhibiting bronchospasm (the tightening of the muscles around the airways) provoked by exercise.

Time Factors

- Prevention of exercise and allergen-induced symptoms occurs within fifteen minutes after inhalation.
- Cromolyn provides maximum long-term protection against inflammation between one and six weeks after starting daily treatment.

Table 15. Cromolyn and Nedocromil

Generic Name	Brand Name	Form
cromolyn	Intal	CDN, MDI
nedocromil	Tilade	MDI

- Nedocromil starts to prevent inflammation in three days.

Possible adverse effects

- Some people dislike the taste of nedocromil, but this sensation can be reduced by using a holding chamber or taking a sip of water or eating a mint before or after inhalation.

Dosage of Cromolyn

- The usual dose delivered by nebulizer is more effective than that delivered by MDI.
- The starting dose is the same for people of any age (see Table 16).
- The usual starting dose by nebulizer is 3 to 4 ampules per day, given in two, three, or four sittings.
- Young children use a mouthpiece or a mask to inhale a mist of cromolyn produced by a nebulizer.
- Use of a high-efficiency nebulizer cup fitted with a medicine-retaining valve (like the Pari LC Jet Plus) often produces an excellent effect with 1 ampule twice a day.
- The usual daily dose delivered by metered dose inhaler is 8 puffs in two or three doses. This dose provides adequate protection against inflammation for some people with mild persistent asthma.

Dosage of Nedocromil

- The usual daily dose of nedocromil given by metered dose inhaler is 8 puffs per day. It may range from 4 to 16 puffs per day.
- Initially, many doctors will prescribe the daily number of puffs to be taken in three or four doses, then reduce to two doses.

Comments

- Many people take cromolyn or nedocromil year-round. Others take it only during the season in which they have symptoms, such as winter (the time of respiratory infections) or pollen season in the spring

Table 16. Usual Daily Doses of Cromolyn and Nedocromil

Medicine	Form	Daily Dose
cromolyn	CDN 20 mg per ampule	3–4 ampules (60–80 mg)
	MDI 0.8 mg per puff	8 puffs (6.4 mg)
nedocromil	MDI 1.75 mg per puff	8 puffs (14 mg)

or summer. The timing should be worked out with your doctor.

- Once you stop taking cromolyn or nedocromil, you should restart:
  – four weeks before a threatening season.
  – if your symptoms recur more than two days a week.
- If the doctor reduces your child's cromolyn dose, make sure you monitor your child closely for the next month.
- During an episode, albuterol can be added to the cromolyn to be delivered by CDN. To save time, use 0.25 cc to 0.5 cc of the concentrated albuterol solution, rather than the albuterol that is available in a unit dose (3.0 cc). The total medicine volume will be 2.25 cc or 2.5 cc instead of 5.0 cc. The lower volume of the concentrated medicine will cut the treatment time in half.
- Cromolyn and nedocromil are of no help in treating an asthma episode. However, you should continue using them during an episode so that their antiinflammatory effects are not lost, unless taking the medicine causes significant cough. If cromolyn or nedocromil is stopped and restarted, it may take the usual time to become fully effective again.
- For a discussion of using nedocromil or cromolyn to prevent symptoms with exercise, see Table 7.

LONG-ACTING BETA$_2$-AGONISTS

These controller medicines help prevent asthma symptoms by keeping the airways open for up to twelve hours. These long-acting bronchodilators help eliminate asthma symptoms when added to antiinflammatory treatment (inhaled steroids, nedocromil, or cromolyn). Beta$_2$-agonists work mainly by relaxing the smooth muscles around the airways but possibly also by inhibiting the release of chemicals involved in inflammation.

Because these bronchodilators act slowly, they will not provide emergency relief during an asthma episode. However, since they help control daytime and nighttime symptoms, long-acting beta$_2$-agonists can reduce your need for quick relief medicines. They can also enable you to reduce your dose of an inhaled steroid, but they should not be used as a substitute for it.

There are two types of long-acting beta$_2$-agonists available: one is inhaled, and the other is a tablet. Salmeterol is an inhaled medicine that has been available in the United States since 1994. Its chemical structure is similar to albuterol but modified so that it attaches to smooth muscle cells in the lungs longer and repeatedly stimulates bronchodilation for twelve hours. The other type is an oral albuterol preparation made as an extended-release tablet. This specially-designed tablet releases its dose of albuterol gradually over twelve hours.

Table 17. Long-Acting Beta$_2$-Agonists

Generic Name	Brand Name	Form
salmeterol	Serevent	MDI, DPI
extended-release albuterol	Proventil Repetabs	tablet
	Volmax	tablet

Time Factors of Salmeterol

- Salmeterol usually starts to take effect in ten to thirty minutes. It reaches peak effect in three to four hours.
- Bronchodilation effect lasts at least twelve hours after a single dose of 2 puffs of salmeterol by metered dose inhaler (MDI) or 1 puff by dry powder inhaler (DPI).

Time Factors of Long-Acting Albuterol

- Albuterol extended-release tablets start to work in thirty minutes and reach peak effect in four to six hours.
- Bronchodilation lasts at least eight hours and up to twelve hours after taking 4 to 8 mg.

Possible Adverse Effects

- headache
- nervousness
- irregular heartbeat or palpitations; risk may be increased if you are also taking some antidepressants
- skeletal muscle tremors or cramps
- The adverse effects of salmeterol may be increased if it is taken at the same time as some psychoactive medicines.

Dosage of Salmeterol

- Recommended adult dose is 2 puffs by MDI, or 1 puff by DPI, taken in the morning and again in the evening, approximately twelve hours apart.
- Daily dose should not exceed 4 puffs (84 mcg) by MDI or 2 inhalations (100 mcg) by DPI, as higher doses may cause irregular heartbeat.
- If you are taking salmeterol only to pre-vent symptoms with exercise, take it thirty to sixty minutes before exercise.
- The dose for children under four years of age has not been established.

Dosage of Long-Acting Albuterol

- The recommended adult dose is 4 or 8 mg taken every twelve hours. This dose should be sufficient for most people. (Proventil Repetabs are available in 4 mg tablets; Volmax, in 4 and 8 mg tablets.)
- If the usual dose does not bring relief of symptoms, it can be gradually increased up to a maximum of 16 mg every twelve hours. The dose should never exceed 32 mg in one day. Any increase in dose should be made cautiously under close supervision by your doctor.
- Extended-release tablets must be swallowed whole (not chewed or crushed) for the extended-release mechanism to function properly.
- The dose for children under the age of 6 years has not been established.

Cautions on the Use of Salmeterol

- If you are already taking salmeterol daily to control asthma, do not take additional doses to prevent symptoms with exercise.
- Salmeterol can be used as a supplement to inhaled steroids, not as a substitute for them.
- Use of salmeterol should not be started in a person whose asthma is worsening significantly.

LEUKOTRIENE MODIFIERS

Leukotriene modifiers are a new type of controller medicine. They act by interfering with the formation or action of certain chemi-

Table 18. Usual Doses of Long-Acting Beta₂-Agonists

Medicine	Form	Usual Dose	Maximum Daily Dose
salmeterol	MDI 21 mcg	two puffs, twice per day	four puffs (84 mcg)
	DPI 50 mcg	one inhalation, twice per day	two inhalations (100 mcg)
albuterol (long-acting)	extended-release tablet (4 or 8 mg)	4 or 8 mg, twice per day	32 mg (in two doses)

cals (leukotrienes) in the airways which trigger inflammation and cause bronchoconstriction. Leukotriene modifiers can improve airflow, reduce symptoms, and reduce the bronchoconstriction that occurs in response to allergens, exercise, and especially aspirin.

Leukotriene modifier medicines are very useful in some patients who have not achieved adequate control of their symptoms using a moderate dose of an inhaled steroid. These medicines may reduce the need for a high daily dose of an inhaled steroid or the need to take multiple inhaled medicines. They also offer some people with mild asthma the convenience of once-a-day therapy. Leukotriene modifiers should not be used to bring rapid relief of asthma symptoms during an asthma episode.

Three leukotriene modifiers are available as tablets in the U.S.: montelukast (Singulair), zafirlukast (Accolate), and zileuton (Zyflo). Montelukast and zafirlukast act by blocking the action of leukotrienes that have already formed in the airways. Zileuton works by blocking the formation of leukotrienes during the asthma reaction.

Time Factors

- It may take a few days to a week for a patient to benefit from the antiinflamma-

tory effects of leukotriene modifier medicines.

- The bronchodilation effect may begin within hours of starting the medicine.

Possible Adverse Effects

The adverse effects experienced by patients in clinical trials have differed for each medicine. Leukotriene modifiers have been shown to inhibit the activity of certain liver enzymes that may be needed to metabolize (break down) other medicines in your body. Make sure your doctor knows what other medicines you are taking so she can check if they call for special consideration (monitoring, reduced dose, or change of medicine). Some medicines of concern are erythromycin (an antibiotic) and phenytoin and carbamzapine (antiseizure medicines), but this list is not exhaustive. A very small number of patients taking zafirlukast or montelukast have developed a rare but very serious vascular disorder, Churg-Strauss syndrome. Many experts think that the disorder became apparent when a patient's oral steroid dose was reduced after starting a leukotriene modifier, rather than caused by the medicine itself.

MONTELUKAST

- May interfere with the metabolism of phenobarbital, rifampin, or related medicines. Your doctor should monitor you more closely for the adverse effects of these medicines when starting treatment with montelukast.

ZAFIRLUKAST

- Headache (more frequent), nausea (less frequent).
- Increase in respiratory infections in patients over the age of 55.
- May interfere with the metabolism of warfarin (Coumadin). Your doctor should monitor your prothrombin times and reduce the warfarin dose as needed.
- May interfere with the metabolism of aspirin or theophylline. Your doctor should monitor you for adverse effects of the-ophylline.

ZILEUTON

- Elevated liver function tests, which can indicate impairment of liver activity, were seen in about 3 percent of patients studied. Liver function should be monitored in all patients using zileuton, particularly during the first year of use.
- Upset stomach, nausea (more frequent); abdominal pain, weakness (less frequent).
- Not to be used by people with existing liver conditions or alcohol problems.
- May interfere with the metabolism of warfarin (Coumadin) or propanolol (a beta-blocker). Your doctor should monitor you for possible adverse effects of these medicines.

Dosage

- Refer to Table 19, "Usual doses of leukotriene modifiers."

Comments

- Continue to take your usual dose of an inhaled or oral steroid during treatment with leukotriene modifiers, unless your doctor changes the dose.

Table 19. Usual Doses of Leukotriene Modifiers

Medicine	Form	Age	Usual Daily Dose
montelukast* (Singulair)	5 mg	6 to 14	one tablet, in the evening (5 mg)
	10 mg	15 and over	one tablet, in the evening (10 mg)
zafirlukast† (Accolate)	20 mg	12 and over	one tablet, twice per day (40 mg)
zileuton** (Zyflo)	600 mg	12 and over	one tablet, four times per day (2400 mg)

*Montelukast can be taken with or without food.

†Zafirlukast should be taken either one hour before or two hours after meals because food in the stomach reduces the absorption and effect of the medicine.

**Zileuton should be taken at regular intervals throughout the day.

- A leukotriene modifier will not provide emergency relief during an asthma episode. However, if you are taking this medicine daily, you should continue to take it during an asthma episode.
- Patients who are sensitive to aspirin should continue to avoid aspirin and other nonsteroidal antiinflammatory drugs (NSAIDs) even though a leukotriene modifier may decrease their sensitivity.

THEOPHYLLINE

Theophylline is a bronchodilator of mild-to-moderate strength and has some antiinflammatory properties. In the 1970s and '80s, it was the medicine most widely used to treat asthma. Its use has decreased greatly since then, because inhaled steroids are more effective as controllers and inhaled beta$_2$-agonists are faster, safer, and more effective quick relief medicines. Theophylline is now usually used as an add-on controller medicine in combination with inhaled steroids. If you are taking a high dose of an inhaled steroid to control your asthma, adding theophylline to your daily routine may allow you to reduce your inhaled steroid dose.

Theophylline helps maintain asthma control and prevent symptoms by relaxing the smooth muscles around your airways, allowing them to open more completely. It also increases the ability of the airways to clear mucus and of the diaphragm muscle to contract. Because the effects of long-acting theophylline last for eight to twenty-four hours, this medicine is particularly useful for controlling nighttime asthma symptoms.

Theophylline is a medicine with a low therapeutic index, which means that there is a narrow window within which the dose is both effective and safe. The safe and effective blood level is between 5 and 15 micrograms of medi-

cine. Circumstances that alter the way your body eliminates theophylline will change your blood level (see "Dosage" section). Your doctor must monitor your blood concentration levels to make sure you are taking a dose low enough to be safe. However, now that theophylline is used in smaller doses than before, there is less risk of blood levels being too high. Ask your doctor how frequently your level should be checked. Expert opinion varies. It may need to be checked every six to twelve months.

Time Factors

- Sustained-release, also known as extended-release or long-acting theophylline preparations, start to work in about an hour and reach full effect about two hours after you take the second dose.
- If theophylline doses are taken too close together, the amount of the medicine in your blood may reach high levels and cause adverse effects.
- If doses are taken too far apart, asthma symptoms may reappear.
- Children under 12 years of age should not take once-a-day theophylline preparations because their bodies may eliminate it quickly, resulting in an ineffective low blood level for part of the day.

Possible Adverse Effects

- Theophylline is a safe medicine, but it must be used with care because adverse effects occur at a dose close to the effective dose.
- Liquid preparations or fast-release tablets produce more adverse effects than the sustained-release forms and should not be used.
- Adverse effects are most prominent during the first few days of use and then de-

crease. For this reason, treatment is often started with a low dose.

- The most common adverse effects are hyperactivity, nervousness, insomnia, upset stomach, nausea, vomiting, loss of appetite, and headache.
- You may experience adverse effects with one brand but not with another.
- It may cause gastric reflux.
- Toxic adverse effects such as convulsions, coma, and death have occurred when theophylline blood levels are too high. (See "Medicines and Conditions that Can Raise Theophylline Levels in Your Blood.")

Dosage

- Take theophylline at regular intervals to ensure that the amount in the blood is both effective and safe. It is usually taken every eight to twenty-four hours, depending on the brand.
- Establish a set routine, though occasional deviation from the schedule of an hour or two will not cause a problem.
- Swallow tablets whole or split as indicated, since chewing destroys the extended-release properties of the product. Capsules containing beads can be opened and the beads mixed with applesauce or ice cream.
- Sustained-release preparations are available as capsules and tablets (see Table 20).

Many children 8 years or older can swallow theophylline tablets without difficulty.

- Each sustained-release theophylline preparation has its own advantages and disadvantages, including absorption characteristics, ease of administration, dosage form, dose amount, how long the effect lasts, degree of stomach irritation, and effect of food on medicine absorption.

Doses are individualized, but a common starting dose is 3 to 5 milligrams (mg) per pound of patient weight or 200 mg per day, whichever is lower. The dose can then be increased every three days either until it is effective in controlling symptoms or a blood level of 12 to 15 mcgs per ml is reached. If you experience adverse effects, skip a dose, or take an extra dose of theophylline by mistake, consult your doctor for advice.

WHEN THE DOSE IS TOO HIGH   When your body eliminates theophylline more slowly than usual, the amount of the medicine in your body will increase. This will raise your blood theophylline level, which can cause adverse effects if your dose is not reduced. Viral illnesses, including upper respiratory infections and fever, may slow the elimination of theophylline from your body. For this reason, asthma experts recommend that your theophylline dose be reduced by 50 percent

Table 20. Commonly-Used Extended-Release Theophylline Preparations

Brand Name	Form	Doses Available (mg)	Duration (Length of Effect)
Slo-bid Gyrocaps	capsules	50, 75, 100, 125, 200, 300	12 hours
Theo-Dur	tablets	100, 200, 300, 450	12 hours
Theo-24*	capsules	100, 200, 300, 400	24 hours
Uni-Dur	tablets	400, 600	24 hours
Uniphyl	tablets	400, 600	24 hours

*May produce toxic blood levels if taken within one hour of a high-fat meal.

(one half) or stopped completely under these circumstances.

In addition, taking medicines for other conditions can affect how your body handles theophylline because they compete for processing by your liver. If your liver is occupied metabolizing another medicine (or alcohol), it may be unable to break down theophylline at its usual rate. This can raise the amount of theophylline in your bloodstream and cause adverse effects. (See "Medicines and Conditions That Can Raise Theophylline Levels in Your Blood.")

WHEN THE DOSE IS TOO LOW   If your body eliminates theophylline more quickly than expected, the amount left in your blood will be too low and therefore less effective in controlling asthma symptoms. (See "Medicines and Conditions That Can Lower Theophylline Levels in the Blood."

Comments

- If you develop nausea, vomiting, a severe headache, or irritability, stop taking theophylline immediately. Then contact your doctor to discuss what changes should be made in your treatment plan.
- A small number of my patients take theophylline to reduce their need for a high dose of inhaled steroids.

MEDICINES AND CONDITIONS THAT CAN RAISE THEOPHYLLINE LEVELS IN YOUR BLOOD

- Erythromycin (Ilosone, EES, Pediazole) and other macrolide antibiotics, e.g., clarithromycin (Biaxin), troleandomycin (Tao)
- Quinolone antibiotics, e.g., cipro-floxacin (Cipro), enoxacin (Penetrex), perfloxacin
- Cimetidine (Tagamet), used to treat gastrointestinal problems
- Propranolol (Inderal), used for high blood pressure or migraine
- Allopurinol (Zyloprim), used for gout
- Ticlopidine (Ticlid), used to reduce blood clotting
- Oral contraceptives
- Tacrine (Cognex), used to treat Alzheimer's disease
- Thiabendazole (Mintezol), used to treat for parasites
- Mexiletine (Mexitil), used for life-threatening irregular heartbeat
- Fluvoxamine (Luvox), antidepressant
- Viral infections, especially when accompanied by high fever
- High-carbohydrate diet
- Age: Infants and people older than 60 years of age clear theophylline from their blood 30 percent more slowly than other people.
- Liver failure, cirrhosis
- Consumption of alcohol

MEDICINES AND CONDITIONS THAT CAN LOWER THEOPHYLLINE LEVELS IN YOUR BLOOD

- Smoking cigarettes or marijuana
- High-protein diet
- Charcoal-broiled food
- Phenytoin (Dilantin), phenobarbital, or carbamazepine (Atretol, Tegretol, Epitol), used for seizure control
- Rifampin (Rifadin, Rimactane), an antibiotic
- Moricizine (Ethmozine), used for life-threatening irregular heartbeat

- Theophylline preparations are convenient because they are taken by mouth one to three times a day.
- Do not use theophylline to treat an asthma episode.

Quick Relief Medicines

BETA$_2$-AGONISTS

Beta$_2$-agonists are the medicines of choice for bringing quick relief during an asthma episode and for preventing asthma symptoms related to exercise. Beta$_2$-agonists rapidly relax the smooth muscles around the airways, causing the air passages to open (dilate). For this reason, they are commonly called bronchodilators. Doctors also call them quick relief medicines or rescue medicines.

Beta$_2$-agonists can be inhaled directly into the airways, taken by mouth, or given by injection. The inhaled form acts most rapidly and is least likely to cause adverse effects. Albuterol liquid (syrup) is rarely recommended because the same effect can be achieved by using the inhaled form with a lower risk of adverse effects.

Beta$_2$-agonists are known by many names, including beta-adrenergics and adrenaline-like medicines. I will call them beta$_2$-agonists because that is the name most health professionals use. There are several types of beta$_2$-agonists used in the United States for treating asthma episodes: albuterol, levalbuterol, pirbuterol, and terbutaline. Only albuterol has been approved for patients under 12 years of age, and since albuterol is the most widely prescribed beta$_2$-agonist, I will often refer to beta$_2$-agonists by that name.

In the past, doctors commonly prescribed beta$_2$-agonists to be taken daily for relief of asthma symptoms. Some of the asthma stories you read in Chapter 1 showed patients regularly using albuterol three or four times a day.

Recent studies have shown that people who have mild or moderate persistent asthma gained no additional benefit from taking albuterol daily compared to using it only when they felt symptoms. They can maintain excellent asthma control by taking a controller medicine daily and using albuterol as needed. This "as-needed" approach requires that you and your doctor define which situations call for you to use the medicine.

My patients use albuterol prior to exercise or exposure to cold air and to treat asthma episodes (whether mild, moderate, or severe). They also take it to open their airways before inhaling a controller medicine if their peak flow scores are in the yellow zone. If you are using more than one canister of albuterol per month, or having asthma symptoms more than two times in a week, then your asthma is not under control. Your treatment plan needs to be changed.

Beta$_2$-agonists are related to adrenaline, which causes the airways to dilate, the heart to beat rapidly, and the hand or leg muscles to develop tremors. The beta$_2$-agonist medicines were designed to act mainly in the lungs. They achieve the good effects of adrenaline but with fewer adverse effects on the heart and skeletal muscles.

Beta$_2$-agonists cause the fewest adverse effects when they are inhaled. Sheryl McEnaney discovered that oral and inhaled albuterol had very different effects on her 7-year-old son, Patrick. She wrote this account.

I used to live in fear of Patrick's asthma attacks. He is high strung. Liquid albuterol and theophylline made him feel like crying because he was so shaky. What made it worse, the medicine did not help him much. When he started kindergarten, the frequent colds along with the dry heat and dusty air in the school set off his wheezing.

We went to see a new asthma specialist who recommended that we give the albuterol by compressor driven nebulizer. This brings Patrick fast relief without the shakiness he had with the liquid albuterol. The specialist said Patrick should only use albuterol when his peak flow falls into the yellow zone. He showed Patrick how to use a holding chamber and reminded him that he must inhale slowly and then hold his breath for 10 seconds after he inhales. Patrick likes to count ten pink elephants to measure the time. Patrick no longer sees himself as a wimp or a crybaby. He is now a social boy and a secure student. When I send him out into the cold, I don't worry like I used to.

Almost everyone who received emergency treatment for an asthma episode twenty years ago remembers the epinephrine (adrenaline) shot. This shot dilates the airways and improves breathing within ten minutes. The effect lasts from one to four hours. Side effects of epinephrine include pain on injection, anxiety, restlessness, shakiness, headache, and rapid, pounding, or irregular heartbeat. In the past, some children have been so afraid of getting an injection of epinephrine that they have not told their parents they were having an asthma problem. This led to delay in treatment and an episode that was more difficult to treat. The 1997 NHLBI *Guidelines* recommend giving inhaled beta$_2$-agonist medicines instead of epinephrine shots because the inhaled medicine works faster, lasts longer, and causes fewer adverse effects.

Time Factors

- Inhaled beta$_2$-agonists begin to work within one to five minutes and reach peak effect in thirty to sixty minutes.
- The effect lasts three to six hours.
- If the bronchodilator effect does not last at least three hours, it means that either your

inhaler is empty or dirty (the medicine exit hole is blocked), your technique is incorrect, or your asthma is not well controlled. You should consult your doctor.

Possible Adverse Effects

- Headache, shakiness, rapid or pounding heartbeat, a temporary increase in blood pressure, nervousness, throat discomfort, and nausea are common adverse effects that are generally not dangerous. Research has found that these "common" effects occur in less than 10 percent of patients studied.
- An irregular heartbeat, chest pain, or any other symptom that worries you should be discussed with your doctor.
- Adverse effects may occur with one kind of beta$_2$-agonist medicine, yet not with another.

Dosage

- The dose of albuterol varies with the situation.
- Two puffs is a common dose, although some people get full relief with a single puff.
- If you are having symptoms, wait one to three minutes between puffs. This will allow time for your airways to dilate so more medicine will travel deeper with the next puff.
- Your doctor may prescribe a larger and more frequent dose for use in the low yellow or red zones.
- To prevent symptoms due to cold air, take 2 puffs one to fifteen minutes before exposure.
- To prevent symptoms due to exercise, inhale your beta$_2$-agonist medicine at least fifteen minutes before starting. (Some benefit still occurs if the medicine is in-

haled even one minute before exercise.) A single dose of 1 or 2 puffs is often adequate. Protection for vigorous exercise lasts two hours.

- Use frequent and larger doses of albuterol to relieve symptoms that accompany a severe viral respiratory infection or exposure to an allergen.
- If you need to take more than 6 puffs of albuterol by MDI at once, consider taking medicine by nebulizer instead to save time.
- When giving children cromolyn and albuterol by nebulizer, mix the medicines to save time. Use the concentrated solution of albuterol instead of the unit dose.

- Begin to discontinue beta$_2$-agonist medicines once your peak flow scores have been in the green zone for twenty-four hours. One way of doing this is to first drop the frequency of use to three times a day. If your peak flow score remains in the green zone all day, cut the number of puffs in half for a day. If you remain in the green zone, discontinue the beta$_2$-agonist the next day. Restart if needed.
- It is rare that an extra dose of an inhaled beta$_2$-agonist taken by mistake will cause a significant problem.

Table 21. Beta$_2$-Agonists

Generic Name	Brand Names
albuterol	Ventolin, Proventil, Proventil HFA
levalbuterol	Xopenex
pirbuterol	Maxair
terbutaline	Brethaire, Brethine, Bricanyl

Table 22. Usual Doses of Beta$_2$-Agonists

Medicine	Form	Dose Available
albuterol	MDI	90 mcg/puff
	DPI	200 mcg/inhalation
	nebulizer solution*	unit dose or concentrated solution
	tablets	2 mg, 4 mg
	syrup	2 mg per 5 ml
levalbuterol	nebulizer solution	unit dose
pirbuterol	breath-activated MDI	200 mcg/puff
	MDI	200 mcg/puff
terbutaline	MDI	200 mcg/puff
	tablets	2.5 mg, 5 mg

*Available in plastic or glass vials containing 2.5 mg of albuterol in 3.0 cc of liquid or as a concentrated solution in multidose containers that can be given in a variety of strengths (see Table 23).

Table 23. Dose of Albuterol in Specific Volumes of Concentrated Solution

Volume of Liquid	Dose of Medicine
1.0 cc	5 mg
0.5 cc	2.5 mg (equivalent to unit dose)
0.25 cc	1.25 mg
0.125 cc	0.62 mg

Comments

- If you use more than one canister (200 puffs) of a beta$_2$-agonist medicine in a month, you are taking too much. This usually means that the inflammation in your airways is out of control. You need an antiinflammatory medicine. Discuss a change in treatment with your doctor.
- If your beta$_2$-agonist inhaler does not provide the usual relief, it may be empty or dirty, or you may need to reduce the triggers in your environment.
- If you have mild or moderate persistent asthma, using your beta$_2$-agonist medicine only as needed for symptoms is as effective or more effective than regularly scheduled use.
- If you are taking a beta$_2$-agonist, you should not take a beta-blocker medicine. These two medicines have opposite effects that may cancel out the therapeutic benefits of both. Your doctor may recommend using an alternative to beta-blockers. If this is not possible, she may recommend that you take ipratropium instead of a beta$_2$-agonist as your quick relief medicine.
- Most doctors no longer recommend metaproterenol, an inhaled beta$_2$-agonist, for the treatment of asthma because it is more likely to cause irregular heartbeat than other beta$_2$-agonist medicines.

- Levalbuterol (Xopenex) is a purified form of albuterol.
- Some nebulizer solutions contain preservatives (editate disodium [EDTA] or benzalkonium chloride [BAC]), which may cause bronchoconstriction with repeated use.

Comments on Inhaled Epinephrine (Adrenaline)

- I recommend use of inhaled epinephrine only if you are in an emergency situation and cannot obtain a safer and longer-acting quick relief medicine (a beta$_2$-agonist).
- Epinephrine is more likely to cause shakiness and irregular heart rhythm than beta$_2$-agonist medicines are.
- Epinephrine will relieve asthma symptoms, but only for one to three hours.
- Epinephrine should not be taken during pregnancy, because it can cause the unborn baby to be deprived of oxygen. It also should not be used during breast-feeding, as the medicine will pass through breast milk and may have adverse effects on an infant.
- Epinephrine is available by MDI without a prescription as Primatene Mist, Bronkaid Mist, AsthmaHaler, Bronitin-Mist, Medihaler-Epi, and Primatene Mist Suspension.

SHORT-ACTING BETA₂-AGONIST TABLETS

Beta₂-agonist medicines should be given in tablet or liquid form only in special cases, because the oral form takes longer to work and is more likely to cause adverse effects than the inhaled medicine. This is because the oral dose contains about ten times more medicine than two puffs from a metered dose inhaler. However, if an oral preparation causes adequate bronchodilation without adverse effects, it may be used. Some people use the tablet because it is more convenient to take than the MDI.

Time Factors

- The tablet takes twenty minutes to work, and the effect lasts six to eight hours.

Dosage

- Albuterol is available as 2 and 4 mg tablets. Terbutaline is available as 2.5 and 5 mg tablets.
- An adult can take up to 8 mg of albuterol every six to eight hours around the clock during an episode. The total daily dose should not exceed 32 mg per day. Terbu-

taline can be taken in doses of up to 15 mg per day. Elderly adults should use lower doses to reduce the possibility of irregular heart rhythm.

ANTICHOLINERGICS

Anticholinergic medicines are inhaled bronchodilators, generally taken as add-on quick relief medicines. The most commonly used anticholinergic is ipratropium bromide (Atrovent). It dilates the airways quickly, but not as rapidly as beta₂-agonists do. When taken together with a beta₂-agonist, ipratropium provides additional bronchodilation with minimal adverse effects. When taken alone, ipratropium acts more slowly and less effectively than the beta₂-agonists, so it is not usually recommended as the primary treatment for asthma episodes. Although the U.S. Food and Drug Administration has not specifically approved ipratropium for use in asthma, it is useful as a supplementary quick relief medicine or as a substitute when beta₂-agonists cannot be used (see "FDA Approval of Drugs," page 279).

Used alone, ipratropium is particularly helpful as a quick relief medicine for people with asthma who need to take a beta-blocker medi-

---

Table 24. Usual Doses of Short-Acting Oral Beta₂-Agonists (Tablets)

	Medicine	Amount	Times Per Day	Maximum Per Day
Adults				
	albuterol	2–4 mg	3–4	32 mg
	terbutaline	5 mg	3	15 mg
Children				
	albuterol (ages 6–12)	2 mg	3–4	up to 24 mg
	terbutaline (ages 12–15)	2.5 mg	3	7.5 mg

cine for heart disease, high blood pressure, or glaucoma. Beta-blockers and beta$_2$-agonists should not be taken at the same time because they can cancel each other's effect. Ipratropium may also be useful for people who experience unacceptable adverse effects from beta$_2$-agonist medicines.

Ipratropium relieves asthma episodes through a different mechanism from beta$_2$-agonists. It blocks signals to the smooth muscles that have tightened around the large- and medium-sized airways, enabling the muscles to relax. Since very little of the medicine is absorbed into the bloodstream, adverse effects from ipratropium are rare.

Time Factors

- Bronchodilation begins within five to fifteen minutes, but ipratropium takes one to two hours to reach its peak effect.
- The effect usually lasts from three to four hours, but may last longer.

Possible Adverse Effects

- The most common adverse effects are cough, dry mouth, and unpleasant taste.
- If medicine is sprayed accidentally in the eyes, it can cause temporary glaucoma with symptoms of pain, irritation, and blurred vision. Use a holding chamber to reduce the possibility of ipratropium entering your eyes. When giving ipratropium by nebulizer, use a mouthpiece or a mask with a tight seal.
- Rare adverse effects include dermatitis, swelling of the face, lips, or eyelids, skin rash, and hives.
- People who are allergic to legumes (peanuts, soy products) should not take ipratropium by MDI because it contains soya lecithin and may cause an allergic reaction in sensitive individuals. The nebulizer solution contains no soya lecithin.

Dosage

- The doses listed in Table 25 are usually taken in addition to a beta$_2$-agonist medicine.

Comments

- The amount of bronchodilation produced by ipratropium varies from person to person.
- Ipratropium may be more effective than beta$_2$-agonist medicines for some people over 40 years of age who have a long history of smoking.
- Use of tacrine (Cognex), taken for Alzheimer's disease, may reduce the effectiveness of ipratropium.
- Ipratropium is an important medicine for treating people with Chronic Obstructive Pulmonary Disease (COPD), a severe respiratory condition.

Table 25. Usual Doses of Ipratropium

Form	Unit	Usual Daily Dose
MDI	18 mcg/puff	Adult: 1–4 puffs, 4 times per day
		Child under 12: 1–2 puffs every 6–8 hours, as needed
CDN	0.02% solution	Adult: 500 mcg (2.5 cc) every 6–8 hours, as needed
		Children 5–12: 125–250 mcg (0.6–1.2 cc) every 4–6 hours, as needed

Table 26. What to Do If You Miss a Dose of Medicine

Controller Medicine	What to Do
cromolyn or nedocromil	take dose now and resume schedule
inhaled steroid	take dose now and resume schedule
long-acting beta$_2$-agonist	take dose now and resume schedule
leukotriene modifier	discuss with your doctor
theophylline	discuss with your doctor
Quick Relief Medicine	
beta$_2$-agonist	take dose now and resume schedule
ipratropium	take dose now and resume schedule
Oral Steroids	
oral steroid	take dose now and resume schedule

Table 27. What to Do If You Take an Extra Dose of Medicine

Controller Medicine	What to Do
cromolyn or nedocromil	continue on regular schedule but do not exceed your usual dose for the day
inhaled steroid	continue on regular schedule
long-acting beta$_2$-agonist	continue on regular schedule but do not exceed your usual dose for the day
leukotriene modifier	discuss with your doctor
theophylline	discuss with your doctor
Quick Relief Medicine	
beta$_2$-agonist	continue on regular schedule
ipratropium	continue on regular schedule
Oral Steroids	
oral steroid	continue on regular schedule

Quiz on Asthma Medicines

Accurate knowledge about the medicines used to treat asthma will allow you to communicate better with your doctor. It also provides the foundation for you to work out an effective treatment plan and acquire the skills you need to manage most asthma episodes at home. This quiz helps you test your knowledge of asthma medicines. You should be able to give the correct answer to every question that applies to a medicine you take.

Match the type of medicine with the descriptions listed below.

(C) Controller   **(QR)** Quick relief medicine
(OS) Oral steroids

____ acts rapidly to relax muscles that have tightened around the airways.

____ taken daily to reduce and prevent inflammation in the airways.

____ added to daily medicine routine to boost control of symptoms.

____ taken in short "bursts" to relieve severe asthma episodes or long-term for some cases of severe persistent asthma.

Using the same letters as above, identify each of the asthma medicines by type.

____ inhaled steroids
____ cromolyn / nedocromil
____ theophylline
____ long-acting beta$_2$-agonist medicine
____ leukotriene modifiers
____ fast-acting beta$_2$-agonist medicines
____ ipratropium
____ oral steroids

Answer True or False to the following statements:

____ Medicines taken by inhalation are less likely to cause adverse effects because they are effective in small doses.

____ Different inhalers may contain different amounts of medicine in each puff.

____ Inhaled steroids are the most effective medicine taken daily to prevent inflammation in the airways.

____ Cromolyn is the safest medicine taken daily to prevent inflammation in the airways.

____ A long-term beta$_2$-agonist medicine (salmeterol, extended-release albuterol) will not bring rapid or adequate relief during an asthma episode.

____ Taking inhaled albuterol "as needed" means that you take this quick relief medicine under circumstances worked out in advance with your doctor.

____ Reducing your exposure to asthma triggers can reduce the amount of medicine you need to achieve excellent asthma control.

____ When oral steroids are taken for less than two weeks a year, the adverse effects are usually minor and serious effects are rare.

____ If you need more than two short bursts of oral steroids in one year, your treatment plan may need to be changed.

Short answer questions.

1. Why should you give medicine early to treat an asthma episode? _____

_____

_____

_____

2. How long should you take a quick relief medicine for an asthma episode?_____

_____

_____

3. When do you need to use an oral steroid to treat an asthma episode?_____

_____

4. A "short course" or "burst" of an oral steroid means that you take it for _____ days or less. Adverse effects are more likely if you take an oral steroid for longer than _____ days, or take more than two short courses in one year.

5. What medicines do you (or your child) take?

Medicine	Strength	Action	Time to reach full effect	How long effect lasts

ANSWERS

Match the type of medicine with the descriptions listed below.

(**C**) Controller (**QR**) Quick relief medicine
(**OS**) Oral steroids

QR *(Quick relief medicine)* acts rapidly to relax muscles that have tightened around the airways.

C *(Controller)* medicines are taken daily to reduce and prevent inflammation in the airways.

C *(Controller)* medicines are also added to daily medicine routine to boost control of symptoms.

OS *(Oral steroids):* Oral steroids are in a class of their own. They are taken in short "bursts" to relieve severe asthma episodes. They may also be taken long-term as a controller medicine by a person with severe persistent asthma.

Using the same letters as above, identify each of the asthma medicines by type.

C__ inhaled steroids
C__ cromolyn / nedocromil
C__ theophylline
C__ long-acting beta$_2$-agonist medicine
C__ leukotriene modifiers
QR fast-acting beta$_2$-agonist medicines
QR ipratropium
OS oral steroids

Answer True or False to the following statements:

T Medicines taken by inhalation are less likely to cause adverse effects because they are effective taken in smaller doses.

T Different brands of inhalers may contain different amounts of medicine in each puff.

T Inhaled steroids are the most effective medicine taken daily to prevent inflammation in the airways.

T Cromolyn is the safest medicine taken daily to prevent inflammation in the airways.

T A long-acting beta$_2$-agonist medicine (salmeterol, extended-release albuterol) will not bring rapid or adequate relief during an asthma episode.

T Taking inhaled albuterol "as needed" means that you take this quick relief medicine under circumstances worked out in advance with your doctor.

T Reducing your exposure to asthma triggers can reduce the amount of medicine you need to achieve excellent asthma control.

T When oral steroids are taken for less than two weeks a year, the adverse effects are usually minor and serious effects are rare.

T If you need more than two short bursts of oral steroids in one year, your treatment plan may need to be changed.

Short answer questions.

1. Why should you give medicine early to treat an asthma episode? *It is easier to stop swelling and mucus secretion early on in an episode.*

2. How long should you take a quick relief medicine for an asthma episode? *Until all asthma signs and symptoms have disappeared and peak flow scores have been in the green zone for two full days, unless your doctor says otherwise.*

3. When do you need to use an oral steroid to treat an asthma episode? *When your peak flow or asthma signs score is "stuck" in the low yellow or red zone. (See Chapter 7, "Asthma Treatment.")*

4. A "short course" of an oral steroid means that you take it for 7 days or less. Adverse effects are more likely if you take an oral steroid for longer than 14 days, or take more than two short courses in one year.

5. What medicines do you (or your child) take? *Review this chapter to learn more about each medicine.*

Chapter Four

Devices for Inhaling Asthma Medicines

You must work closely with a competent doctor to control your asthma safely and effectively. To make sure you are getting full benefit from your inhaled medicines, ask your doctor or nurse to check your inhalation technique at each visit.

Devices that people with asthma use to inhale medicine look simple. The directions in the package insert describing their use also seem simple. But the truth is that it takes some work to learn how to use these devices correctly. It takes serious instruction, demonstration, practice, and regular review. With the proper guidance, almost everyone can use these devices effectively and get full benefit from their asthma medicines.

As you will learn in this chapter, several different classes of devices are available for inhaling your asthma medicine: metered dose inhalers (MDIs), holding chambers and spacers used with MDIs, MDIs with special features, dry powder inhalers (DPIs), and compressor driven nebulizers (CDNs) and ultrasonic nebulizers (USNs). Not all medicines can be delivered by each device.

Be aware that the correct technique for using one kind of device may be exactly the wrong technique for using another. My niece Jessie discovered this fact when she switched from a metered dose inhaler to a dry powder inhaler. She called me from Washington, D.C. last year because she started having asthma symptoms when she caught a cold. Jessie generally doesn't have trouble with colds because she takes an inhaled steroid daily. Three weeks earlier, she had told her allergist that she didn't like taking her inhaled steroid with a holding chamber because it was too bulky. The allergist had solved that problem by prescribing the Pulmicort Turbuhaler. The Turbuhaler is a dry powder inhaler, containing an inhaled steroid, that is put directly in the mouth.

Jessie called me to see what she could do to eliminate her symptoms. I asked her to pretend she was using her Turbuhaler while I listened on the phone. She inhaled for five seconds, then held her breath for ten seconds. This was perfect technique for using a metered dose inhaler with holding chamber. But no one had explained to Jessie or to her mom that this technique wouldn't work when using the

Turbuhaler. Proper technique for the Turbuhaler is a rapid, deep breath in. No breath hold is needed. After I explained the proper technique to Jessie, she practiced a few times while I listened. A few days later she was getting the full benefit of her new medicine.

Like Jessie, most people with asthma take their asthma medicines by inhaling them. For an asthma medicine to work, it must come into contact with cells that line your airways. In almost every case, inhaling an asthma medicine accomplishes this faster and more safely than taking a capsule, a pill, or liquid. Even in most emergency situations, inhaled medicines are as effective as injections. They are less painful, work faster, and have fewer adverse effects.

When you inhale a medicine, it can go directly into your airways and begin to act. If you swallow a medicine, it must first go to your stomach, then be absorbed into your bloodstream, then circulate in your blood throughout your body. By the time the medicine reaches your lungs, most of it has been absorbed by other parts of the body. Because only a small amount of the swallowed medicine actually reaches the lungs, you must take a much larger dose of medicine to get the same benefit.

For example, you can swallow albuterol as a pill or liquid or inhale it from a metered dose inhaler (MDI) or dry powder inhaler (DPI). An adult usually takes 2 puffs or about 200 micrograms (0.2 mg) by MDI. When you take it as a pill of 4 mg, you are using twenty times as much medicine to get the same result. This makes adverse effects more likely, explaining why you get shakes that are worse and last longer after you swallow a standard dose of albuterol than when you inhale it. (The inhaled dose may cause no shakes at all.) This dose factor also applies to steroids and is the major reason why inhaled steroids are safer than oral steroids.

Controller medicines such as inhaled

SUMMARY OF DEVICES FOR TAKING ASTHMA MEDICINE

Metered Dose Inhaler (MDI)
- pressurized canister of medicine in a plastic sleeve
- delivers reliable, consistent dose of medicine
- open mouth technique recommended

Holding Chamber with MDI
- delivers medicine more effectively than MDI alone
- reduces adverse effects of inhaled steroids
- with mask, useful for young or very sick patients

Dry Powder Inhaler (DPI)
- activated by inhalation
- difficult for young or very sick patients to use
- contains no propellant

Compressor Driven Nebulizer (CDN) and Ultrasonic Nebulizer (USN)
- Useful for young or very sick patients
- More convenient than an MDI, or MDI with holding chamber, for taking more than six puffs of medicine at a time
- Best way to give cromolyn to children

steroids, cromolyn, nedocromil, and salmeterol are available in inhaled form, as are quick relief medicines (see Table 28). Some asthma medicines, such as leukotriene modifiers, long-acting albuterol, and theophylline, are available only as a pill or capsule. Under some circumstances, a pill or capsule may be more convenient or effective for you, even when an inhaled form is available.

Table 28. Asthma Medicines Available in Inhaled Form

Medicine	Forms Available*
cromolyn	MDI, CDN, USN
inhaled steroids	MDI, DPI, CDN, USN
nedocromil	MDI
salmeterol	MDI, DPI
fast-acting beta$_2$-agonists	MDI, DPI, CDN, USN
ipratropium	MDI, CDN, USN

*Some devices are available for specific preparations only.

Inhaling Asthma Medicine Deep into Your Airways

Unfortunately, much of the medicine you inhale does not reach your lower airways, where it can help your asthma; it is trapped in the mouth. Some medicine gets caught on surfaces of the tongue, palate, throat, and voice box and is absorbed from there into the bloodstream. Inhalation devices create tiny droplets or powder particles that range in diameter from 1 to 40 microns. (A micron is a millionth of a meter.) Only the particles between 1 and 5 microns are small enough to enter the lower airways that are affected by asthma.

The larger particles will not produce any good effects in your lungs, but may cause adverse effects throughout your body. A holding chamber helps keep the large medicine particles out of your mouth. Under ideal conditions, about 15 to 30 percent of the medicine in an inhaled dose will reach your lower airways. Certain medicines and devices are better than others at making particles of the correct size. If you use your medicine devices properly, you inhale as many of the small particles and as few of the larger particles as possible.

The Right Medicine the Wrong Way

People generally come to see me because they have been unable to gain control of their asthma through their previous treatments. Each person's story is different, but in my years as an asthma specialist, I have seen the same problem over and over again. People are usually taking effective medicines but not getting much benefit because they are taking them the wrong way. Many times, a patient only needs proper instruction in how to use an inhalation device, and asthma symptoms disappear in the next few weeks.

Juan's story is typical. Juan first came in with his mother for a consultation when he was 11 months old. His primary care doctors had been hesitant to make a diagnosis of asthma despite Juan's bouts of bronchitis, pneumonia, and coughing. He had been treated with inhaled albuterol (quick relief medicine) in the doctor's office and in the hospital. It didn't take long for us to work out an effective plan. His parents gave him oral steroids for the first week of treatment to clear up the inflammation in his airways and continued treating him with 4 ampules of cromolyn daily by nebulizer. For the first month, they added albuterol to the cromolyn solution. Taking cromolyn daily kept Juan out of asthma trouble for the next few years.

I didn't see Juan again in the office for three years, since his family moved to Boston. His doctor there changed his daily medicine from cromolyn to an inhaled steroid, which Juan was to take by holding chamber with mask. Soon after, Juan started having asthma trouble again. He had four colds in three months, and each cold triggered an asthma episode that lasted for two weeks.

Concerned that his asthma had gotten worse, Juan's parents brought him back to see me. During the visit, I asked his mom to show me how she gave Juan the inhaled steroid using the holding chamber with mask. She began correctly, placing the mask so it made a good seal with Juan's face. Then she squeezed a puff of inhaled steroid into the chamber, and Juan breathed it in. But two seconds later she gave him another puff. She gave a total of four puffs of medicine in eight seconds. No one had told her that it would take 20 seconds for Juan to empty each puff of medicine from the chamber.

After learning this, Juan's mother used the holding chamber with mask perfectly. It took about twenty seconds for him to take six breaths. His mother then waited thirty seconds before squeezing the next puff into the chamber. I made no further change in Juan's treatment. One month later, his mother called me to let me know that Juan had no asthma symptoms at all.

There are several possible reasons why patients take medicines the wrong way:

- No one taught them how to take the medicine.
- Someone taught them the wrong way.
- Someone showed them the right way but didn't check that they did it properly.
- They learned the proper technique but lost the skill over time because the technique was not reviewed at subsequent office visits.

When you finish reading this chapter, you will have the knowledge you need to work with your doctor to get the best effect from inhaled medicines. After you learn the proper technique, it is important to work with an observer who can give you feedback. Once you get the procedure right, you should pay attention to your technique each time you take your medicine.

Metered Dose Inhalers (MDIs)

Metered dose inhalers are safe and convenient devices for taking inhaled medicines. Most people with asthma use an MDI, which consists of a metal medicine canister that fits inside a plastic sleeve (See Figure 14). When you press down on the canister, a valve opens and propellant forces medicine into the air as a spray. As this spray exits through a tiny hole in the mouthpiece, the propellant evaporates in a fraction of a second and leaves the small medicine particles to be inhaled. If you use your MDI correctly, about 15 to 30 percent of the medicine will reach your lower airways.

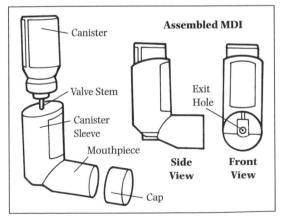

Figure 14. Metered Dose Inhaler (MDI)

PROPER USE OF A METERED DOSE INHALER

There are four main aspects to the proper use of an MDI, which is called "open mouth technique":

- *Position.* You should hold the MDI one to two inches away from your mouth.
- *Hand-breath coordination.* You should already be breathing in when you press the canister down in the MDI sleeve to release the medicine.
- *A slow breath in.* Inhalation of medicine should take three to five seconds.
- *A breath hold of five to ten seconds.* My patients count "one green elephant, two green elephants" for ten seconds, because "one-one thousand, two-one thousand" takes too little time.

Position. Position the MDI one to two inches away from your mouth. This allows the large medicine particles to drop out of the mist before the rest of the medicine enters your mouth, thereby reducing adverse effects in the mouth and throat and throughout the body. (Large particles are unable to reach your lower airways and, if inhaled, are absorbed into your bloodstream.) A second benefit is that less propellant will enter your mouth. In addition, the medicine mist has time to slow down, allowing it to make the sharp turn down into your trachea (windpipe) more easily.

Hand-breath coordination. Press down on the medicine canister just after you start to breathe in. If you press down on the canister before you start to inhale, all of the medicine particles will hit the air sitting in your mouth and bounce back out. Watch someone use an inhaler this way, and you will see the medicine mist spill back into the room. You can check your own technique by using an MDI in front of the mir-

ror. If you see medicine coming out of your mouth, you know it didn't get into your lungs. You should correct your technique and repeat the dose.

Slow breath in. Breathing in slowly helps the medicine move down into your airways instead of getting stuck to the back of your throat. As you continue to breathe in as fully as you can, the medicine is drawn deep into your airways, where it can do its job.

Ten-second breath hold. Hold you breath for 5 to 10 seconds once you have inhaled the medicine mist. Remember that the tiny particles of medicine must touch the cells lining your airways in order to have a good effect. It takes time for them to settle out of the mist and stick to the airway lining. By holding your breath at least five seconds, ten seconds if possible, you give the medicine time to deposit. If you breathe out too quickly, you will simply exhale much of the medicine back into the room.

Check your MDI technique by following these step-by-step instructions:

1. Stand up and remove cap.
2. Make sure that the canister is inside the plastic sleeve, with the valve stem pointing toward the mouthpiece.

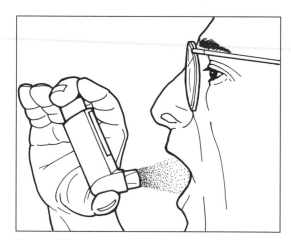

Figure 15. Proper Inhaler Position

3. Shake your inhaler hard for two seconds (with a finger over the top of the canister so it doesn't fall out).
4. Position the mouthpiece one to two inches from your lips. (Some people use three fingers pressed together as a measure. Remove your fingers after you have positioned the MDI.)
5. Open your mouth wide.
6. Breathe out naturally.
7. Start to breathe in slowly through your mouth.
8. As you start to breathe in, squeeze the medicine canister down to release the medicine.
9. Breathe the medicine mist in slowly for three to five seconds.
10. Hold your breath for five to ten seconds.
11. If you are taking your daily controller medicine or pretreating before exercise, wait thirty seconds before taking another puff of medicine.
12. If you are having asthma symptoms, wait one to three minutes between puffs of a quick relief medicine (albuterol) and between the quick relief medicine and any other inhaled medicine. (The wait allows your airways to open further, so more medicine from the next dose can reach deep into your lungs.)
13. Prime your MDI by releasing one puff of medicine into the room before you use a new canister for the first time.

Some children can use an MDI effectively, but most cannot. It is not easy for a child to perform good MDI technique. I have seen some parents resort to what I call "blow-by" technique, which is not effective. The parent points the inhaler at her child's mouth and presses the canister down. A mist of medicine moves toward the mouth. But the timing will be off and the breath hold will be too short. Your child is much better off using an MDI with holding chamber, or an MDI with holding chamber with mask. I will describe both of these devices later in the chapter.

COMMON ERRORS

People who are just learning how to use an MDI, or who have not been properly guided in its use, make some common errors. They release the medicine too early, instead of just after beginning to breath in. They put the MDI into their mouth, instead of positioning it one to two inches away. Most often, they breathe in too quickly, instead of taking three to five seconds to inhale, and do not hold their breath for five to ten seconds. Each of these errors will reduce the amount of medicine that reaches the lungs. Because it is easy for technique to become sloppy as time passes, ask your doctor or nurse to check your technique at each office visit.

THE CLOSED MOUTH TECHNIQUE

The closed mouth technique was widely used before the open mouth technique was developed but it is less effective. In closed mouth technique, you place the MDI mouthpiece directly in your mouth and close your lips snugly around it. The rest of the technique is the same as open mouth.

Problems with this technique are:

- Large medicine particles end up in your mouth and are absorbed into the bloodstream, causing increased adverse effects.
- Smaller particles move so fast that they strike the back of your throat, so less medicine reaches your lower airways.
- It is impossible for an observer to see if you have good hand-breath coordination.

The Maxair Autohaler

One type of MDI is specially designed to be used with closed mouth technique: the Maxair Autohaler, which contains pirbuterol, a quick relief medicine (see Figure 16). The mouthpiece is placed directly in your mouth. It contains a special device that triggers release of medicine when you inhale with sufficient force. There is no need to press down on the canister. People with arthritis have found this breath-activated system easier to use than standard MDI. Another advantage of this design is that you do not have to coordinate your breathing with activating the MDI.

TAKING CARE OF YOUR MDI

To clean your MDI, first remove the medicine canister from the plastic sleeve by pulling gently on the canister. Wash the plastic sleeve in warm, soapy water for thirty seconds, rinse thoroughly, shake off excess water, and allow to air-dry before you put the medicine canister in again. Don't wash the medicine canister. It is a good idea to clean the sleeve once a week, especially if you are using an MDI with HFA propellant (see below). The exit hole in the

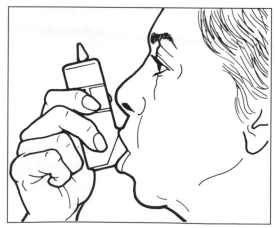

Figure 16. Maxair Autohaler. This device is used with closed mouth technique.

mouthpiece of an HFA inhaler is smaller than that in other inhalers. It may become clogged if you do not wash it regularly.

The performance of an MDI is also affected by temperature extremes. If it is too cold, the MDI may not deliver a reliable dose of medicine to your airways. If it is exposed to extreme heat, the canister could explode. MDI manufacturers recommend that you do not expose your MDI to temperatures greater than 120 degrees Fahrenheit, a condition that could occur in a closed car during the summer. To insure that your MDI functions properly, follow the storage recommendations found in the package insert, or ask your pharmacist for information.

PROPELLANTS USED IN MDIs

All metered dose inhalers contain propellants to disperse the medicine from the canister. Until 1998, the only propellants available were chlorofluorocarbons (CFCs). These chemicals are nontoxic, nonflammable, and evaporate almost instantly once they force medicine out of the MDI canister. Unfortunately, they have been found to damage the stratospheric ozone layer, a crucial part of the earth's atmosphere that screens out harmful ultraviolet radiation from the Sun. Therefore, the production and sale of CFCs have been banned by international agreement. Temporary exemptions for medical uses will last until alternative propellants are developed. An alternative propellant, hydrofluoroalkane (HFA), is currently available for some medicines.

HOW CAN YOU TELL WHEN YOUR INHALER IS EMPTY?

The most reliable way to keep track of the medicine in your MDI is to calculate the "discard date" each time you start to use a new inhaler. Check how many puffs (metered inhalations) of medicine are in the full canister.

The number of puffs in inhalers varies: it may be 80, 100, 112, 200, 240, or 400. The number is printed on the canister label. Divide this number by the number of puffs you take in a day. The result is the number of days your inhaler will last.

For example, let's say your MDI contains two hundred puffs of medicine. If you take 8 puffs every day, your MDI will last for twenty-five days. Calculate the discard date and write it on the canister label and in your asthma diary. If you start using this inhaler on September 5, you should throw it away on September 30. If your treatment plan calls for you to take six puffs every day, this inhaler will last for thirty-three days, with a discard date of October 8.

We used to estimate how much medicine remained in an inhaler by seeing how well it floated in a container of water. This test was not always reliable and caused medicines like cromolyn and nedocromil to clog in the inhaler valve stem. The discard date method is the simplest and most reliable way to keep track of an inhaler you use daily.

Quick relief medicines like albuterol are not taken regularly, so there is no way to calculate ahead of time how long your MDI will last. You can record each albuterol dose on a label taped to your MDI or in your asthma diary. Alternately, you can purchase an electronic dose counter (Doser) for about $30 (see Figure 17). This device looks like the face of an electronic watch. It is connected to a short, rubber sleeve that attaches snugly onto the top of your MDI canister. Each time you press on the canister to release a dose of medicine, the Doser counts the puff. It keeps track of how many doses you have left as well as the number of doses taken that day. This device is particularly helpful for an inhaler that you use intermittently.

Once you have used up the number of puffs

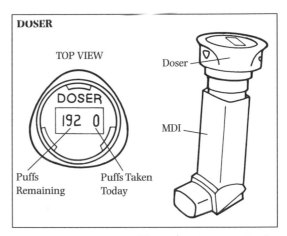

Figure 17. The Doser. This device keeps track of how many puffs of medicine are left in your MDI.

listed on the canister label, two things happen inside the MDI. First, the pressure drops, and any remaining medicine won't mix properly with the propellant. Second, the tiny cup that measures the medicine dose fails to fill properly. For both these reasons, you won't get a proper dose of medicine from an MDI that is used past its puff total. You should discard your inhaler once you have used the number of puffs listed on the label.

Do not try to figure out whether your inhaler is empty by using the "shake" test. When you have used up the total number of full puffs, you will still hear some medicine sloshing inside. However, the remaining medicine will not generate a reliable dose on its own. The mother of one of my patients used to think that as long as she could hear some medicine in the MDI when she shook it, there was enough left to treat her son. Then he developed a bad asthma episode while using a depleted inhaler. Now she counts the doses by recording them in an asthma diary and always knows when to start a new inhaler.

Holding Chambers

Holding chambers help people of all ages get full benefit from their MDI while reducing possible adverse effects. These devices are used in combination with an MDI and let you deliver inhaled medicines more effectively than by open mouth or closed mouth technique. Holding chambers hold the medicine mist released from a metered dose inhaler so you can breathe it in more slowly. Other names for holding chambers are "spacers" or "extenders."

A holding chamber has a body with two openings: a mouthpiece and a place to insert the MDI. Holding chambers come in various shapes and sizes (see Figure 18). Some look like a tube, some look like a ball, some look like a box, and some are shaped like a pear. Two fold up like an accordion. The most effective holding chamber has the following attributes:

- a volume of at least 5 ounces
- a valve that holds the medicine until you breathe it in and prevents you from exhaling into the chamber
- a flow monitor to indicate when you breathe in too fast

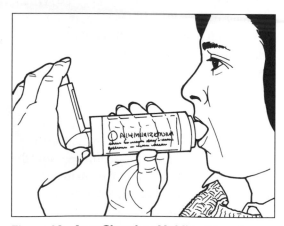

Figure 18. AeroChamber Holding Chamber

A collapsible holding chamber is in effect an effort monitor that tells parents their child is taking a good breath in.

A holding chamber makes MDI technique much simpler and can increase the benefit you get from the medicine. When your MDI is inserted into the holding chamber, it is the proper distance from your mouth. When you press down on the medicine canister in your MDI, the medicine is released into the chamber and is held there until you inhale. Therefore, you don't need to coordinate the timing exactly, although you should start to breathe in within one second. Since you can inhale the medicine more slowly from the chamber, more of it gets deep into your small airways.

Holding chambers can also reduce the possible adverse effects from medicine. Many of the medicine particles that would be too large to enter the small airways drop out of the airstream and stick to the wall of the chamber. Since they never enter the mouth, they cannot be absorbed by the body and thus cause no adverse effect. Also, since the medicine is mixed with air as it is inhaled, the bad taste is reduced.

A holding chamber is designed for taking only one puff of medicine at a time. If you put several puffs into the holding chamber at the same time, the small particles of medicine will clump together and will be too big to reach your small airways. As a result, you will get less medicine from two or three puffs together than you would from one puff.

In general, a holding chamber should be washed every one to two weeks with warm water and detergent, and it should be allowed to air-dry overnight. About once a month, you should take it apart to clean it more thoroughly. Consult the package insert from your holding chamber for specific instructions.

A makeshift holding chamber, such as a paper tube, is inexpensive and convenient for improving delivery of a quick relief medicine taken away from home.

HOLDING CHAMBERS WITH MASK

Holding chambers with masks became available in 1993 (see Figure 20). They are particularly helpful for infants or small children who cannot make a good seal around the mouthpiece with their lips or hold their breath after inhaling medicine.

The holding chamber with mask works like a regular holding chamber except it does not require a person to breathe in slowly or hold her breath. After one puff of medicine is released into the chamber, the child (or adult) breathes in and out normally into the mask. It generally takes twenty seconds of normal breathing for a person of any age to fully inhale one puff of medicine from a holding chamber. The next puff of medicine can be released into the chamber thirty seconds after the first puff has been completely inhaled. A mask must be the right size to make a good seal with the person's face if it is to deliver medicine properly. A well-designed mask has a valve that allows the user to breathe out normally while holding the medicine inside the chamber.

WHEN TO USE A HOLDING CHAMBER

It is most important to use a holding chamber when you take an inhaled steroid by MDI. Using a holding chamber every time you use your MDI will give you full benefit from the medicine at the lowest effective dose. Using a holding chamber reduces the risk that you might develop the long-term adverse effects of growth retardation, osteoporosis, cataracts, or glaucoma. It also reduces the possibility of the short-term effects of hoarseness and a yeast infection in the mouth. It is still important to

rinse with water and spit out after taking an inhaled steroid to reduce adverse effects. Most of my patients take inhaled steroids only once or twice a day, so they don't have to carry their holding chambers with them.

WHICH HOLDING CHAMBER SHOULD YOU USE?

Since most people with asthma take several medicines, it makes sense to buy a holding chamber that works with any type of MDI. The holding chamber should be easy to use, easy to clean, and strong enough to last at least a year. Several holding chambers have an intake valve that prevents medicine from entering your mouth unless you are inhaling. This reduces the risk of adverse effects. This valve also prevents an accidentally exhaled breath from entering the chamber. Some chambers have a flow-rate monitor, which makes noise if you breathe in too quickly. An effort monitor is helpful for parents of small children, since it shows if the child is actually breathing medicine in through her mouth. In Tables 29 and 30, I summarize the qualities of five holding chambers to help you choose which one suits your needs best.

AeroChamber Holding Chamber (Monaghan Medical Corp.)

The AeroChamber is suitable for most patients. Because it is so reliable and effective, it is the holding chamber most often used in scientific studies of asthma medicines. The AeroChamber has an intake valve and also a flow monitor that whistles if you breathe in too fast. Since it is made of clear plastic, you can observe how your child is breathing in the medicine mist. Illustrations and instructions for use are printed on the device. If you hear a whistling sound while you are breathing in, you have inhaled too quickly to get full benefit

Table 29. Design Characteristics of Five Holding Chambers

Chamber	Valve	Flow Monitor	Collapsible	Mask
AeroChamber	Yes	Yes	No	Yes (3 sizes)
EasiVent	Yes	Yes	No	No
E-Z Spacer	No	No	Yes	Yes (1 size)
InspirEase	No	Yes	Yes	No
Space Chamber	Yes	No	No	Yes (4 sizes)

Table 30. Approximate Yearly Cost* of Five Holding Chambers

Chamber	Purchase Cost	Replacement Time	Approximate Yearly Cost
AeroChamber	$34**	more than one year	$34
EasiVent	$22	more than one year	$22
E-Z Spacer	$20**	months–1 year†	$20–60
InspirEase	$28	months–1 year†	$45–62
Space Chamber	$27**	more than one year	$27

*Prices are based on retail sales in New England. They may vary by region.
**Price for holding chamber without mask. Purchase with mask will cost more.
†Depends on frequency of use. Torn bags must be replaced.

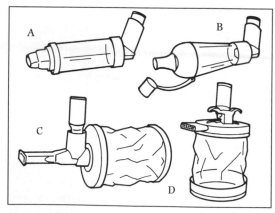

Figure 19. Four Holding Chambers. A: Aero-Chamber, B: EasiVent, C: InspirEase, D: E-Z Spacer. The Space Chamber (not pictured here) is similar in shape to the AeroChamber.

from your medicine. The AeroChamber is a 5-inch-long tube that cannot be folded or compressed, so it will not fit in your pocket. Since my patients take their controller medicines at home, they do not need to carry an AeroChamber with them. It does fit well into a fanny pack, purse, or briefcase, and it is very durable and easy to clean.

INSTRUCTIONS FOR USING THE AEROCHAMBER
1. Stand up and place MDI mouthpiece (without cap) inside the hole at the end of the AeroChamber.
2. Shake MDI and holding chamber hard for two seconds (holding on to both).
3. Exhale fully through your mouth.

4. Place the mouthpiece of the AeroChamber on your tongue (behind your teeth, like a Popsicle).
5. Close your lips snugly around the AeroChamber mouthpiece.
6. Spray one puff of medicine into the chamber.
7. Breathe in slowly, taking three to five seconds to inhale the medicine.
8. Hold your breath for ten seconds.
9. Wait thirty seconds before taking another puff of medicine. Wait one to three minutes after taking a puff of quick relief medicine if you are having asthma symptoms.

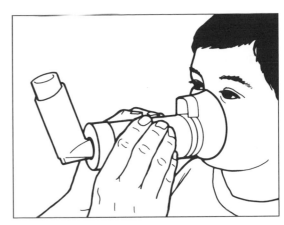

Figure 20. AeroChamber with Mask

Inhaling slowly helps the medicine reach deep into your airways.

AeroChamber with Mask

The AeroChamber with mask is available in three sizes: infant, young child, and standard (adult). It is designed to be used with relaxed normal breathing, so no flow or effort monitors are needed. This device is excellent for young children or anyone who cannot breathe in slowly or hold her breath for ten seconds. It also is helpful for anyone who has difficulty making a good seal around the holding chamber mouthpiece or coordinating inhalation with MDI activation. You can empty one puff of medicine from the chamber in twenty seconds of normal breathing.

INSTRUCTIONS FOR USING THE AEROCHAMBER WITH MASK

Follow the instructions printed on the device. Place the mask over your child's nose and mouth. The mask must fit snugly over your child's face, leaving no gaps between the mask and the skin. Check with your doctor to make sure the fit is good, especially as your child grows.

Once the mask is in place, spray one puff of medicine into the chamber. Allow the child to breathe in and out normally for twenty seconds for each puff of medicine. Adults should also breathe in and out for twenty seconds. Because this chamber has a valve, your child will be able to exhale comfortably without displacing the mask. You should still wait thirty seconds after each puff of a controller medicine or a quick relief medicine. If your child is having symptoms, wait one to three minutes after each puff of a quick relief medicine.

EasiVent Holding Chamber (Dey Laboratories)

The clear, cone-shaped EasiVent has a valved mouthpiece that prevents you from exhaling accidentally into the chamber. Basic instructions for use are printed on the chamber, and a flow monitor will sound if you inhale too quickly. The chamber can be opened easily, which is convenient for cleaning and allows you to carry or store your MDI inside the chamber. This hard plastic device should last a year or more with normal use.

Instructions for using the EasiVent are identical to those for the AeroChamber. No masks are available for use with the EasiVent.

Space Chamber Holding Chamber
(Pari Respiratory Equipment, Inc.)

The Space Chamber is a clear plastic cylinder, somewhat larger than the AeroChamber. The standard model can be used with any of four available masks (infant, pediatric, adult regular, and large). It has an intake valve, but it does not have a flow monitor. The valve in the chamber ensures that the mask does not lift off your child's face during exhalation. The plastic is durable and can be cleaned in the dishwasher.

Instructions for using the Space Chamber are identical to those for using the AeroChamber.

InspirEase
(Key Pharmaceuticals, Inc.)

I call this collapsible holding chamber "the accordion" because it makes a musical sound if you breathe in too fast. When parents see the bag collapse, they know their child is taking in a good breath of medicine. The InspirEase requires a slow breath in and a breath hold of five to ten seconds to be most effective. This may be difficult for children under 4.

The InspirEase has two main components: a collapsible plastic bag and a hard plastic mouthpiece. The InspirEase is not as durable as the hard plastic holding chambers, but it is easier to carry. If the bag has even a small hole or tear, it will be less effective and must be replaced. The manufacturer recommends replacing bags every two to three weeks, but the bag can last up to three months if you use it with care. The mouthpiece is detachable and can be washed with warm water daily.

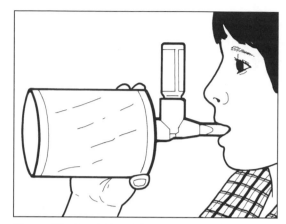

Figure 21. InspirEase Holding Chamber

INSTRUCTIONS FOR USING THE INSPIREASE

1. Assemble the mouthpiece and bag as directed in the package insert and expand the bag.
2. Place the MDI valve stem directly into the InspirEase plastic receptacle.
3. Stand up and shake the MDI and InspirEase hard for two seconds (holding on to both).
4. Exhale fully through your mouth.
5. Place the mouthpiece on your tongue (behind your teeth, like a Popsicle) and close your lips snugly around it.
6. Release one puff of medicine into the chamber.
7. Breathe in slowly for three to five seconds. The bag should collapse completely and not make a musical sound.
8. Hold your breath for five to ten seconds.
9. After inhaling a puff of medicine, wait at least thirty seconds before taking another puff. Wait one to three minutes after taking a puff of quick relief medicine if you are having asthma symptoms.

E-Z Spacer
(WE Pharmaceuticals, Inc.)

The E-Z spacer is a collapsible holding chamber similar to the InspirEase, but it does not make a sound if you breathe in too quickly. The mouthpiece is small and built into the top plate of the collapsible bag. Like the InspirEase, the E–Z spacer does not have a valve that prevents you from exhaling into the bag by mistake.

Because the device is only one piece, it is even more compact than the InspirEase. However, you must replace the whole spacer when the bag tears or wears out. It is easy to clean, since the end plate is removable. The entire device can be washed by submerging it in warm water weekly or more often, if use requires. A small mask for children aged 2 to 5 is available.

Instructions for using the E-Z spacer are similar to those for the InspirEase.

Dry Powder Inhalers (DPIs)

The medicine in these inhalers comes out as a powder, instead of the aerosol produced by a metered dose inhaler (MDI). To use this device, you place the mouthpiece directly in your mouth. Breathing in forcefully draws the powder into your lungs. This fast, deep inhalation provides the force needed to disperse the medicine throughout your airways.

Currently, four medicines (two inhaled steroids, salmeterol and albuterol) are available in powder form (see Table 31). I discuss the Turbuhaler and the Diskus as examples here. The Rotahaler delivers powdered albuterol from a capsule, and the Rotadisk delivers a powdered inhaled steroid from multidose packets. Other dry powder inhalers (DPIs) will be available soon.

Dry powder inhalers offer several advantages. The propellant-free design means that the performance of a dry powder inhaler is not reduced by cold temperatures, as with an MDI. And unlike an MDI, it is easy to tell when a dry powder inhaler is empty. Because they are breath-activated, the coordination of releasing medicine and inhaling occurs automatically. Finally, because they release no CFCs, dry powder inhalers do not damage the earth's stratospheric ozone layer.

Dry powder inhalers also have some drawbacks. First, because the mouthpiece goes directly in your mouth, much of the powdered medicine lands inside your mouth and throat, increasing the possibility of adverse effects. For this reason, it is particularly important to rinse your mouth with water and spit out after each dose. Second, delivering a reliable dose of medicine from one of these inhalers depends on the force of your inhalation. Poor effort or inability to breathe in quickly enough may reduce the

Table 31. Asthma Medicines Available in a Dry Powder Inhaler

Device	Medicine	Dose (per inhalation)
Pulmicort Turbuhaler	budesonide	200 mcg
Flovent Rotadisk	fluticasone	50, 100, 250 mcg
Serevent Diskus	salmeterol	50 mcg
Ventolin Rotahaler	albuterol	200 mcg

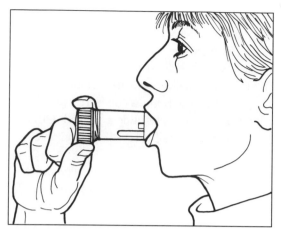

Figure 22. Using a Turbuhaler Dry Powder Inhaler

dose of medicine you receive. You also must be sure to place the mouthpiece on your tongue, behind your teeth (the Popsicle position).

The powdered medicine must stay dry to prevent it from clumping together (caking). Keep it sealed in its container until just before you are ready to take a dose. To prevent caking, do not wash any dry powder inhaler that contains medicine.

USING A DRY POWDER INHALER CORRECTLY

If you are used to taking inhaled medicine by MDI, you will have to adjust your technique to use a DPI properly. Each dry powder device has a different design and specific instructions for use. For all of them you should turn your face away from the mouthpiece to exhale before taking medicine so you don't blow any powder out of the device. Then, put the mouthpiece in your mouth and take a fast breath in to pull the medicine into your airways.

Some DPI package inserts instruct you to hold your breath after inhaling medicine, while others do not. Holding your breath for five to ten seconds will not cause a problem and may lead to an additional benefit from the medicine. Because the dose of medicine contained in a single inhalation from a DPI may be different from the dose of medicine in one puff from an MDI, you may take a different number of doses per day.

Many aspects of using a dry powder inhaler are completely the opposite from what you have learned to do with your MDI. For example, you should never shake a dry powder inhaler, because you can scatter the medicine powder and lose part of the dose. For the same reason, you need to hold a DPI oriented as the instructions specify while you are using it. This means holding it so the mouthpiece faces up or sideways.

Pulmicort Turbuhaler (Astra USA)

The Turbuhaler contains budesonide (an inhaled steroid) as a fine powder. This torpedo-shaped device is about the size of a roll of quarters and has no removable parts except for the dome-shaped cover. It should be stored with the cover on to prevent moisture from causing the powder inside to cake. Each dose in a Turbuhaler contains 200 mcg of an inhaled steroid. The specific amount of medicine you get from each dose depends on how fast you breathe it in.

The device comes preloaded with two hundred doses. Below the mouthpiece you will see a small "dose indicator" window. When you have twenty doses left, a red mark will appear at the top of the window. When this red mark reaches the bottom of the window, your Turbuhaler is empty and should be discarded.

INSTRUCTIONS FOR USING THE TURBUHALER
The first time you use a new Turbuhaler, you need to prime it once:
1. Hold the device with the mouthpiece up.
2. Turn the brown grip on the bottom to the right, then back to the left until it

clicks. Turn it to the right and the left again.

3. Now this Turbuhaler is ready to use.

For daily use:

1. Hold the Turbuhaler with the mouthpiece up. Remove the cover by holding onto the brown disk at the bottom, then twist and pull the cover upward.
2. To load a dose, twist the brown grip at the bottom to the right as far as it will go. Then twist it to the left until you hear a click.
3. Shift the Turbuhaler to the horizontal position.
4. Turn your face away from the device and breathe out comfortably through your mouth. (If you do blow into the device by accident, twist the Turbuhaler again. This will replace the spilled dose with a new one.)
5. Place your mouthpiece on your tongue (between your teeth, like a Popsicle) and close your lips around it.
6. Breathe in once forcefully and deeply through your mouth. You do not need to hold your breath.
7. Rinse your mouth with water and spit out.
8. If your doctor has prescribed more than one dose, repeat this process.
9. When you are finished, replace and twist the cover to keep the powder dry.

Serevent Diskus (Glaxo Wellcome)

The Diskus contains salmeterol, a long-acting beta$_2$-agonist medicine. This disk-shaped device is approximately 3 inches in diameter, about the same size as a compact make-up kit. There are no removable pieces. It comes already loaded with sixty sealed packets, or blisters, of salmeterol powder. Before you can inhale medicine, you need to pierce a blister. This is done by rotating a small lever on the device. The activation also causes a counter to register the dose activated to keep track of how many doses you have left. When you have used up the sixty blisters, you must buy a new Diskus. It cannot be reloaded.

The Diskus device contains the same medicine found in the salmeterol MDI. However, one inhalation from the Serevent Diskus contains twice as much medicine as one puff from the MDI.

INSTRUCTIONS FOR USING THE DISKUS   Hold the device level (horizontal) with the "Serevent Diskus" label facing up during all the following steps. The package insert contains illustrated instructions for use.

1. Rotate the thumb grip counterclockwise while holding onto the case. (This will expose the mouthpiece, a small lever, and the dose counter.)
2. Hold the mouthpiece toward you but a few inches from your mouth.
3. Press the small lever all the way over to the dose counter until you hear it click. This punctures the medicine blister.
4. Turn your head away from the Diskus and exhale comfortably.
5. Put the mouthpiece in your mouth (on your tongue, like a Popsicle), and close your lips around it.
6. Breathe in steadily and deeply through your mouth.
7. Remove the Diskus from your mouth and hold your breath for ten seconds.
8. Close the Diskus by rotating the thumb grip clockwise.

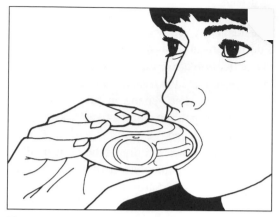

Figure 23. Using A Diskus Dry Powder Inhaler

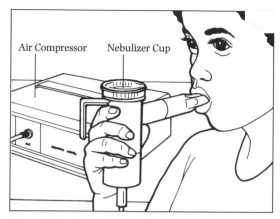

Air Compressor   Nebulizer Cup

Figure 24. Compressor Driven Nebulizer

Compressor Driven and Ultrasonic Nebulizers

Nebulizers create a medicine mist by two different mechanisms. In a compressor driven nebulizer (CDN), a machine (the compressor) produces air under pressure, which flows at a steady rate. The air passes from the machine through a tube into a plastic nebulizing cup that contains liquid medicine. The air is then forced through this specially designed cup, creating a fine mist of medicine particles. Finally, the mist flows out of the cup through an exit tube, into a mouthpiece, and then into your mouth and lungs. For infants or children who cannot use the mouthpiece, the exit tube can be attached to a mask.

An ultrasonic nebulizer (USN) produces mist by using a sound wave to agitate the liquid medicine inside the chamber. I will use the term "nebulizer" to refer to both compressor driven and ultrasonic devices.

For many years, nebulizers have been used to treat asthma in hospitals and emergency rooms. They are popular and effective because they require little cooperation and no special technique for the patient to benefit from the medicine. The effectiveness of a nebulizer is due

to the large dose of medicine it delivers, not to anything special about the device itself. The dose of albuterol given by nebulizer is seven to fourteen times greater than the standard dose given by MDI. Two puffs from an MDI contain 180 mcg of albuterol, while the usual dose given by nebulizer is 1,250 to 2,500 mcg.*

In the 1980s, nebulizers played a very prominent role in the home treatment of hundreds of thousands of people with asthma. Doctors recommended these devices for anyone who was too sick, too young, or otherwise unable to use an MDI with a holding chamber.

Fortunately, preventive care has improved dramatically in the past few years, reducing the need for nebulizers. The use of inhaled steroids makes it possible for almost all people with persistent asthma to achieve excellent control of their asthma. With such control, people need to treat acute asthma episodes by nebulizer less frequently. In addition, the holding chamber with mask allows a person of any age to inhale asthma medicine effectively. Before the holding

---

*The actual amount of albuterol placed in the nebulizer cup is 2,500 to 5,000 mcg. About one-half of this medicine is lost to the room when the mist escapes out the top of the cap, so the inhaled dose is 1,250 mcg to 2,500 mcg.

chamber with mask became available, the nebulizer was the only device that could deliver inhaled medicines effectively to patients unable to hold their breath. Now, a parent can choose which of these two devices to use for a small child. (Nebulizers are still very helpful devices for managing asthma in the hospital, the doctor's office, and at home, but fewer people with asthma need to own one.)

If you (or your child) have been in the hospital or emergency room or have received urgent treatment in a doctor's office for asthma more than once, you should consider purchasing a nebulizer for home use. You will need it until you work out an effective asthma treatment plan with your doctor. If, after you have a good asthma treatment plan, your breathing problems still develop quickly, it makes sense for you to have a nebulizer at home. Also, if you have a child under 4 who takes cromolyn, you should deliver it with a nebulizer. (The full daily dose can be given in two sittings per day.)

USING A NEBULIZER AT HOME

If you and your doctor decide it is best for you to have a nebulizer at home, you need to understand how to assess your asthma status, how the machine works, and what medicines are to be taken. Before your doctor sends you home with the nebulizer, he should make sure that you:

- use a peak flow meter properly or know the four signs of asthma trouble
- understand your asthma medicines
- are willing to keep an asthma diary
- have been trained in the use of the nebulizer
- have a written home treatment plan for your asthma

You can learn how to use a nebulizer from your doctor, a nurse, a respiratory therapist, or other health professionals. Home care companies can provide instruction in your home, and insurance companies sometimes cover their charge for services. Much of the information you need about using a nebulizer is contained in this book, but a health professional must observe you using the device to make sure your technique is correct. You can buy a nebulizer without a prescription, but don't rely on a salesperson to teach you how to use it.

Before you start to use a nebulizer at home, you must know when it is safe to give treatment at home and when to seek medical help during an asthma episode. Taking a quick relief medicine by nebulizer can provide temporary relief from asthma symptoms, but if your peak flow score drops or your symptoms return in less than four hours after a treatment, you should consult your doctor for advice. Taking a quick relief medicine more than six times in twenty-four hours may be dangerous.

The danger is not in giving too much medicine, but in the fact that you haven't been able to control your asthma with a treatment that is usually effective. This often means that the inflammation in your airways must be treated with oral steroids to bring the episode under control. You may also need to make changes in your environment. *It is not safe to give more than six treatments within 24 hours without consulting your doctor.*

USING A NEBULIZER PROPERLY

When you receive your first nebulizer treatment in the office, the nurse should describe each step to you. Ideally, you should set up the second treatment yourself while the nurse stands by to comment and to answer questions. I lend a nebulizer to patients so they can continue treatment at home for the duration of an asthma episode. If they require a loaner nebulizer a second time, I suggest they buy one.

There are three parts to good nebulizer technique:

- The medicine mist must flow freely into your mouth.
- Your breathing rate must be slowed down.
- Breathing in should take longer than breathing out.

Medicine must flow freely into your mouth. For your medicine to help you, it must leave the nebulizer cup, enter your mouth, and be breathed into your lungs. This happens most effectively when you use a mouthpiece rather than a mask. The mouthpiece must be placed on the tongue, behind the teeth (the Popsicle position), with your lips sealed around it. When you use a mouthpiece you pull all the medicine mist into your mouth as you breathe in. In contrast, most masks are designed with two holes that allow you to breathe out comfortably. As you breathe in, a large amount of room air passes through these holes into your mouth. Much of the medicine mist stays behind, never entering your mouth.

Many infants can take asthma medicine effectively from an infant-sized mouthpiece. Your child may kick and cry, especially when you first try to use a mouthpiece. But after she cries, she must breathe in, and she will draw some medicine into her lungs. After you've treated her for several days, she will struggle less because she is used to the procedure and knows that her struggle won't keep you from giving her the medicine.

Though a good seal around the mouthpiece leads to the best results, your child does not have to close her lips around it to benefit from the medicine. Place the mouthpiece between her open lips. Make sure that the mouthpiece is pointed toward the throat, not at her cheek or the roof of her mouth. To give a medicine treatment to a sleeping child, rest the mouthpiece or the top of the nebulizer cup on the child's lower gum without waking her. Some medicine will escape, but she will breathe much of it into the airways.

People who breathe only through their noses (usually children), rather than through their mouths, should use a mask or wear nose clips. If you and your doctor decide to give medicine with a mask, make sure that the mask fits well so no medicine escapes around the sides. Simply holding the mask close to the nose and mouth is not an effective way to deliver medicine.

Your breathing rate must be slowed down. Nebulizers are easier to use than an MDI, because you don't have to hold your breath after you inhale. However, the medicine does need some time to settle onto your airway lining to do its job most effectively. The more slowly you breathe, the more time the medicine has to settle. If we assume breathing in and breathing out take an equal amount of time and you breathe 20 times per minute, each breathing cycle (breathing in plus breathing out) takes three seconds. In this case, breathing in takes one and a half seconds — that's how much time there is for the medicine to attach to your airway lining. If you breathe 30 times a minute, the medicine will have only one second to settle, and more of it will be exhaled into the room.

I have noticed that many people start breathing faster as soon as a nebulizer mouthpiece is put into their mouths. I have been able to gradually talk most people ages 2 and older down to a rate of 10 to 20 breaths per minute. At this slower breathing rate, treatment is much more effective.

Breathing in should take longer than breathing out. An important part of nebulizer technique is to take longer to inhale than to exhale. Many healthy people do this naturally, but during an asthma episode that pattern often changes. As your airways narrow, breathing out becomes difficult and takes more time. During a severe episode, breathing out may take twice as long as breathing in. If you can deliberately take more time to breathe in, your medicine will benefit you more, your treatment will start to work faster, and its effect will last longer.

To get the best effect from your treatment with a nebulizer, first work on slowing down your breathing rate, and then work on taking longer to breathe in. It is a good idea to practice while you are feeling fine, just to get the hang of it. That way it will require less thought and effort during an asthma episode. Some people find that holding their breath for five seconds every fifth breath increases the effectiveness of their treatment.

"Blow-by" technique is a much less effective way to give medicine by nebulizer. It involves holding the nebulizer mouthpiece close to your child's mouth. Some medicine enters her mouth but most of it disappears into the room. You may have seen this method used in the emergency room, hospital, or in a doctor's office. Health professionals often use it because it doesn't require any cooperation from the patient. But in order to get an effective dose of quick relief medicine into the patient, they often give multiple or continuous doses. This is safe only in a hospital environment, where doctors and nurses can monitor the patient closely to see that the dose is both effective and safe.

Blow-by is not an effective technique to use at home.

Do not give cromolyn or inhaled steroids by blow-by technique. Your child needs a full dose of these controller medicines each day to receive the cumulative benefit of treatment. Blow-by technique will not deliver a full dose.

To make sure the treatment is effective and safe, you must observe your child taking her medicine with a nebulizer. Treatment using an efficient nebulizer cup should take less than five minutes. For safety, you should watch your child while she uses a mask; it is possible for a child to vomit during a treatment. If this occurs, the mask must be removed immediately to prevent inhalation of vomit into the airways. For maximum effectiveness, you should continually observe any child under 6 using a nebulizer. Check that she is breathing slowly and maintaining a good seal either around the mouthpiece or between the mask and her face. Otherwise, she may get only a fraction of the medicine produced by the nebulizer.

Occasionally, the dense mist produced by a nebulized medicine may cause a cough. This usually can be eliminated by breathing in more slowly.

The instructions for using an ultrasonic nebulizer are similar to those for a compressor driven nebulizer. You can adjust your intake of medicine by your breathing rate or depth, pro-

Table 32. Comparison of Three Techniques for Delivering Medicine By Nebulizer

	Mouthpiece	Mask	Blow-by
Medicine goes	into mouth	into mouth and nose	mostly into room
Effective	most	medium	least
Cooperation required	most	medium	least
Comment	can be used by young children	less enters lungs since nose removes medicine	never use to deliver controller medicines

longing inspiration, or holding your breath after a certain number of inspirations. Some ultrasonic nebulizers have a control that allows you to adjust the flow of medicine. A slow flow is less likely to produce cough.

WHAT KIND OF NEBULIZER MACHINE SHOULD YOU USE?

If you and your doctor decide that you should use a nebulizer at home, you have a choice about which kind to purchase. Most nebulizers sold in the U.S. are powered by an air compressor. These machines vary in size, shape, weight, the noise they produce, and cost. Some get their power from a wall outlet. Others are powered by a wall outlet and a battery and/or a car lighter plug. A high-quality compressor driven nebulizer (the ProNeb or ProNeb Turbo by Pari Respiratory, or the PulmoAide by Sunrise-DeVilbiss) costs less than $90 when purchased by mail. Portable units are more expensive. Nebulizers may cost more when you buy one in a drugstore or if instruction from a respiratory therapist is included in the purchase price. Some health insurance policies cover the expense of a nebulizer. For a nebulizer used daily, replacement of non-durable parts will cost less than $30 per year.

Ultrasonic nebulizers are quieter, lighter, and often smaller than compressor driven nebulizers. They are also more expensive and more fragile. You may prefer using an ultrasonic nebulizer in an office, library, or other place where the noise of the usual compressor driven nebulizer might be disturbing. Prices range from $265 to $400 and are comparable to those of a portable compressor driven nebulizer. If the machine is used daily, replacement parts cost between $15 and $30 per year.

WHAT KIND OF NEBULIZER CUP SHOULD YOU USE?

The most important part of the compressor driven nebulizer is the cup that produces the medicine mist. The various nebulizer cups available fit any compressor, so you can buy the one that suits your needs, no matter which air compressor you own. Some nebulizer cups are disposable and last a few weeks. Others are made to last for a year and come with a six-month warranty. Their costs range from $10 to $17.

More than a dozen nebulizer cups are commercially available, and they vary widely in how well and how fast they deliver medicine. You should consider several factors when selecting a nebulizer cup. To be most effective, a nebulizer should create a mist of medicine particles that are small enough to reach deep into the lungs. A few nebulizer cups do this much better than others.

An efficient nebulizer cup should:

- nebulize 2.5 cc of medicine in less than five minutes.
- provide more than fifty percent of this output as particles that can reach the lower airways (1 to 5 microns).

In a study of seventeen nebulizer cups conducted in 1995, only the Pari Jet and the Pari LC Jet met these criteria. The exact time it takes to deliver medicine will depend on the kind of compressor you use.

A nebulizer makes mist continually during a treatment. Almost all nebulizers lose about half of this medicine to the room while you are exhaling. A new generation of nebulizer cups, for example, the Pari LC Plus and the Pari LC Star, has a valve system that solves the medicine escape problem (see Figure 25). A valve in the nebulizer cup closes when you exhale. It traps the medicine mist in the cup until you are ready to inhale again, so more medicine gets from the nebulizer cup to your lungs. The valve in Pari cups can be removed.

Make sure that your doctor knows if you are using a cup with a medicine-retaining valve. Doctors usually prescribe medicine given by nebulizer based on the fact that nebulizer cups lose half of the medicine during exhalation. When a doctor prescribes 4 amplues of cromolyn daily, he knows that 2 amplues will be lost into the room. If you are using a medicine-retaining cup, you will receive twice as much medicine as your doctor intended unless he reduces the dose. If you are giving a quick relief medicine, such as albuterol, along with the cromolyn treatments, the dose of albuterol should be reduced as well.

I recommend that parents use the valved nebulizer cup to give cromolyn to their child. Since hardly any medicine is lost during expiration, your doctor can reduce the dose of cromolyn from 4 ampules to 2 ampules per day. The lower dose saves money but the treatment time remains the same. The cost of giving 4 ampules of cromolyn per day is approximately $85 to $90 per month. If that dose is cut in half by using a medicine-retaining cup, a family can save $40–45 per month. That adds up to $480–$540 per year.

If you are giving only a quick relief medicine by nebulizer, you have a choice. You can remove the medicine-retaining valve and give the usual dose of quick relief medicine. Or, you can keep the valve in the cup and ask your doctor to recalculate the dose. If you or your child are taking ipratropium by nebulizer, use the medicine-retaining valve to keep the medicine away from your eyes.

Another way to reduce loss of medicine is to use a flow interrupter, a simple vent for air located below the medicine chamber of the nebulizer cup. (It can be a separate piece or part of the nebulizer tubing.) When you cover the vent with your thumb or finger, you force air into the medicine cup, creating the fine medicine mist. When you uncover the vent, air coming from the compressor flows out before it reaches the medicine, so no medicine mist is made. If you cover the vent only when you are inhaling, you will lose less medicine.

When purchasing a nebulizer cup, consider durability, reduction in cost of medicine, time saved in giving medicine, and purchase price.

In Summary

When you take medicine by inhalation, you maximize the amount of medicine that reaches

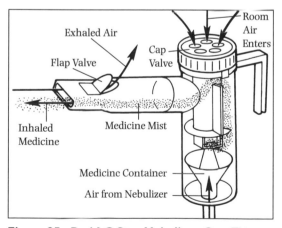

Figure 25. Pari LC Star Nebulizer Cup. This cup has a removable cap valve at the top to prevent medicine mist from escaping during exhalation.

your lungs, while reducing adverse effects. In addition, inhaled quick relief medicines start to work faster than when taken as a pill or liquid. To achieve full benefit from your inhaled medicines, you must take them using proper technique. Make sure your doctor or another health professional teaches you how to use each of your asthma medicine devices and then checks your technique regularly.

Chapter Five

Peak Flow

You must work closely with a competent doctor to control your asthma safely and effectively. Peak flow monitoring will make little sense until you know your personal best peak flow score.

Your "peak expiratory flow rate" (PEFR), or peak flow, is the most accurate way for you to measure how your airways are doing. Almost all my patients use it to manage their asthma at home.

Peak flow measures how fast you can move air out of your lungs in a fraction of a second; it is your fastest flow. Peak flow is high when your large airways are clear: it is lower when they are narrowed or blocked. Since your scores often drop before you are aware of any asthma symptoms, you can use peak flow as an early warning system. Monitoring peak flow will help you start treatment early and avoid serious problems. Anyone with persistent asthma or who has had a severe asthma episode will benefit from using peak flow to learn about and manage asthma.

Peak flow is measured with an inexpensive, portable meter about the size of a flashlight (see Figure 26). Meters come in many shapes: cylinders, boxes, and triangles. When you give a hard, fast blow of air through the mouthpiece, a marker on the meter moves along a numbered scale. The marker stops at your peak flow score. This score is an objective measure of your airflow that you — as well as doctors, parents, relatives, teachers, friends, and others — can use to manage asthma. Once you have a solid understanding of your asthma, peak flow can provide a reliable guide for asthma treatment. Peak flow scores also help by reinforcing your perception of asthma symptoms, making them easier to quantify and harder to ignore.

Peak flow meters allow you to reduce the uncertainty that can be so frightening with asthma. If your asthma is not well controlled, an episode may come on suddenly and your symptoms may worsen quickly. This sudden onset can be especially alarming. Will an episode respond to the usual home treatment? Will it require a visit to the doctor or the emergency room? What will happen then? Your peak flow scores can provide the answers.

The fact is that a full-blown asthma episode almost always comes on slowly, but its onset

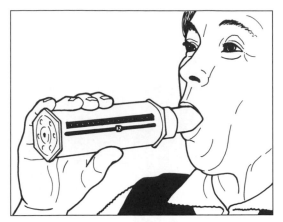

Figure 26. Mini-Wright Peak Flow Meter

might seem sudden if you miss or ignore a series of early signs of trouble. Many people do not notice any symptoms until a great number of their airways have been blocked. Others ignore their symptoms as long as possible because they don't think that they have an asthma problem or they want to avoid the hassle of dealing with asthma. If these people had measured the airflow from their lungs, many of them would have seen a drop in their peak flow scores before they noticed any symptoms. If they had started treatment early, they could have reduced the intensity and duration of the episode. With a peak flow meter, almost everyone 5 years old and older can do exactly that.

Spirometry (pulmonary function testing) and peak flow monitoring are complementary tools in the diagnosis and management of asthma. Peak flow is done at home with an inexpensive meter and measures the fastest rate that air is leaving the lungs. In contrast, spirometry is done in the doctor's office and requires a more elaborate machine that can measure the rate of airflow throughout exhalation and inhalation. Doctors commonly use a spirometer to measure your FEV_1 (forced expiratory volume for one second) score. This is most air you can blow out in one second. This FEV_1 score can provide accurate and helpful information about the extent of inflammation and bronchoconstriction in your airways. However, since affordable FEV_1 meters for home use are not yet available, these measurements are done only in a doctor's office.

Spirometry is particularly useful in diagnosing asthma, distinguishing asthma from other lung problems, and checking lung function until asthma is under excellent control. For a person with moderate asthma, spirometry should be done about once a year after excellent control is established. If asthma is more severe, or if particular difficulties exist, more frequent spirometry may be necessary.

Using Peak Flow at Home

To manage your asthma at home, you must first master the four steps of peak-flow based treatment:

1. Learn how to blow a peak flow and read the score from the meter.
2. Learn to assign that score to a peak flow zone: green, yellow, or red.
3. Carry out the proper treatment for that zone.

 FOUR STEPS OF PEAK FLOW BASED TREATMENT

- Learn to use the peak flow meter
- Identify the asthma treatment zone
- Carry out proper treatment for the zone
- Monitor response to treatment

4. Monitor how well your airways respond to treatment by checking your peak flow and recording the scores in a peak flow diary.

After you read this chapter, you will understand how to take each of these four steps, in cooperation with your doctor. The Asthma Peak Flow Diary (Chapter 6) and a written Home Treatment Plan (Chapter 7) will help you learn to apply this knowledge to controlling your asthma.

Peak flow is more than a monitoring tool. It is your best asthma teacher. When your peak flow score drops, you know to look in your environment for asthma triggers. When you remove asthma triggers from your environment and take your asthma medicine, you can see your peak flow scores rise. If you have symptoms and your peak flow score doesn't increase after you take a quick relief medicine, you know that your airways are probably narrowed by inflammation. This means you need treatment with an antiinflammatory medicine.

Your peak flow scores also allow you to communicate more effectively with your doctor during an office visit and over the phone. Your doctor will be able to interpret the combination of peak flow scores and symptoms more accurately than she can judge symptoms alone. This means you can get better advice from your doctor. For parents of a child with asthma, peak flow scores can provide all of your child's caregivers with a useful guide for assessment and treatment. Audrey Eldred wrote this account of how peak flow enabled her family to take control of asthma.

Dan's Story
Audrey Eldred
First visit in the 1990s

Dan is a much happier and healthier 5-year-old this winter. It's been many months since I've heard his sad, discouraged little voice saying "I hate having asthma." Using the peak flow readings has also made our family life much calmer. We're not anxiously trying to assess how sick he is or making guesses about whether he needs the doctor or the ER. Now peak flow readings tell us when there's trouble, and the rest of the time we can relax.

Dan has had four respiratory infections since September. With each one, his peak flow readings fell dramatically. When this happened, we adjusted his medicine and kept him almost completely free of asthma symptoms. No scary middle-of-the-night wheezing or trips to the ER so far this winter.

Last winter, before we were using the peak flow meter, we kept Dan indoors during much of the cold weather because the cold air seemed to make his asthma worse. He was miserable because he loves to play in the snow. This year we've done peak flow readings before and after he goes outside, and have figured out that he can even exercise in quite cold weather without difficulty, unless he has a cold. He is having so much fun this year! He gets to go outside at recess with his friends, and he gets to go sledding like everyone else. We've used this same peak flow routine with sports and determined that he doesn't have to miss basketball or soccer unless he is acutely ill.

Dan usually stays in the green zone. I will let him go to school or participate in activities away from home in the high yellow zone. In addition to his individual scores, I look at the trend of his peak flow scores, his symptoms and how easily my husband or I can be reached at work that day. My judgment is getting pretty good, so we have no surprises. On a couple days when Dan's condition appeared marginal, I went to the school at noon, measured his peak flow, and gave him albuterol by nebulizer instead of a puffer.

Our relationship with our pediatrician has changed. He has always been supportive and concerned. However, because I was terrified that Dan would die of asthma I felt dependent on the doctors and the emergency rooms. The pediatrician referred us to you for a consultation. Now that we have a better understanding of asthma and have peak flow readings to guide us, Dan hasn't been to the ER at all.

In the five months since our first visit to you I have taken Dan to the pediatrician only once for asthma. I wanted his opinion on my treatment plan. Instead of telling me what to do, he asked me what I thought and then he said, "Carry on." Having seen the changes in Dan and in our family, our pediatrician told me he is now using peak flow meters and parent education with all his kids with asthma.

I like the peak flow meter because it's a step towards Dan managing his own asthma. He's beginning to know what the numbers mean and to respond to them, rather than struggling with me. He understands that under 200 means he must stop to use his puffer before going outside. He can be annoyed or disappointed, but the issue is between him and the score, not between us. I know that this is an important step for any kid with a chronic illness. Because of our understanding of asthma and peak flow monitoring, Dan is healthier, we are all happier, and asthma is no longer running our family.

Measuring Peak Flow

You need to understand how to use the peak flow meter and how to read it before you can benefit from using it. Although it is possible to make an error, most people have no trouble doing peak flow reliably. Before you start monitoring peak flow at home, a health professional should demonstrate proper technique to you and then watch as you demonstrate.

Most people can learn the basics of using a peak flow meter in a few minutes. It may take some practice before your technique is satisfactory. Your doctor or a staff member should check your technique regularly.

To use a peak flow meter properly:

1. Remove gum or food from your mouth.
2. Move the pointer on the peak flow meter to zero.
3. Stand up and hold the meter horizontally.
4. Make sure your fingers are away from the vent holes and the marker.
5. Breathe in as much air as you can.
6. Quickly place the mouthpiece on your tongue behind your teeth.
7. Close your lips snugly around the mouthpiece and blow out as fast as you can — a short, sharp blast. (You don't need to get all of the air out of your lungs. The meter only measures the first fraction of a second.)
8. Observe where the marker has stopped: this is your peak flow score.
9. Move the pointer to zero and wait at least 15 seconds.
10. Blow two more peak flow scores.
11. Take the highest of the three tries as your peak flow score.
12. Record that score in your asthma diary.

Generally, whenever you do peak flow, you should make three good attempts. Three attempts allow you to correct any problems with technique or effort so that your peak flow score accurately shows how open your large airways are. Take the highest value you get as your peak flow score; do not average them. Peak flow is like the high jump. You get three tries to make your best score.

If you usually cough after you blow a peak flow, it means that your asthma is not well controlled and your doctor needs to change your treatment.

When you are quite sick, exhaling forcefully may trigger a bout of coughing or wheezing. In this case, just blow once. Base your treatment on this single reading. Under these circumstances, it is likely that your score will be in the low yellow zone or red zone.

COMMON ERRORS

There are some common problems that cause peak flow scores to be low. Most people blow out too slowly when they are first learning. Remember that your peak flow attempt should be a fast blast. It will sound like a huff. Also, if your lips are not sealed well around the mouthpiece or the mouthpiece doesn't fit well, air will escape without being measured. Some people forget to breathe in fully before starting their peak flow. Do not pause between inhalation and the fast blast. Occasionally, a physical problem, such as an inflamed eardrum, will cause pain when you blow and reduce the effort exerted.

Several techniques cause you to produce an artificially high peak flow score:

- coughing during a fast blast
- spitting while blowing, especially if your meter has a small mouthpiece
- blowing with pursed lips on the mouthpiece, like a trumpet player
- allowing your cheeks to balloon out before blowing (the chipmunk maneuver)

While you are learning, it is likely that your scores will vary widely. However, if a health professional guides you properly, you will be able to correct any problems with technique and blow reliable, consistent scores. Your score will improve with instruction and practice. If you blow a score far above your personal best (see below), don't count it, check your technique and repeat the attempt.

Once you have learned the proper technique and have blown reliable peak flow scores, never attribute a low score to poor effort. If you can't move the marker on the peak flow meter or have a very low score, you may have an extremely serious problem and should call 911 immediately. Go to the emergency room if you do not have 911 service.

A peak flow score less than 50 percent of your personal best that does not improve after inhaling a quick relief medicine also calls for you to see your doctor or go to the emergency room right away.

The Personal Best Peak Flow Score

If you are healthy, your peak flow score should always be close or equal to your personal best peak flow score. The personal best is the highest number you have blown when you are having no signs or symptoms of asthma and your airways are completely clear. If you blow a low peak flow score, it doesn't necessarily mean that you are not as healthy as someone with a high score. The important thing is how close your score is to the best you can blow.

Peak flow score has a lot to do with the size of your lungs. Scores vary between people by height, age, sex, and race. A taller person will generally have a higher personal best peak flow score than a shorter person. Girls generally have slightly lower peak flow scores than boys, and African-Americans have slightly lower peak flows than white Americans and Mexican-Americans. However, the difference in the peak flow scores of one individual during an asthma episode is much greater than the differences between individuals due to height, race, or sex.

You may have heard that your peak flow score is "normal" if it is equal to or higher than the average peak flow for someone your age and height. This is not always true. The average is calculated for a particular group of healthy people of a given height, which may be further grouped by age, sex, or race. It is impossible to predict whether your score will be higher, lower, or the same as the average score. In fact, the average score is not very helpful. What you really need to know is the best score you can blow when your airways are completely clear of inflammation and bronchoconstriction. For some people, the best will be higher than the average, while for others, it will be lower.

My 12-year-old patient Sage blew a peak flow score of 480 at her first visit. The average peak flow for girls her height (5'7") is 470. It would seem that her peak flow score was normal. Yet, Sage complained of having a tight chest during gym class and swim meets. After taking albuterol (a quick relief medicine) in my office, her score increased to 565. With additional treatment, she blew a score of 610 two weeks later. This was her personal best score, much higher than the average score on the table for a girl her height.

Another patient, Sarah, was 5'8" tall and a competitive long-distance runner. The average peak flow for a young woman her height is 480. You might expect an athlete to exceed the average peak flow score, but after achieving excellent asthma control, Sarah's best peak flow score was 400. Her airways were clear, she had no asthma symptoms, and she became an All-American runner in college.

Sarah certainly had healthy lungs that could support hard training. So why was her personal best lower than the average? She had long legs and a short torso. A short torso means smaller lungs and a lower peak flow score.

DETERMINING YOUR PERSONAL BEST PEAK FLOW SCORE

At your first asthma visit, it is unlikely that your doctor will be able to determine your personal best peak flow. She will take the average peak flow score from a chart, or use the best score you can blow at that visit, whichever is higher. For example, if you blow a score of 300 at your first office visit, and the average for someone your height is 350, your doctor should use the higher number. If the average score is 350 and you blow a score of 400, your doctor should use the 400 as your personal best. You and your doctor do not want to set your expectations too low.

Since I base the asthma treatment plan on the personal best peak flow score, I make sure that my patients really achieve their best. To do this, they must have clear airways. I prescribe seven days of prednisone (an oral steroid) and inhaled albuterol (a quick relief medicine) to reduce or eliminate inflammation and asthma symptoms. If patients prefer not to take prednisone, taking a moderate dose of an inhaled steroid daily for one month usually will have the same effect. Clearing the airways is necessary to determine the personal best peak flow score in almost all people who have symptoms several times a week. People who have had uncontrolled asthma for many months or years will need to take an oral steroid for more than seven days to clear their airways.

After a patient has cleared his airways and learned how to blow peak flow correctly, I take the highest score he can blow on two separate days as his personal best (even if it is below the average). I tell the patient to reset his personal best whenever he blows a higher score on two separate days.

Table 33. Average Personal Best Peak Flow Scores by Height and Age

Women

Age	Height (inches)				
	55	60	65	70	75
20	390	425	460	495	530
25	385	420	455	490	525
30	380	415	450	485	515
35	375	410	440	475	510
40	370	400	435	470	500
45	365	395	430	465	495
50	360	390	425	455	490
55	355	385	420	450	480
60	350	380	415	445	475
65	345	375	405	440	470
70	340	370	400	430	460

Men

Age	Height (inches)				
	60	65	70	75	80
20	555	600	650	695	740
25	545	590	635	680	725
30	530	575	620	665	710
35	520	565	610	650	695
40	510	550	595	635	680
45	500	540	585	620	665
50	485	525	570	605	650
55	475	515	555	595	635
60	465	500	540	580	620
65	450	490	530	565	605
70	440	475	515	550	585

Scores are rounded to the nearest interval of five.
Adapted from Leiner, GC, et al., 1963.

Using Peak Flow to Guide Asthma Treatment

Asthma specialists agree that the most reliable way to guide treatment at home is to follow the zone system based on your personal best peak flow score. These asthma zones correspond to the colors of a traffic light. Green means "Go: no additional medicine needed" and includes scores of 80 to 100 percent of your personal best. Yellow means "Caution: time to intensify treatment" and includes scores ranging from

Table 34. Children and Adolescents: Average Peak Flow Scores by Height

Boys

Height in Inches	Average Score	Range*
40	150	110–190
42	170	120–220
44	190	135–245
46	210	150–270
48	230	165–295
50	250	180–320
52	270	195–345
54	300	215–385
56	330	240–420
58	360	260–460
60	390	280–500
62	415	300–530
64	445	320–570
66	480	345–615
68	515	370–660
70	550	395–705

Girls

Height in Inches	Average Score	Range†
40	170	125–215
42	190	140–240
44	210	155–265
46	225	165–285
48	245	180–310
50	265	195–335
52	290	210–370
54	310	225–395
56	330	245–415
58	360	265–455
60	380	280–480
62	405	300–510
64	435	320–550
66	460	340–580
68	480	360–600

Scores are rounded to the nearest interval of five.
*Includes 95 percent of white males age to 20 years.
†Includes 95 percent of white females age to 20 years.
Adapted from Hsu, K., et al., 1979.

50 to 80 percent of your personal best. Red means "Stop! Danger! Time for emergency action" and includes all peak flow scores falling below 50 percent of your personal best.

The yellow zone is divided into two parts — the high yellow and the low yellow zones — to allow for more individualized treatment. An asthma episode in the high yellow zone can be treated without an oral steroid, while an episode in the low yellow zone often requires several days of treatment with an oral steroid. The red zone signals a severe asthma episode requiring medical attention right away.

I recommend that you base your asthma treatment on peak flow scores blown before inhaling a quick relief medicine (bronchodilator) such as albuterol. This prebronchodilator score gives you a better idea of how vulnerable your airways are. A low score lets you know that your airways are blocked by inflammation and bronchoconstriction and are extra-sensitive to asthma triggers. If you check peak flow only after you inhale a quick relief medicine, you will miss important information about your asthma condition. By checking your peak flow score both before and after taking the quick relief medicine, you can adjust your treatment most effectively.

The exact zone boundaries are arbitrary, but they work well for almost all of my patients. In some cases, we modify them to improve their usefulness. I will discuss zone adjustment later in this chapter.

SETTING UP YOUR ASTHMA TREATMENT ZONES

Once you know your personal best peak flow score, you can figure out your asthma treatment zones by calculating them or by using the numbers in Table 38. Let's say that your personal best peak flow is 500. This means that scores between 400 and 500 fall into your green zone. Scores between 325 and 400 are in your high yellow zone; between 250 and 325, in your low yellow zone. A score below 250 falls in your red zone (see Figure 27). You can place colored stickers or markers right on your peak flow meter to show the boundaries of each zone. Enter your zones in Table 35, based on your personal best peak flow score.

HOW OFTEN SHOULD YOU CHECK PEAK FLOW?

The frequency with which you check your peak flow will change as you learn about your asthma and bring it under control. For the first month, you should check your peak flow before and after taking asthma medicine in the morning, and again in the afternoon or evening. In each case, wait one to ten minutes after you take your quick relief medicine (albuterol) to blow the second peak flow score. If you are not

Table 35. Asthma Treatment Zones Based on the Personal Best Peak Flow Score

Treatment Zone	Percent of Personal Best Peak Flow Score	Example: Personal Best = 500	Your Zones: Personal Best = _____
green	80–100%	400–500	_____
high yellow	65–80%	325–400	_____
low yellow	50–65%	250–325	_____
red	less than 50%	less than 250	_____

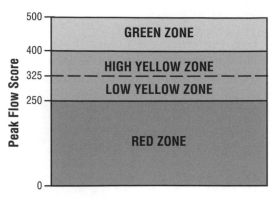

Figure 27. Peak Flow Zones. These zones are the basis for asthma treatment. Here they are based on a personal best score of 500.

Getting asthma under control:
- for about two months, take your peak flow every morning and evening

Fine-tuning asthma control and asthma learning:
- for the next two months, take peak flow every morning

Maintaining excellent asthma control:
- continue to take peak flow two mornings a week or as often as helpful

Return to daily peak flow readings if you:
- have symptoms
- are entering a threatening season (e.g., pollen) or environment (e.g., cat)
- are changing medicine or dose
- have a doctor's appointment next week

If you have had poorly controlled asthma for a long time, it may take more than two months of treatment to bring your asthma under control.

If your doctor has prescribed a quick relief medicine, take peak flow readings before and after your treatment each time. If your score before taking medicine is in the green zone, there is no need to blow another score after medicine. Remember to take the best of three attempts each time.

taking a quick relief medicine, you only need to check your peak flow once in the morning and once in the afternoon or evening.

Until your asthma is under excellent control, continue monitoring your peak flow in the morning and evening. After using an effective plan for two months, my patients generally find that checking peak flow only in the morning gives them all the information they need. If they start having symptoms or need to adjust their medicines, they will return to checking peak flow in the afternoons or evenings as well.

After following proper asthma treatment for a few weeks or months, you will probably find that your peak flow scores are in the green zone most of the time. When you go for a full month with less than five of your daily prebronchodilator peak flow scores in the high yellow zone, you are ready to reduce your readings to twice a week. After another month or two I recommend that you use peak flow as often as you find it useful in learning about and managing your asthma.

I have a few patients (usually athletes in their teens and twenties) who are so tuned in to their symptoms and airway status that they can predict a peak flow score before they blow it. These patients need to check their peak flow scores only when they have symptoms, change their medicine routines, or during the week before they see me.

Interpreting Your Peak Flow Scores

Once you have mastered peak flow technique, your peak flow meter will provide an objective measure of the condition of your large airway. Learning how to relate your scores and symptoms to your asthma management will take some more time. When you have learned this, you will be able to manage your asthma confidently at home most of the time and know when to go for help. Table 36 guides you in judging the severity of an asthma episode based on peak flow scores and asthma treatment zones.

THE GREEN ZONE

A peak flow score between 80 and 100 percent of your personal best means that you are in the green zone. You should be having only occasional signs or symptoms of asthma. When you are in the green zone, a mild asthma trigger may not cause symptoms. If asthma symptoms do occur in this zone, they usually come on slowly and give you adequate warning to begin treatment.

A peak flow score steadily in the green zone almost always means that your asthma is under control. However, if you are having asthma symptoms or asthma signs, you should pay at-

tention to them. It may be that you have outgrown your personal best peak flow score. If so, scores that used to be in your green zone are now in your high yellow zone. This often happens as children and adolescents grow taller. Each inch of growth generally produces a 10 to 15 L/min increase in peak flow scores.

Stacey, a sixth grader with asthma, noticed that she was wheezing when her peak flow score was 320, which I had set as the lower limit of her green zone. Because of her symptoms, she concluded that her personal best score must be higher than the 400 she had blown six months before. We rechecked her personal best and found that she could blow 450 after her airways were cleared.

If you have symptoms when you are in the green zone, you may have inflammation in your small airways, which peak flow does not measure. In this case, you should follow your high yellow zone plan.

If you frequently notice asthma symptoms before your peak flow score drops into the yellow zone, and a pulmonary function test (spirometry) shows that your small airways are clear, your doctor might consider reducing the size of your green zone to better reflect your asthma status. For example, the bottom of the green zone can be raised so that the zone lies

Table 36. Judging the Severity of an Asthma Episode

Treatment Zone	Percent of Personal Best Peak Flow Score	Severity of Episode
green	80–100%	no episode*
high yellow	65–80%	mild episode
low yellow	50–65%	moderate episode
red	less than 50%	severe episode

*If only the small airways are affected, a mild episode can exist without lowering peak flow scores into the yellow zone. Monitoring of asthma signs and symptoms will identify this situation.

between 90 and 100 percent of the personal best peak flow score, instead of 80 and 100 percent. The high yellow zone would then stretch from 70 to 90 percent and the low yellow zone from 50 to 70 percent. The red zone would remain the same. You should no longer experience symptoms in this smaller green zone.

THE HIGH YELLOW ZONE

If you blow a peak flow score in your high yellow zone (65–80 percent of personal best), it means that you are having a mild asthma episode. You know that your airways are partially blocked, but not too severely. Your treatment plan will call for avoiding triggers, not exercising strenuously, and increasing your asthma medicines.

THE LOW YELLOW ZONE

If you blow a peak flow between 50 and 65 percent of your personal best, you are in the low yellow zone. This occurs when you are having a moderate asthma episode. You should not engage in strenuous physical activity, and you may have to leave work or school. You can determine your need for additional asthma medicines by inhaling albuterol or another quick relief medicine, and seeing whether your peak flow score improves. Rapid improvement that lasts for four hours generally means you do not need to take an oral steroid to clear up the episode. If you do not improve, or your improvement lasts less than four hours, treatment with an oral steroid is necessary.

THE RED ZONE

The red zone is the danger zone where your peak flow score is less than 50 percent of your personal best. This is a sign of a severe asthma episode. Your treatment plan will instruct you to take an inhaled quick relief medicine immediately. If your peak flow scores are "stuck" in the red zone, you need to take an oral steroid and seek emergency help right away. You are stuck in a zone if you can't get out and stay out of that zone for four hours after inhaling four puffs of albuterol. If you are stuck, a phone call to the doctor is *not* enough.

If you can barely blow a peak flow, your respiratory muscles are exhausted from the work of breathing through blocked airways. Tired muscles simply can't produce a fast blast. They can't move air well. As a result, your wheezing will decrease and your retractions may appear less severe. In this situation, *you are in serious trouble and need medical help immediately, even though your signs appear to be improving.*

Never blame a peak flow attempt which barely moves or fails to move the marker on poor technique or poor effort. You should be able to correct effort or technique problems in two minutes. If you truly cannot move the marker on the peak flow meter, your respiratory muscles may be exhausted. *This is a life-threatening emergency. Call 911 or go to the emergency room immediately.*

PEAK FLOW SCORES THAT CHANGE BETWEEN MORNING AND AFTERNOON (EVENING)

Most people with asthma will blow a higher peak flow score in the afternoon than in the morning. The daily fluctuation in peak flow scores is called "diurnal variation," and some variation is normal. For some people, daily variation increases as an asthma episode develops. Thus, it provides them with an additional early signal to change their asthma treatment.

A PEAK FLOW SCORE ABOVE YOUR PERSONAL BEST

The best peak flow score you can blow after the first week of treatment is often close to the personal best. Whenever you blow a higher number on two separate days, you can consider that score your new personal best. I specify two days to make sure that the higher peak flow score is not a freak event.

Your best score may continue to increase in the early weeks of treatment as you improve your peak flow technique and get the full benefit of your medicines. Even though my patients take an oral steroid for seven days after their first visit, many have had inflammation for weeks or months and need longer treatment to completely clear their airways. As the inflammation disappears, their peak flow scores increase.

Your asthma treatment zones must be based on your personal best peak flow score to be effective. My patient Max Stewart, age 16, had never blown a score higher than 450. The average score for someone of Max's height, sex, and age is 480, so I used the higher number (480) as his estimated best score. Based on this number, Max's green zone was between 390 and 480 (see Figure 28a). Most of his peak flow

scores during the week before his visit had been in the green zone. But because he still had trouble biking in cold weather and had asthma symptoms with colds, I prescribed an inhaled steroid to be taken daily.

Three weeks later, Max blew a peak flow score of 530 several times, establishing that as his actual personal best score. This meant that his green zone was really between 430 and 530. When I regraphed his peak flow record using 530 as his personal best, it became clear that Max had actually been in the high and low yellow zones when he was having symptoms (see Figure 28b).

Now that Max takes an inhaled steroid daily, his airways are clear. He can bike in all weather conditions and does not have asthma symptoms with a cold. Since he is in the middle of a growth spurt, his personal best score continues to increase. Whenever he blows a higher peak flow score on two separate days, we consider that score to be his personal best and recalculate his treatment zones.

RELATING YOUR PEAK FLOW SCORES TO ASTHMA SYMPTOMS

For many years we believed that a person with asthma could detect a change in breath-

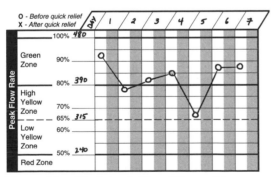

Figure 28a. Max's Peak Flow Diary with a Personal Best Score of 480. Max's peak flow scores seemed to be mostly in the green zone, but he had asthma symptoms.

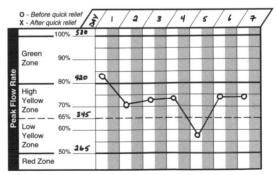

Figure 28b. Max's Peak Flow Diary with a Personal Best Score of 530. Using his true personal best score, we realized that Max's peak flow scores had been in the high and low yellow zones.

ing only after their airflow had dropped by 25 percent or more. Now it is clear that some people can perceive a change of less than 10 percent, while others do not notice a change even when their airflow has dropped by 50 percent. Using a peak flow meter, you can detect a drop in airflow that an experienced doctor using a stethoscope will often miss.

Symptoms are important, too. Some people who have learned to be sensitive to the signs and symptoms of their asthma can tell that an asthma episode is starting even before their peak flow scores change. If you have just been diagnosed with asthma, or have lived for a long time with poorly controlled asthma, it may be difficult for you to recognize the signs of early changes in your airways. Peak flow is therefore your most reliable tool for monitoring your asthma. Later, you may become much more perceptive about your symptoms. As your asthma control improves, you may begin to notice the cough that you used to ignore, or to feel tightness in your chest much earlier.

Usefulness of Peak Flow

PEAK FLOW CAN HELP OTHER ADULTS MANAGE YOUR CHILD'S ASTHMA

Peak flow is an objective measure of your child's airflow. Once your child or teenager knows how to blow peak flow properly, he can do it anywhere. Peak flow meters are light, portable, and durable, and along with a written treatment plan, can accompany your child to school or on a trip. If your child develops symptoms, the school nurse, a sports coach, or the parent of a friend can follow a treatment plan based on peak flow scores without having to know a lot about your child's asthma. Monitoring peak flow helps adults feel more competent

and comfortable having a child with asthma in their care. A nursing professor wrote this account.

As a sponsor of our church's high school ski trip, I was concerned about Mike, a teenager with a difficult case of asthma. His mother was worried that he would get into trouble on the trip. I told her that I was willing to take him if he would learn to use a peak flow meter. Mike started measuring his peak flow regularly about a month before the trip. During the trip, I would check in with him periodically to see how his score compared to his personal best. Since we had his nebulizer and medicines with us I felt confident that we could take whatever action he needed. Mike went through the entire week with only a couple of minor asthma problems.

CHECKING YOUR PEAK FLOW SCORE WILL HELP YOUR DOCTOR

Your doctor can use peak flow to diagnose asthma. The diagnosis is almost certain if your peak flow score increases more than 15 percent after you take an inhaled quick relief medicine (albuterol) using a holding chamber or nebulizer. A drop of 15 percent in peak flow after strenuous exercise can also confirm the diagnosis of asthma.

Peak flow scores can guide treatment in the doctor's office. In the case of a severe episode, peak flow provides more reliable information on the response to treatment than do symptoms or signs. Peak flow can also be used to adjust your long-term treatment plan. A doctor who analyzes peak flow scores while reducing your medicine dose can make sure that you are getting the desired benefit from your medicines at the lowest possible dose.

CHECKING YOUR PEAK FLOW
SCORE WILL HELP IN THE
EMERGENCY ROOM AND HOSPITAL

If you go to the emergency room, a nurse can evaluate your condition with peak flow right away to decide whether you need immediate treatment or can wait a few minutes. Once treatment has been started, the response of your peak flow scores will help the doctor decide whether more intensive treatment is needed. Peak flow can help the doctor determine whether to admit you to the hospital for further treatment. When your peak flow scores improve rapidly and then remain stable, you can probably continue treatment at home.

During hospitalization, the staff can evaluate the effect of each treatment with inhaled albuterol by checking your peak flow before and after giving it. This helps them decide whether you need a change in treatment, such as more frequent inhalation of medicine, a course of oral steroids, or antibiotics. If you monitor your own peak flow in the hospital, you can provide helpful information to your doctor. You should continue monitoring peak flow after discharge from the hospital to make sure that your improvement is steady.

Learning from Peak Flow

Peak flow can teach you much of what you need to know about your asthma and the medicines used to treat it. As you follow your peak flow scores, you will learn to look for triggers in the environment that cause your peak flow to drop. You will also see how your airways respond to different medicines. Some inhaled medicines work in a minute, and others take days or weeks to have an effect. Peak flow clarifies this. And as you track peak flow during an episode, you will learn how long it takes for you to get better and how episodes vary depending on what triggers them.

LEARNING ABOUT ASTHMA
MEDICINES

Peak flow can help you and your doctor figure out if your medicines are working properly. You will see how long it takes each kind of medicine to take effect and how long those effects last. During an asthma episode, you can see how well you respond to your quick relief medicine. When you start to take a controller medicine, a steady increase in your peak flow scores will show that you are benefiting from daily treatment. Once you have achieved excellent asthma control, your doctor can try to gradually reduce your medicine dose to the lowest effective amount. During this step-down procedure, monitoring peak flow enables you to make sure that the reduced medicine dose is adequate to maintain asthma control.

Controller Medicines

Using peak flow, you will see that controller medicines take time to work. At your first asthma visit, your doctor will probably prescribe an inhaled steroid. You may hope to feel better the next day, but the medicine doesn't work that fast. It may take days to weeks for inflammation in your airways to clear completely. We call this period the run-in time.

It also takes time for the effects of a controller medicine to decrease or disappear from your body after you reduce the dose or stop taking it. After your doctor reduces your inhaled steroid dose, you may continue to have some benefit from the original (higher) dose for two to four weeks. After that period, you will know that the lower dose is adequate if symptoms don't recur and your peak flow score does not drop.

If an inhaled steroid alone does not bring you to excellent asthma control, your doctor may prescribe an additional controller medicine, such as nedocromil, a long-acting beta$_2$-agonist, a leukotriene modifier, or theophylline. Each controller medicine has its own specific run-in time. An inhaled long-acting beta$_2$-agonist medicine starts to act in twenty minutes and reaches full (peak) effect in three to four hours. Nedocromil starts to prevent inflammation in three days. Leukotriene modifiers start to take effect in three to twelve hours but may take a week or more to reach full effect. Theophylline begins to act in an hour and reaches full effect two hours after the second dose (about fourteen hours total).

Your asthma symptoms should decrease and your peak flow scores increase as the controller medicine takes effect. If you observe no improvement in your peak flow scores after the run-in time has passed, review the situation with your doctor.

Quick Relief Medicines

Quick relief medicines have a rapid "onset of action," the time it takes a medicine to work after you take it. You will be able to see the effect that a quick relief medicine has on your airways by checking your peak flow score before and then shortly after you inhale it (see Figure

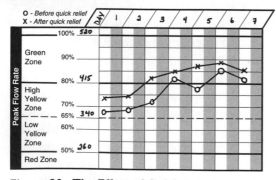

Figure 29. The Effect of Quick Relief Medicine. Karen's diary shows that her peak flow scores increased each time she inhaled albuterol.

29). Quick relief medicines like inhaled albuterol and other inhaled, fast-acting beta$_2$-agonists dilate your airways in a few minutes. Ipratropium, a different kind of bronchodilator, starts to act in five to fifteen minutes, reaching its full effect in thirty minutes. Quick relief medicines work much faster than controller medicines, but their effects last only a few hours. By checking your peak flow at intervals after inhaling a quick relief medicine, you can see when it begins to have the desired effect and how long the benefit lasts.

Oral Steroids

Oral steroids relieve obstruction of the airways by rapidly reducing airway inflammation, but they take six to twelve hours to begin working. If you have a large amount of airway inflammation, it may take one to several days for oral steroids to work.

USING PEAK FLOW TO LEARN ABOUT ASTHMA TRIGGERS

As you already know, you can reduce your asthma symptoms and need for medicine by avoiding asthma triggers. Peak flow can help you figure out what your triggers are and how you respond to each of them. In some cases, you may feel symptoms right away after exposure, while in other situations, a trigger may not cause trouble for several hours. Some triggers will cause an abrupt drop in peak flow scores, while others will cause a gradual decline. By writing down possible triggers and recording your peak flow scores in your asthma diary, you can figure out how your airways respond.

For several of my young patients, peak flow has helped to identify and resolve problems with the indoor environment at school. Poor indoor air quality can trigger symptoms in people with asthma, but its causes may be difficult to define. One mother was able to convince the school principal that something in the classroom was triggering her son's asthma when she showed him that her son's peak flow score dropped by 20 percent in the hour after entering his classroom. Similarly, adults can use peak flow to identify problem areas in a work environment.

Do Peak Flow Scores Always Tell You What Is Going On in Your Lungs?

In some circumstances, peak flow scores are not reliable. Once you know what these are, you can avoid them. Peak flow scores are unreliable if you are rushed or using poor technique. This can be remedied by proper instruction and observation by a qualified health professional. Peak flow scores also may not be reliable if you use an unreliable peak flow meter. You should use a meter that gives consistent readings.

Some people will make errors in reading a peak flow meter. Others make errors in reading a thermometer. In both cases, the errors have nothing to do with the reliability of the device. Let's say you read your temperature at home as 104. When you come in to the doctor's office, the nurse takes your temperature and asks you to read the thermometer. You look and say, "One hundred and four, exactly what I got at home." In fact, it is 100.4.

Does the fact that you made an error mean that thermometers are unreliable and shouldn't be used? No. You need instruction in order to use the thermometer correctly, but you can learn what you need to know in a few minutes. Peak flow meters are similar. You can learn the basics in a few minutes at an office visit. It takes additional practice and coaching to learn how to blow your best score, and more instruction, experience, and thought to learn

how to interpret readings as a basis for managing your asthma at home.

Since a peak flow meter does not measure airflow in the small airways, inflammation in those airways will not reduce your peak flow score. You may experience symptoms even though your peak flow score is in the green zone. If this causes confusion about what treatment you need, your doctor can perform a pulmonary function test (with a spirometer) to determine the status of your small airways as well as your large airways. However, serious asthma trouble will almost always cause obstruction in both your small and large airways, in which case it will be reflected in reduced peak flow scores.

For a small number of people with asthma, an episode may worsen very rapidly, with peak flow scores dropping from normal to the red zone in less than an hour. These people must be particularly careful about avoiding triggers and monitoring their asthma using both peak flow and the signs and symptoms of asthma.

Does Everyone Agree That Peak Flow Is a Helpful Tool?

My patients have found peak flow to be immensely useful in managing and learning about their asthma, but not all doctors and health professionals are convinced. One of my patients told me of her daughter's visit to such a doctor: "He never looked at the asthma diary. He said, 'Her chest sounds great' and that he did not want to deal with peak flow." This doctor failed to use two tools that are extremely useful in guiding asthma care. I speak to doctors around the country, and I have heard many criticisms of peak flow that I will share with you, along with my responses to them.

A common critique of peak flow is that it relies on patient effort. I respond by saying that breathing also relies on patient effort. Coaching will usually produce a good effort and an accurate peak flow score. If your respiratory muscles are exhausted, you will not be able to produce good effort. This is a serious situation that can lead to death if not reversed. A very low peak flow score warns you of that danger.

Some doctors fear that people may blow a low peak flow score on purpose (malingering). This can happen when a patient stands to gain from blowing a low peak flow. I believe this is rare. If patient effort is questionable, spirometry can be used to determine the status of the airways. The results from a spirometry test are less dependent on effort.

Many doctors say that patients won't check peak flow regularly. It is true that in the past monitoring peak flow was very time-consuming, since most doctors recommended that a person wait twenty minutes after taking his asthma medicines before checking peak flow for the second time. That time commitment was a lot to expect from patients. Now we know that you only need to wait for one or a few minutes after inhaling a quick relief medicine to check whether the medicine has had an effect on your peak flow score. Once your asthma is under excellent control, you no longer need to take a quick relief medicine and check the peak flow afterward. You may need to check peak flow only once or twice a week. Peak flow should not run your life. Instead, it should keep asthma from running your life.

Some doctors say that peak flow is too technical for people to use at home. They say that learning this part of asthma care is too demanding and may make a family overinvolved with asthma. But these doctors don't realize how much fear, anxiety, and disruption uncontrolled asthma causes in a family. Certainly, there is a lot to learn. Yet, my patients are willing to learn about peak flow to improve their health. They would much rather be overinvolved with peak flow monitoring than be overinvolved with an emergency room.

I have learned that when patients check peak flow more frequently than I think necessary, they almost always have a good reason. They have often had a traumatic asthma episode in the past. Parents of a child who has been hospitalized may continue to monitor peak flow scores frequently even though I think that it is safe to check less often. A normal peak flow score may bring the parent peace of mind that is worth the time it takes. People usually reduce their peak flow monitoring once they begin to understand asthma and feel confident that they have achieved excellent control.

Some doctors worry that a patient may make a disastrous error while managing asthma at home because of an improper interpretation of a peak flow score. I know of no report in which a patient who was properly instructed in monitoring his asthma by peak flow and symptoms made a fatal miscalculation. I do, however, know of patients who have died because their doctors failed to check their peak flow or misinterpreted the meaning of a peak flow attempt that did not register on the meter. If a patient has been properly instructed and coached, the peak flow scores he blows are legitimate and should be taken seriously. A doctor should use peak flow scores to help in assessing the patient's situation and determining proper treatment at every visit.

Peak Flow Meters

Your peak flow meter must be accurate and reliable. Here I mention several peak flow meters I have found to be reliable, meaning that they give a consistent score (within five percent) each time you blow into them. You may also want to consider other qualities, such as dura-

A unique "windmill" training device can help both children and adults improve their peak flow technique.

The windmill clips onto the standard or low-range Mini-Wright meter. When you blow through the mouthpiece hard enough, the windmill turns. As you place the windmill farther up the scale, it requires a stronger blast to move it. This feedback can help people of all ages improve technique and peak flow scores.

The Windmill Trainer is especially useful for young children, but it has also helped 40-year-olds. I use it for patients who I think can blow a higher score but who don't improve with my coaching. Your doctor can request Windmill Trainers free of charge from Clement Clarke.

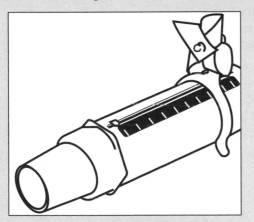

Figure 30. AFS Mini-Wright with Windmill Trainer. The windmill helps you improve peak flow technique and can be used with a standard Mini-Wright meter or the low-range meter pictured here.

bility, ease of use and cleaning, and approximate cost.

A meter should last from one to three years with regular use. Some peak flow meters are available without prescription, while others require one. This may change over the next few years.

All children can use a regular range (60–850 L/min) peak flow meter. Some brands of peak flow meters are also available in a low-range model (50–400 L/min) designed for children. The main advantage of these models is that the scale is larger and easier to read. Because the maximum peak flow score is 400 in the low-range models, these meters are useful as long as your child's personal best is below that score. A child's peak flow score will increase as he grows. Once your child's peak flow reaches 380, you should switch to a standard peak flow meter.

CHOOSING A PEAK FLOW METER

All of the peak flow meters discussed below are well-designed and durable. They vary in shape, size, cost, and range (see Figure 31). For ordering information, see the list of vendors in the Resource Section.

Astech (Dey)

The Astech is a well-engineered peak flow meter. Since it is made of metal, it can withstand hard use. It has movable zone markers that can be reset when your personal best score changes with age.

Mini-Wright (Clement Clarke)

I have used the Mini-Wright in my office for eighteen years and recommend it to most of my patients. It was the first portable peak flow meter manufactured. Asthma specialists who are doing research use the Mini-Wright more often than all other peak flow meter brands combined. My patients find it easy to use and read, and it lasts for several years if not mishandled. One problem my patients have encountered is that the plastic marker may pop out and get

Table 37. Comparison of Peak Flow Meters

Brand	Range (L/min)	Size (inches)	Approximate Cost
Astech	50–800	8 x 1	$25
Mini-Wright	60–800	8 x 2	$30
Mini-Wright AFS	50–400	8 x 2	$20
Pocket Peak	50–720	3.5 x 3.5	$22
Pocket Peak	50–400	3.5 x 3.5	$22
TruZone	60–800	7 x 1	$18

lost. A new marker can be purchased from the company for about a dollar. The low-range AFS Mini-Wright is available for children.

PocketPeak (Ferraris Medical)

The PocketPeak is a compact peak flow meter that can fit into a pocket or purse. It has a reversible mouthpiece that can be used by children or adults. The meter is also available in a low-range model. It comes with small, round stickers that your doctor can attach to the me-

ter to indicate your green, yellow, and red zone boundaries.

TruZone (Monaghan Medical)

I have found the TruZone to be reliable and easy to use. All of the moving parts, including the marker, are inside the body of the meter. You never need to open the meter for cleaning. You also do not need to reset the marker between your three peak flow attempts. Once your doctor has established your personal best

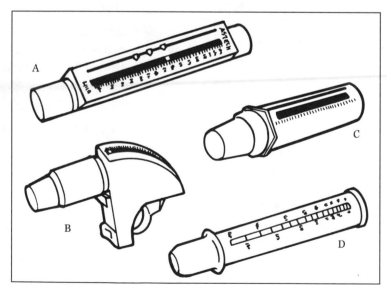

Figure 31. Four Reliable Brands of Peak Flow Meter. A. Astech,
B. Pocket Peak, C. Mini-Wright, D. TruZone

peak flow score, she can place the green, yellow, and red sticker strip on the meter. The strips are designed to identify the peak flow zones for you. The meter fits into a shirt pocket or purse.

TAKING CARE OF YOUR PEAK FLOW METER

Each peak flow meter comes with instructions in the package insert for care and washing. All of the meters mentioned here can be washed safely in the upper rack of the dishwasher or in the sink with mild detergent and hot water. A thorough cleaning involving disassembly may be required each month or few months. Check the package insert for specific instructions.

PEAK FLOW SCORES VARY WITH BRAND OF METER

Peak flow meters that are manufactured by different companies vary in the scores they produce. This is due to differences in design. What you need is a peak flow meter that produces consistent peak flow scores when you use the same meter over and over. The score you blow with another meter may be different. If you buy a new peak flow meter (either the same brand or a different one), your doctor should reestablish your personal best peak flow score. In addition, your doctor should check your technique with the new device.

Even though my patients use a reliable peak flow meter, they may blow a different peak flow score when they use my office meter. For example, a patient may consistently blow a personal best of 400 on his peak flow meter, and a personal best of 420 on mine, even when our meters are the same brand. He always brings his peak flow meter to visits, so we can check his technique and his meter. We set the personal best peak flow score based on his meter (400),

and define the asthma care zones based on that score.

HOW WILL YOU KNOW IF YOUR PEAK FLOW METER IS DEFECTIVE?

The brands that I mention in this book are unlikely to be defective. In rare cases, a new peak flow meter will produce scores that are unusually low, high, or erratic. If this occurs, it is defective and you should exchange it for one that works properly.

USING ZONE MARKERS ON YOUR PEAK FLOW METER

Inside many peak flow meter packages, you will find red, yellow, and green stickers. You or your doctor can attach the stickers to the meter to show where your red, yellow, and green zones are. When you blow a peak flow, you can easily see which zone it falls into. Some of my patients use the stickers for immediate feedback and then refer to their Home Treatment Plan to see what action they should take.

SPECIAL DEVICES TO MEASURE AND RECORD PEAK FLOW

A specialized peak flow device, the AirWatch, records your peak flow scores electronically. The scores can then be transmitted electronically to your doctor. Because of its expense, the AirWatch is used mainly to monitor people with severe asthma problems or for research purposes.

In Summary

As you learn about medicines and asthma triggers with peak flow, you will achieve a much deeper understanding of your asthma. Each person's asthma is different; your doctor will help you learn, but only you can make the daily observations that tell your asthma story. You will become more attuned to your symptoms and learn whether your peak flow scores drop before you feel them. You will find out how much your peak flow scores vary between morning and afternoon. You will learn to match your peak flow scores with the severity of various asthma symptoms. The information you provide will help your doctor understand your asthma better, too.

Each person has an individual pattern of asthma episodes. You will learn what to expect by seeing how quickly and how much your peak flow scores drop. You will soon know how your episodes respond to treatment. The more you know about your asthma, the better you can prevent most asthma symptoms and respond promptly and appropriately when an episode occurs. Most importantly, peak flow will help you learn to tell the difference between an asthma episode you can handle at home and one that needs a doctor's help.

Chapter Six

Using an Asthma Diary

You must work closely with a competent doctor to control your asthma safely and effectively. Use the asthma diary to collect and analyze data, to identify your treatment zones, and to communicate with your doctor.

My patients tell me repeatedly that one of the most useful tools I have developed to help them manage asthma is the asthma diary. Since 1981, I have given diaries to my patients to help them monitor peak flow scores and asthma signs and symptoms, learn about asthma and asthma medicines, and manage asthma more effectively at home. Adults, teenagers, and parents of children age 5 and older use the Asthma Peak Flow Diary (see Figure 32). Parents with children under age 5 use the Asthma Signs Diary (see Figure 39). You can enter all of the information needed to assess your or your child's asthma on a single diary sheet.

An asthma diary enables you to record information about your asthma every day, or as often as is helpful. Recording is particularly important during the first few months that you are learning about asthma and bringing it un-

der control. In the morning and evening, you graph your peak flow scores or total score of asthma signs on the diary. You check off each time you take a dose of asthma medicine, and you record any additional asthma signs or symptoms you observe. A comment section allows you to include other important information, such as exposure to a cat or the beginning of a cold.

All entries for one day go in the same column so you can see all the events that occurred together. Over time, you and your doctor will see relationships between peak flow score, asthma symptoms, medicines, and triggers. One peak flow or asthma signs score provides a "snapshot" of your asthma condition. My asthma diary shows your scores varying over 16 days, like a home video of how your airways are responding to medicines and triggers.

You have read a lot about the three asthma treatment zones — green, yellow, and red — that provide you with a way to guide your treatment. They can help you respond quickly and appropriately to asthma episodes. An asthma diary allows you to actually see the zones and observe how they relate to your asthma. The

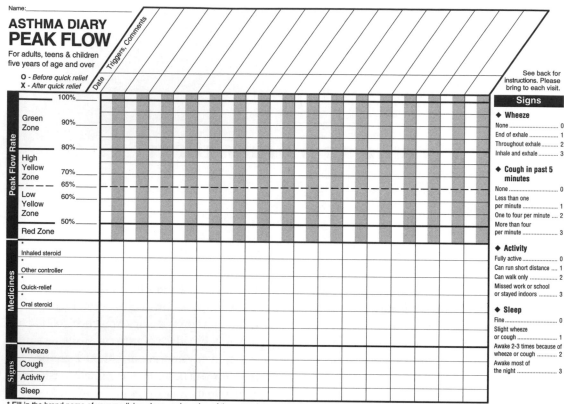

* Fill in the brand name of your medicine, dose, and number of times per day you take it.

Figure 32. The Asthma Peak Flow Diary

goal of asthma treatment is for you to live in the green zone, pursuing full activity and having hardly any signs or symptoms of asthma. Melanie Sanford described how the diary helped her improve her son's asthma control.

![black square]

The Asthma Diary and Me
Melanie Sanford
First visit in the 1990s

My 8-year-old son Chris has had asthma for four years. I'm learning what triggers an episode and how to control it. This makes asthma not as scary. We've been keeping an asthma diary for about five months and it has helped me in so many different ways. I used to have a very hard time remembering exactly when Chris's asthma symptoms started or exactly how much medicine he took during the past week (depending on whether he had an episode or not). Sometime it's hard to tell how much medicine is left in his metered dose inhalers.

The asthma diary has saved me a lot of time and guesswork. I can look at the diary and the answer to my question is right there in front of me. We keep track of Chris's peak flow, so if he starts getting into trouble we know before the episode gets out of hand and then we can control it.

Chris stores his medicines on top of his asthma diary. When he takes a dose he marks it down. He takes two medicines by metered dose inhaler, an inhaled steroid and albuterol. There are 100 puffs of inhaled steroid in the canister. Since he takes 4 puffs a day, I know it will run out in 25 days. I write that date on the canister and in the diary. When that date comes, I throw the canister out. Before, I wasn't sure when the canister was empty. I thought as long as you could hear something splashing around in there it still was usable. I was wrong, though, and he developed an asthma episode while it still splashed. Now I know when to start a new inhaler.

Chris takes albuterol by metered dose inhaler when his peak flow drops into the yellow zone. That doesn't happen very often, so I can't figure the discard date ahead of time. His canister of albuterol holds 240 puffs. He marks each dose down on the diary and we replace the inhaler after he has used the 240 puffs. It lasts about four months.

The diary also helps me to keep a record of all the asthma signs Chris exhibits, such as how many times he had a coughing fit during the night last week or whether he was wheezing while riding his bike yesterday. I can see if there's a pattern developing and then adjust his medicines to control the asthma before it flares up. In addition, the diary has helped me to find certain triggers to stay away from. I can check what Chris was doing the day before he had an episode and see if he has another episode the next time he's doing the same thing. There was one time when I noticed that every time Chris went to play at the neighbors' he came home coughing and wheezing. After I talked to my neighbor I found out that Chris was playing in their barn. Once we figured this out, we told Chris to stay out of the barn.

When we have a doctor's visit, the doctor can look at the diary with us and see exactly what's been happening. He can then evaluate Chris on his day to day activity. I don't have to remember every little detail because all the information is written down. Then we can discuss changes or improvements which will help Chris stay in control of his asthma.

I am glad we learned how to use the diary. It's become like a member of the family. It goes everywhere with us and it always helps me out when I need it. The diary has helped me to understand a lot more about Chris' asthma and to learn how to control it before it controls him. This makes for a lot less sickness and a lot less missed school days. Chris now has more time to just be a normal kid.

An Asthma Diary Helps You Manage Asthma

The asthma diary helps my patients manage their asthma, learn about their medicines, triggers, and asthma patterns, and communicate clearly with me in the office and over the phone. Acquiring skill in using a diary takes some time, and its benefit may not be immediately obvious. But people who use an asthma diary find that it saves them time during an office visit, allows them to avoid emergency visits to the doctor or hospital, helps them talk with a doctor over the phone, and lets them transfer care of a child with asthma confidently to a babysitter or other care provider.

All my patients use diaries in one way or another, but not because I "make" them. I don't have the power to make my patients do anything. I present them with the information that they need to make decisions about their asthma and how it affects their lives. They start keeping a diary because I say it will help them take control of their asthma. When they see that it does, they continue using it. Thousands of doctors now use the Asthma Peak Flow Diary in their practices. I often hear feedback from their patients, such as "I am a 71-year-old lady who has had asthma forever. The Asthma Peak Flow diary [. . .] has been of more help to me than anything I have ever used or taken. It helps me decide when to call my doctor and also helps me to keep down my urge to panic!" After you read about the diary, you can decide whether it is worth a try.

Almost anyone can learn to use an asthma diary. Your doctor or nurse can help you fill it out and teach you how to interpret what you have recorded. I send a diary to my patients and ask them to track their asthma during the week before their first visit with me. They have already read *One Minute Asthma: What You Need to Know* and this book, and they know as much as you now know about asthma, medicines, and peak flow. Most of them are able to fill out the diary without any special instruction from me. The specific information they collect during the week before their visit helps me to understand the severity and frequency of their symptoms. I then can make an initial treatment plan tailored to their needs.

In this chapter, I have included several example diaries filled out by patients before and shortly after they saw me in consultation. First I present the Asthma Peak Flow Diary, which is used by anyone who is able to blow peak flow reliably. Second is the Asthma Signs Diary, which is used by parents of children who have not yet learned to do peak flow. The diaries I use in my practice are identical to the ones in this book, except that they are printed in color (see "Resource Section"). This chapter is based on the diaries I have developed and used over the past eighteen years in my practice.

The Asthma Peak Flow Diary

Peak flow is the best tool currently available for monitoring the state of your airways at home. A drop in peak flow scores gives early warning that asthma trouble is on the way. Tracking peak flow and the signs and symptoms of asthma over time is more useful than looking at a single score. The Asthma Peak Flow Diary helps you to:

- see your asthma treatment zone immediately
- compare your scores over the past days and weeks
- judge if your asthma situation is improving or getting worse
- see how your peak flow score is responding to additional asthma medicine

If your peak flow scores drop rapidly, you know that you should change treatment to head off an asthma episode. If your peak flow scores drop very gradually, it is harder to notice. A peak flow diary will display a trend of decreasing peak flow scores and clarify when you need to change your treatment.

Asthma treatment is based not only on the state of your airways right now, but also on how they were doing yesterday and last week. Without recording, it is very difficult to remember your peak flow scores from morning to night, from day to day, from week to week. When you record your peak flow scores each morning, you can see the big picture of your asthma.

During an episode, you want to know if your morning peak flow scores are improving over the week or getting worse. A trend of improving scores means that treatment is effective and you can expect to be back in the green zone soon. A trend of falling peak flow scores means that your treatment is not adequate, and you need to change it according to your treatment plan or contact your doctor. You will find a full-sized blank copy of the Asthma Peak Flow Diary at the back of the book. You may reproduce it for personal use. My patients use the three-color version (see "Resource Section").

FILLING OUT AN ASTHMA PEAK FLOW DIARY

Filling out the Asthma Peak Flow Diary consists of six steps:

1. Set up your asthma treatment zones.
2. Plot daily peak flow scores.
3. Connect the peak flow scores to see the pattern.
4. Check off the asthma medicines you take each day.
5. Record triggers, events, and other important comments.
6. Score signs and symptoms of asthma.

Your doctor may ask you to do only one or a few of these steps initially, then add others as you master each one. Here I will discuss each step and how my patient, John Mott, completed his diary. In the next chapter, you will follow John during the first few weeks of his asthma care.

Step One: Set Up Your Asthma Treatment Zones

In order for an asthma diary to help you achieve excellent asthma control, it must be set up properly. "Properly" means that you use your personal best peak flow score as the basis for the zones. Figuring out that personal best can be done only when your airways are completely clear of inflammation and you have no symptoms. Most patients who see me have persistent asthma with inflammation in their air-

ways. It may take several weeks of treatment for us to figure out their personal best score.

My patient Jeffrey Wolfman (here identified as John Mott), was 39 years old when he called me for an asthma consultation. He had been a three-sport varsity athlete in high school and very active in college sports. You'll recall from his story in Chapter 1 that he could barely run up a flight of stairs, or push a baby carriage up a hill. I asked John to keep an asthma diary for the two weeks before his first appointment. He figured out his asthma treatment zones using Table 38, based on the best peak flow score he had blown (540). If your score is not listed (for example, 550), use the numbers in the row for the lower score (540).

On his diary, John filled in the numbers for each zone and added scores corresponding to 90 percent, 70 percent and 60 percent to make graphing easier (see Figure 33). Notice that the diary divides the yellow zone in half because the high yellow and low yellow zones call for very different treatment.

Step Two: Plot Daily Peak Flow Scores in the Diary

Each column of the diary corresponds to a day, with unshaded and shaded parts for recording morning and late afternoon (or evening) peak flow scores. Write the date at the top of the column. Use additional columns if you want to record peak flow scores more than twice a day.

Mark a symbol (an "o") at the place in the diary grid that corresponds to your peak flow score. You can estimate where the mark should go for scores that fall between the numbered lines. Remember that when you blow a peak flow score, you should record the highest of three attempts in the diary.

John started recording peak flow scores on

Table 38. Asthma Treatment Zones Based on the Personal Best Peak Flow Score

Personal best

100%	90%	80%	70%	65%	60%	50%
100	90	80	70	65	60	50
120	110	95	85	80	75	60
140	125	110	100	90	85	70
160	145	130	110	105	95	80
180	160	145	125	115	110	90
200	180	160	140	130	120	100
220	200	175	155	145	130	110
240	215	190	170	155	145	120
260	235	210	180	170	155	130
280	250	225	195	180	170	140
300	270	240	210	195	180	150
320	290	255	225	210	190	160
340	305	270	240	220	205	170
360	325	290	250	235	215	180
380	340	305	265	245	230	190
400	360	320	280	260	240	200
420	380	335	295	275	250	210
440	395	350	310	285	265	220
460	415	370	320	300	275	230
480	430	385	335	310	290	240
500	450	400	350	325	300	250
520	470	415	365	340	310	260
540	485	430	380	350	325	270
560	505	450	390	365	335	280
580	520	465	405	375	350	290
600	540	480	420	390	360	300
620	560	495	435	405	370	310
640	575	510	450	415	385	320
660	595	530	460	430	395	330
680	610	545	475	440	410	340
700	630	560	490	455	420	350
720	650	575	505	470	430	360
740	665	590	520	480	445	370
760	685	610	530	495	455	380
780	700	625	545	505	470	390
800	720	640	560	520	480	400

Find your personal best peak flow score on the table. Write the numbers in that row onto the Asthma Peak Flow Diary.

August 9. He recorded his peak flow scores each morning. Because he was taking a quick relief medicine, he checked his peak flow both before and after asthma medicines. He plotted the scores before medicine with an "o." His scores before inhaling a quick relief medicine were in the high yellow zone or low yellow zone during the entire two week period before his first consultation (see Figure 33). After John took his quick relief medicine, he checked his peak flow again and recorded scores with an "x" in the same column. Notice that his scores were consistently higher after the quick relief medicine.

Step Three: Connect the Peak Flow Scores to See the Pattern

As John plotted each new peak flow score, he connected it to scores from previous days. Notice that he connected all the scores blown before quick relief medicine ("o") with one line, and scores blown after quick relief medicine ("x") with another line. These two graphs reveal a pattern of John's changing asthma condition over the two week period.

Step Four: Check Off the Asthma Medicines You Take Each Day

Below the peak flow section of the diary, you will find a list of asthma medicines, each with its own row for recording. Your doctor can write in the brand name of medicines that he prescribes, the dose, and how many times per day you are supposed to take it.

John wrote in the medicines he had been given by his allergist (see Figure 34). He was taking an inhaled steroid, seven puffs at a time, two times per day. He took a quick relief medicine two puffs at a time, up to eight times per day, to relieve symptoms. He was also taking theophylline, 400 mg, two times per day.

John recorded this information in his pre-visit diary and checked off each dose he took. For the inhaled steroid, each check represented seven puffs of medicine, while for theophylline, each check meant one 400 mg tablet.

(It is a little unusual for a patient to take seven puffs of an inhaled steroid at a time. John probably was not taking his medicine properly or was in contact with many asthma triggers in his environment. If John did actually need this dose, his doctor could have switched him to another preparation of inhaled steroid which contained the same dose in fewer puffs of medicine.)

Once John and I have worked out an asthma treatment plan, he will fine tune the amount and type of medicine he takes based on his peak flow scores. The diary will allow him to see how well the new treatment works.

Keeping track of your medicines in a diary is one of the best ways to understand how your medicines work. For example, even though you

Table 39. John Mott's Treatment Zones

Treatment Zone	Percent of Personal Best	John's Zone
green	80–100%	430–540
high yellow	65–80%	350–430
low yellow	50–65%	270–350
red	less than 50%	less than 270

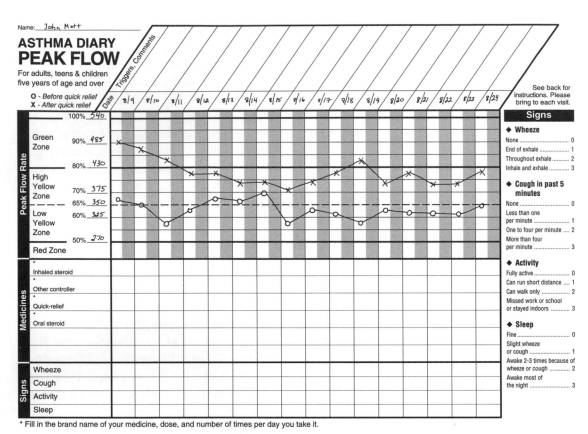

Figure 33. Asthma Peak Flow Diary: Steps One, Two and Three. John recorded peak flow scores each day before and after inhaling a quick relief medicine.

have read in this book that inhaled steroids don't reach their full effect for two to four weeks, you will truly believe it when you see your peak flow scores on the diary start to increase after you have taken an inhaled steroid for a week.

You will soon understand how long it takes each kind of medicine to work. You may have noticed that John was taking an inhaled steroid daily, but his peak flow scores were almost always in the yellow zone. This showed us that there was a problem with his asthma, his treatment, or both. At his first consultation, we were able to figure out the answers.

Step Five: Record Triggers, Events and Other Important Comments

To control asthma, avoiding or reducing your asthma triggers is as important as taking the right asthma medicines. In fact, you can usually reduce the amount of medicine you need if you reduce your exposure to asthma triggers. Of course, to avoid triggers, you have to know what they are.

The asthma diary can help your find a trigger by showing you patterns you might otherwise miss. For example, peak flow scores may drop every time you visit a particular person's

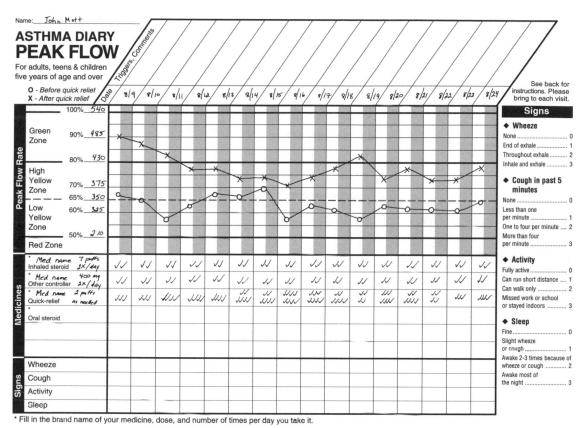

Name: John Mott

ASTHMA DIARY
PEAK FLOW
For adults, teens & children
five years of age and over

O - Before quick relief
X - After quick relief

Triggers, Comments

Date: 8/9 8/10 8/11 8/12 8/13 8/14 8/15 8/16 8/17 8/18 8/19 8/20 8/21 8/22 8/23 8/24

See back for
instructions. Please
bring to each visit.

Peak Flow Rate				Signs
Green Zone	100%	540		**◆ Wheeze**
	90%	485		None 0
	80%	430		End of exhale 1
High Yellow Zone	70%	375		Throughout exhale 2
	65%	350		Inhale and exhale 3
Low Yellow Zone	60%	325		**◆ Cough in past 5 minutes**
	50%	210		None 0
Red Zone				Less than one per minute 1

Medicines				
* Med name Inhaled steroid	7 puffs 2X/day			One to four per minute .... 2 More than four per minute 3
* Med name Other controller	400 mg 2X/day			**◆ Activity** Fully active 0
* Med name Quick-relief	2 puffs as needed			Can run short distance .... 1 Can walk only 2
Oral steroid				Missed work or school or stayed indoors 3

◆ Sleep
Fine 0
Slight wheeze or cough 1
Awake 2-3 times because of wheeze or cough 2
Awake most of the night 3

Signs	
Wheeze	
Cough	
Activity	
Sleep	

* Fill in the brand name of your medicine, dose, and number of times per day you take it.

Figure 34. Asthma Peak Flow Diary: Step Four. John filled in the name and the dose of
his asthma medicines. He checked off each dose he took in the appropriate row.

house or work in a particular environment. A
Comments section provides space above each
daily column for you to record any event that
you suspect may be a trigger. Patients may notice that their symptoms occur simultaneously
with taking a trip to a barn or the zoo, playing
in a hayfield or mowed grass, taking trash to
the landfill, playing soccer during pollen season, vacuuming, or attending welding class.

Look at John's diary (see Figure 35). On August 12, he recorded that he was visiting a
house with dogs. John is allergic to dogs. He
stayed in that house for the next four days. His
peak flow scores after taking a quick relief med-

icine decreased into the high yellow zone for
seven days even though he increased his dose.

My patients use the Comments section in
various ways. They record doctors' visits, concerns, questions, and jubilant words when they
are feeling great. This section is the place to
record anything that you find important about
your asthma.

*Step Six: Score Signs and Symptoms
of Asthma*

If you monitor your asthma signs and
symptoms in addition to your peak flow scores,
you will get important information. I use the

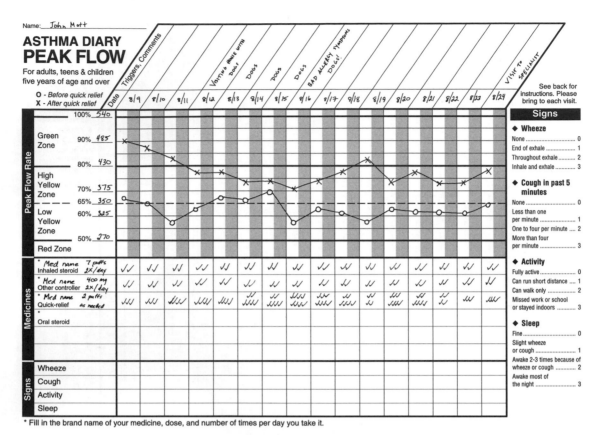

Figure 35. Asthma Peak Flow Diary: Step Five. John recorded triggers, events, and other comments about his asthma in the Comments section.

words "signs" and "symptoms" interchangeably here, not because they mean the same thing, but because you will hear the same concept called by both names.

In the diary I refer to "signs." By recording your asthma signs and your peak flow, you can begin to figure out their relationship. For example, does your peak flow drop before your signs and symptoms appear? Or are you very attuned to your body, noticing symptoms before your peak flow scores begin to change? If you observe and track your signs and symptoms, your awareness will grow.

Record your asthma signs and symptoms in the Signs area at the bottom of the peak flow

diary. Here you can score wheeze, cough, activity, and sleep. The scoring system of 0 to 3 is explained on the front of the diary. When you have achieved excellent control of your asthma, you will almost always score a 0 in all categories. During episodes or before you have developed an effective asthma treatment plan, one, some, or all of the signs and symptoms may appear.

In the two weeks before he saw me, John had a lot of trouble sleeping because of asthma. His diary shows that sleep consistently earned a score of 2, meaning that he was awake two or three times a night (see Figure 36). Asthma also reduced his ability to be active. Despite being in

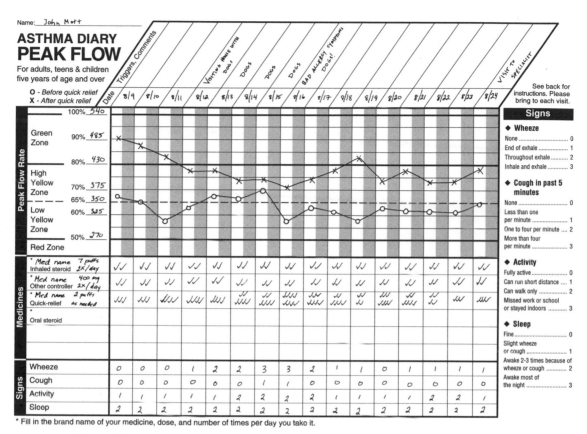

Figure 36. Asthma Peak Flow Diary: Step Six. John recorded his scores for wheeze, cough, activity, and sleep in the Signs section of the diary.

good shape, on some days John could only walk rather than run (score of 2). John frequently wheezed, and for two days he was wheezing throughout his entire breathing cycle (score of 3). John's diary made it clear that his asthma was out of control. When he came in for his consultation, he was eager to get his normal life back.

Sometimes peak flow scores may be in the green zone at the same time a person observes signs and symptom of asthma that indicate a mild asthma episode. This happens most often when the personal best peak flow score is set too low. However, even when the personal best is correct, some people will feel symptoms when their peak flow scores are 85 or even 90 percent of their best. These people will be able to manage their asthma better if their zone boundaries are adjusted to make the green zone narrower (90 to 100 percent, for example). I discuss zone adjustments in Chapter Five, "Peak Flow" (see page 139).

GETTING ASTHMA UNDER CONTROL WITH A PEAK FLOW DIARY

At your first asthma visit, your doctor will work out an initial treatment plan for your asthma. An effective treatment plan should help you achieve daily peak flow scores in the green zone, meaning you will have hardly any symptoms while you are fully active. The asthma diary provides detailed feedback, so your doctor can see what has happened between visits and make any needed adjustments.

At John's first visit, I knew immediately from his diary, as well as his asthma story, that he had both airway inflammation and bronchoconstriction. I was certain that the highest peak flow score he had blown was not his personal best. John is 6 feet tall; the mean peak flow for someone of his age and height is 640, so we decided to use that number until his air-

ways were clear. Using 640 as his personal best, we regraphed the peak flow scores for the previous two weeks. Look at John's initial diary (Figure 33) and see how it compares to the revised one (Figure 37).

When John was using 540 as his personal best, he thought that his peak flow scores were in the yellow or green zones. After increasing our estimate of his personal best, it became clear that John had been living in the low yellow and red zones, particularly after staying in the house with the dogs. No wonder he was having so many signs and symptoms of

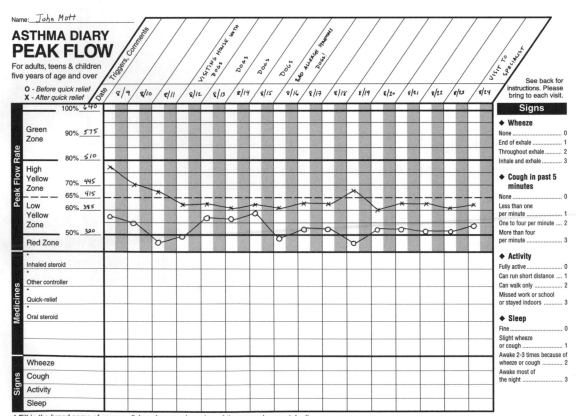

Figure 37. Asthma Peak Flow Diary Using 640 as John's Personal Best.
We regraphed his peak flow scores for the two week period before his asthma consultation.
Compare this diary to the one in Figure 36.

Dr. Tom Plaut's Asthma Guide for People of All Ages

asthma! After a week of taking an oral steroid to clear his airways, John blew a peak flow score of 640 several times. This would serve as his personal best score until he blew a higher score on two separate days.

AFTER THE FIRST ASTHMA CONSULTATION

At John's first asthma visit, he learned how to use his inhalers properly. He added an oral steroid to his daily routine (for seven days), and his symptoms cleared up in three days. His peak flow score increased by more than 200 points during the week (see Figure 38). How did John achieve this remarkable improvement?

In the next chapter, the story of John's asthma visits will illustrate the steps we took to achieve excellent asthma control.

HOW OFTEN SHOULD YOU USE A DIARY?

Initially, you should use the diary every time you check your peak flow. I ask adult patients, teenagers, and parents to keep a diary twice a day. For the first few months that you are learning about asthma and working toward controlling it, the diary will be of great assistance.

Once you have achieved excellent asthma control, you may still want to keep a diary to fine-tune your understanding of asthma and to

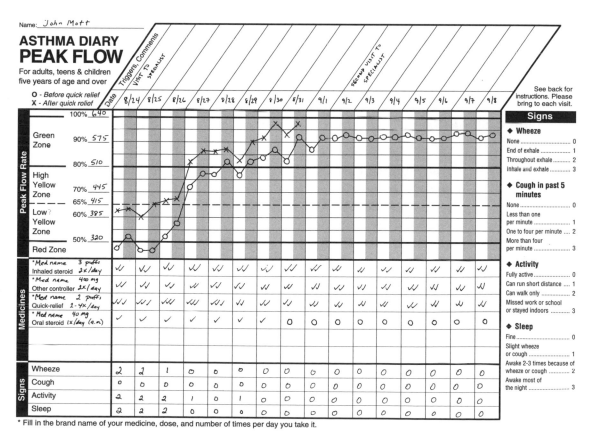

Figure 38. Asthma Peak Flow Diary After John's Asthma Consultation.

monitor the state of your airways. After this point, some patients keep a diary only when they have signs or symptoms, enter an environment that may provoke asthma symptoms, make a change in medicine routine, or encounter a trigger. For example, one patient whom I had not seen in a year came in for a review appointment with her mother. Claire had had three brief asthma episodes during that year. All of the information I needed from the year fit into one diary sheet covering sixteen days. Claire's mother had kept a diary only when she needed it.

Patients who have had a serious episode often wish to continue keeping a daily diary until they are convinced they will not again be caught unawares. In addition, all of my patients keep a diary for the week prior to their appointment with me. It provides me with much of the information I need to assess their asthma.

The Asthma Signs Diary for Children Ages 5 and Under

Many parents can tell that something is wrong when their child is having an asthma episode. They may be seeing some of the signs of asthma or an early clue that is characteristic of their child. These observations are important and become most helpful when they can be quantified. How bad is the episode? How long has it been going on? Is the medicine helping? Should additional medicine be given? A diary based on asthma signs helps parents answer these questions.

If a child is too young to blow a reliable peak flow score, the four signs of asthma are the best way to assess her asthma. When I was a general pediatrician, I taught parents the four signs of asthma during an office visit. If their child was having an asthma episode at the time, the parents could observe the signs before and after treatment with inhaled albuterol, and see how the signs diminished as their child improved. I wanted parents to be able to treat most asthma episodes confidently and safely at home and to know when they needed to see me. I developed the Asthma Signs Diary to help them accomplish this goal (see Figure 39).

Shoshana's story shows how parents use the diary to manage asthma. You will find a full-sized blank copy of the Asthma Signs Diary at the back of the book. You may reproduce it for personal use. My patients use the three-color version ("see Resource Section").

Table 40. How Often and How Long to Keep a Peak Flow Diary

How Often to Record	How Long
twice per day	first two months
once per day	third and fourth months
three days per week	as long as helpful
once a week or less often	ongoing

Shoshana's Asthma Signs Diary
Tamara Barbasch
First visit in the 1990s

We used the Asthma Signs Diary until several months prior to Shoshana's fifth birthday, when she began to use a peak flow meter on a regular basis (see page 24). We found the diary very simple to use, and we often "modified" it by choosing to record information in the way that made the most sense to us. At the beginning of our experience with Shoshana's asthma, we used the diary regularly; then, as we became more proficient at recognizing the somewhat predictable patterns of her asthma episodes, we used it only when she had an upper respiratory infection or other exposure to a significant trigger.

Especially in the beginning of our asthma education, the diary helped us to accurately assess the severity of Shoshana's asthma and communicate this information clearly when asked by health professionals at Shoshana's pediatric office. It helped us identify exactly when we required professional intervention. Later, when we became comfortable with keeping a supply of oral steroid in the house, the diary and home treatment plan helped us to see when to begin administration of this medication. This saved us a trip to the office or a telephone call in the middle of the night. Even after we discontinued regular use of the diary, we occasionally used it to get a clear picture of how bad things actually were when we believed that a severe episode was occurring.

Even more significant to us, however, was the psychological benefit of the diary in helping us feel more in control of the situation by enabling us to track the course of an asthma episode. The times during which Shoshana was experiencing asthma were often stressful and upsetting for all of us. When we were tired and confused, the diary was helpful by acting as a "checklist" to evaluate symptoms. It was comforting to be able to follow an organized and prearranged plan and to be able to consult the diary to determine what was actually happening with Shoshana's lungs. Perhaps it is this aspect of its support and security that has led us to save every single one of those diary sheets in our "asthma file."

FILLING OUT AN ASTHMA SIGNS DIARY

Recording in a diary based on asthma signs differs somewhat from using the Asthma Peak Flow Diary. Follow these steps as you use the diary:

1. Set up the daily column(s).
2. Score each of the four signs of asthma, record each score, and calculate the total score of asthma signs.
3. Plot the total score of asthma signs to determine the asthma treatment zone.
4. Connect daily signs scores to see the pattern.
5. Check off asthma medicines taken each day.
6. Record triggers, events, and other important comments.
7. Score activity and sleep.

Your doctor may ask you to do only one or two of these steps at first, then add more as you master each one. I will discuss how Luke De-Laura's parents filled out the Asthma Signs Diary for their 7-month-old son for the week before they came in for their first visit and for the week after that visit. In the next chapter, you will follow Luke and his parents during their first few months of asthma care.

Name: _____

ASTHMA DIARY
SIGNS
For children under
five years of age
O - Before quick relief
X - After quick relief

Triggers, Comments

Date

See back for
instructions. Please
bring to each visit.

SIGNS		

◆ **Cough in past 5 minutes**
None 0
Less than 1 per minute 1
1 - 4 per minute. 2
More than 4 per minute 3

◆ **Wheeze**
None 0
End of exhale 1
Throughout exhale 3
Inhale and exhale 5

◆ **Sucking in chest skin**
None 0
Barely noticeable 1
Obvious 3
Severe 5

◆ **Breathing faster**
None 0
Slight increase 1
Up to 100% increase 2
Over 100% increase 3

DAILY ROUTINE

◆ **Activity**
Fully active 0
Runs less 1
Plays quietly 2
Sleeps during day 3

◆ **Sleep**
Fine 0
Slight wheeze or cough 1
Awake 2 - 3 times because
of wheeze or cough 2
Awake most of the night 3

SIGNS
- Cough
- Wheeze
- Chest skin
- Breathing faster
- TOTAL:

ZONES
Green Zone	0
	1
HighYellow Zone	2
	3
	4
	5
Low Yellow Zone	6
	7
	8
Red Zone	9

MEDICINES
- Cromolyn
- Inhaled steroid
- Quick relief
- Oral steroid

DAILY
- Activity
- Sleep

* Fill in the brand name of your medicine, dose, and number of times per day you take it.

Figure 39. The Asthma Signs Diary

Step One: Set Up the Daily Column(s)

The columns are designed to hold a lot of information while still being easy to read. Record the date at the top of the column or columns you use each day. Notice that each column has two parts, one clear and one shaded.

Use the clear half of the column to record scores observed before giving a quick relief medicine (albuterol), and the shaded half to record scores observed afterward. If your child is taking a quick relief medicine, it is most helpful if you score asthma signs before and after giving medicine, in the morning and again in the afternoon or evening. This is because albuterol opens the airways, which usually low-

ers (improves) the signs score. Asthma treatment is based on the score before taking the medicine. If the response to the medicine is not adequate, additional medicine must be given.

If your child is not taking a quick relief medicine, you can score signs once in the morning and once in the afternoon. In this case, you can use the clear half of the column for morning scores and the shaded half for afternoon scores. Of course, you should organize the columns in a way that makes sense to you. Luke's parents used a whole column for each part of the day during the week before their first visit (see Figure 40). Because they had not yet learned the importance of observing asthma signs both before and after giving albuterol, they recorded signs on the diary (with "o") only before giving medicine. This information was still very helpful during the office visit.

Step Two: Score the Four Signs of Asthma

To use the diary effectively, you must learn how to score the four signs of asthma accurately. Chapter 2, "The Basics of Asthma," discusses the four signs and explains how to score them. The front of the Asthma Signs Diary outlines the same system.

- *Cough* earns a score (0–3) based on how many times your child coughs each minute for five minutes.
- The *wheeze* score (0–5) depends on where in the breathing cycle the wheeze occurs.
- *Sucking in the chest skin* (retractions) is scored (0–5) by how severe it appears.
- An *increase in breathing rate* is scored (0–3) based on the magnitude of the increase.

Wheeze and retractions are weighted more heavily because they indicate a more serious asthma problem.

Occasionally, the scoring system of the diary needs to be modified. A slim child may suck in (retract) her chest skin somewhat during normal breathing. If the parents and doctor observe her doing this, they can change the retraction score for slight "sucking in" to 0 (instead of 1). As the parent, you are the best observer of what is normal for your child. You can provide your doctor with the information he needs to adjust the scoring system.

RECORD EACH SCORE AND CALCULATE THE TOTAL SCORE OF ASTHMA SIGNS

Luke's mother, Wendy, started to record asthma signs on March 23, one week before her first visit with me (see Figure 40). She had read *Children with Asthma: A Manual for Parents*, and scored Luke's signs based on what she had learned. On the morning of March 23, Luke was coughing between one and four times every minute. This earned a score of 2 for cough. He had no other signs, so his mother recorded 0s in the other boxes. Luke's total score of asthma signs was 2.

By the afternoon, Luke's signs had become worse. He was coming down with a cold. He was coughing more than four times per minute (score of 3), wheezing at the end of exhalation (score of 1), sucking in his chest skin a little bit (score of 1), and breathing at twice his usual rate (100 percent more, score of 2). His total score of asthma signs was 7. Wendy recorded this score in the next column.

You can use the total score of asthma signs to assign a zone to your child's condition (see Table 41). The total score ranges from 0 to 16: 0 means that your child has no signs. When the signs score increases, it means that your child's condition is worsening. The asthma zone then guides you in following your written home treatment plan. Your doctor will make

Table 41. Judging Severity of an Asthma Episode Based on the Total Score of Asthma Signs

Zone	Asthma Signs Score	Episode Severity
green	0	no episode
high yellow	1–4	mild episode
low yellow	5–8	moderate episode
red	9–16	severe episode

sure you are scoring your child's signs accurately.

By recording asthma signs scores each day, you can see how your child is doing from day to day and week to week. The score of asthma signs tends to be higher (worse) in the morning and lower (better) in the afternoon. During an episode, you can look at morning scores over a period of days and see if the trend is improving or worsening. An improving trend means that the treatment plan is effective. A trend of increasing (worsening) signs scores means that treatment is not adequate. In this case, you need to change treatment according to your written plan or see your doctor.

Step Three: Plot the Total Score of Asthma Signs to Determine the Asthma Treatment Zone

After you have scored your child's asthma signs and calculated the total score, graph the total in the Zones section of the diary. Use an "o" to graph scores observed before giving a quick relief medicine and an "x" to record scores observed afterward.

When Wendy graphed Luke's scores on the afternoon of March 23, she realized that he was having an episode in the low yellow zone. Although she had read about asthma zones, she did not yet have a written treatment plan to guide her in responding to Luke's episode. So she continued to give Luke his usual daily medicines and fortunately Luke's episode did not get worse.

Step Four: Connect the Daily Signs Scores to See a Pattern

As Wendy recorded a new score each morning and afternoon, she connected the "o" with the previous score. This showed her the trend of

Luke's changing airway condition. She could see that he was living mostly in the high yellow zone and had dipped into the low yellow zone three times.

Step Five: Check Off Asthma Medicines Taken Each Day

Below the Zones section of the diary you will find a list of asthma medicines, each with its own row for recording information. Your doctor can write in the brand name of medicines that he prescribes, including the dose and how many times per day you are supposed to give it to your child.

Wendy wrote in the medicines that she had been instructed to give Luke: cromolyn, 1 ampule, three times per day by compressor driven nebulizer (a total of 3 ampules per day); albuterol, a quick relief medicine, 0.25 cc with each cromolyn dose. Each time she gave a dose of medicine, Wendy made a check in the column for that day. You can see from the diary in Figure 41 that Luke received each medicine three times per day (one dose in the morning, two in the afternoon or evening).

Step Six: Record Triggers, Events, and Other Important Comments

Helping your child avoid or reduce exposure to asthma triggers will help control asthma as much as giving your child the right asthma medicines. But it can be difficult to figure out what your child's triggers are. Children may keep playing even if they are not feeling completely well. Young children may not be able to explain to you that they feel bad around the neighbor's cat or after a trip to the zoo.

The signs diary can help you identify your child's triggers more easily. When you see the signs score dropping below the green zone, you

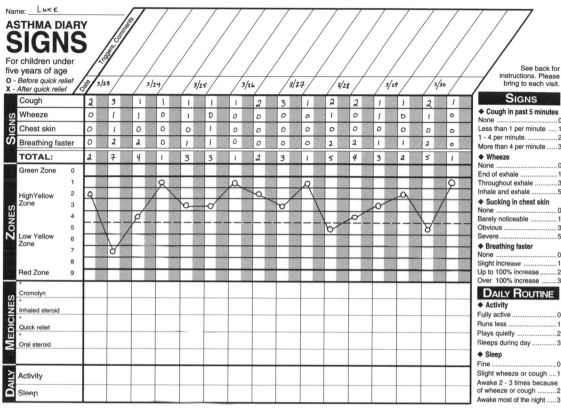

Name: Luke		3/23		3/24		3/25		3/26		3/27		3/28		3/29		3/30	
SIGNS	Cough	2	3	1	1	1	1	1	2	3	1	2	2	1	1	2	1
	Wheeze	O	1	1	O	1	D	O	O	O	O	1	O	1	O	1	O
	Chest skin	O	1	O	O	O	1	O	O	O	O	O	O	O	O	O	O
	Breathing faster	O	2	2	O	1	1	O	O	O	O	2	2	1	1	2	O
	TOTAL:	2	7	4	1	3	3	1	2	3	1	5	4	3	2	5	1

ASTHMA DIARY
SIGNS
For children under five years of age
O - Before quick relief
X - After quick relief

See back for instructions. Please bring to each visit.

ZONES: Green Zone 0; 1; HighYellow Zone 2, 3, 4, 5; Low Yellow Zone 6, 7, 8; Red Zone 9

MEDICINES: Cromolyn; Inhaled steroid; Quick relief; Oral steroid

DAILY: Activity; Sleep

* Fill in the brand name of your medicine, dose, and number of times per day you take it.

SIGNS
◆ Cough in past 5 minutes
None 0
Less than 1 per minute 1
1 - 4 per minute. 2
More than 4 per minute 3
◆ Wheeze
None 0
End of exhale 1
Throughout exhale 3
Inhale and exhale 5
◆ Sucking in chest skin
None 0
Barely noticeable 1
Obvious 3
Severe 5
◆ Breathing faster
None 0
Slight increase 1
Up to 100% increase 2
Over 100% increase 3

DAILY ROUTINE
◆ Activity
Fully active 0
Runs less 1
Plays quietly 2
Sleeps during day 3
◆ Sleep
Fine 0
Slight wheeze or cough 1
Awake 2 - 3 times because of wheeze or cough 2
Awake most of the night 3

Figure 40. Asthma Signs Diary: Steps One Through Four. Wendy scored each of Luke's asthma signs, added them and graphed the total each day for the week before his first asthma visit.

know to look for a recent trigger. For example, you may find that your child's asthma signs scores are worse after coming home from a friend's house in the winter. It may turn out that the friend's parents heat their house with a wood stove, which triggered your child's asthma.

At the top of each column in the diary, a Comments section provides you with space to record possible asthma triggers, such as a respiratory infection, contact with a cat, or exercise in cold air. In Luke's diary of March 23, his mother recorded that he was "very raspy,

maybe getting a cold" (see Figure 42). By the afternoon that day, Luke's total signs score had dropped into the low yellow zone. The diary shows that colds are an asthma trigger for Luke, as they are for many children his age.

Parents use the Comments section in many ways. They often record additional asthma symptoms such as changes in a child's behavior, or observations like "laughing causes cough." I encourage them to record anything that they think may be important about their child's asthma, environment, or medicines.

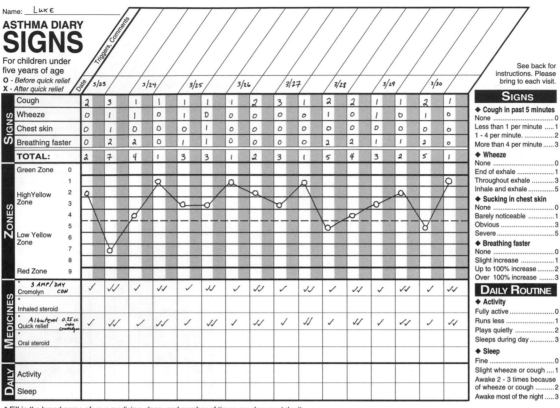

Figure 41. Asthma Signs Diary: Step Five. Wendy wrote the name of each medicine, the dose, and the number of times per day the doctor had instructed her to give it. Every time she gave Luke medicine, she checked off one dose.

This part of the diary adds helpful pieces to the asthma puzzle that we are trying to solve.

Step Seven: Score Activity and Sleep

At the bottom of the Asthma Signs Diary you can record your child's daily activity level and how well she is sleeping through the night (see Figure 42).

HOW OFTEN SHOULD YOU USE THE DIARY?

I ask parents to keep a diary twice a day while they are learning about asthma and working toward controlling it. This phase usu-ally lasts two or three months. Once their child has achieved excellent asthma control, they may still want to keep a diary to fine-tune their understanding and management of their child's asthma.

After this point, some parents keep a diary only when they make a change in medicine routine or when their child has asthma signs or symptoms, enters a threatening environment, or encounters a trigger. Parents of children who have been hospitalized or had a serious episode often wish to continue keeping a daily diary so they will be able to recognize and treat an episode as early as possible. This will enable

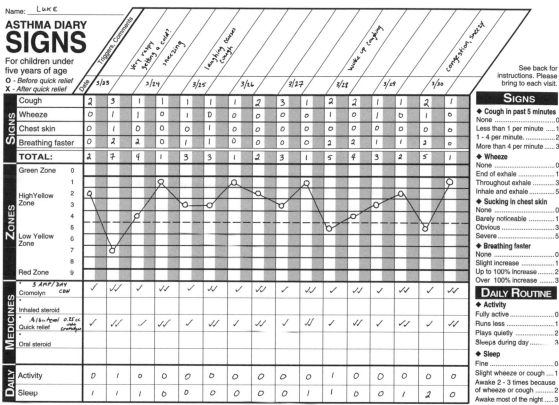

Name: LUKE

ASTHMA DIARY
SIGNS
For children under
five years of age
O - Before quick relief
X - After quick relief

See back for instructions. Please bring to each visit.

Figure 42. Asthma Signs Diary: Steps Six and Seven. Wendy wrote additional information about Luke's asthma triggers in the Comments section of the diary. She also scored Luke's activity and sleep in the Daily section of the diary.

them to prevent another uncontrolled episode. Parents of all my patients keep a diary for the week prior to an appointment with me. It provides me with much of the information I need about their child's asthma.

LUKE'S FIRST VISIT TO THE ASTHMA SPECIALIST

When Luke, his mother, father, and two grandparents came in for their first visit (April 1), they brought the diary shown in Figure 42. I could see that Luke's asthma was poorly controlled. He had been in the high and low yellow zones during most of the week. The diary told a story of inflamed and constricted airways that were vulnerable to even one asthma trigger. Yet his parents were already giving him 3 ampules of cromolyn along with albuterol every day. Did they need to give more medicine? What else could they do?

At the first visit, I suggested several changes in Luke's treatment. I prescribed seven days of an oral steroid (prednisolone) to clear up the inflammation in Luke's airways. This inflammation was blocking the cromolyn from reaching into his lungs and doing its job of preventing

Using an Asthma Diary

Table 42. How Often and How Long to Keep a Signs Diary

How Often to Record	How Long
twice per day	first two months
once per day	third and fourth months
three days per week	as long as helpful
once a week or less often	ongoing

asthma episodes. (I prescribe seven days of an oral steroid for all of my patients to clear the airways when they start cromolyn.)

I also increased Luke's cromolyn dose to 4 ampules per day (from 3), to be given in two sittings. This schedule was more convenient for his parents. In addition, after observing Wendy giving Luke a treatment of cromolyn and albuterol with the compressor driven nebulizer, I made some suggestions about nebulizer technique to improve the effectiveness of treatment. I also suggested that she score Luke's signs before and after giving medicine, to see whether he improved with the albuterol treatment.

After the visit, Wendy recorded Luke's asthma signs in the diary each day and sent me a completed diary one week later (see Figure 43). She recorded asthma signs before giving albuterol with an "o" in the clear half of the column. Asthma signs scored after medicine are recorded with an "x" in the shaded half of the column. Each day took up two columns. Luke's scores almost always improved after taking albuterol.

On the day of his first visit, Luke's total score of asthma signs had been in the lower part of the high yellow zone (score of 4) before he took albuterol. After taking medicine, his asthma signs were still in the high yellow zone (score of 1). This showed that Luke was having a mild asthma episode.

On April 2, Wendy started to give Luke an oral steroid each morning and began to administer the higher dose of cromolyn with albuterol as we had discussed (see the Medicines section of Luke's diary). Four days after starting his new medicine treatment (April 6), Luke was in the green zone before taking albuterol. Because Luke had no asthma signs, Wendy did not need to score signs again after giving medicine.

Luke stayed solidly in the green zone for the next two weeks, until he had a bad cold. At that point, Wendy was ready to respond with additional medicine. I discuss the story of Luke's first few months of treatment in the next chapter.

For members of Luke's family, the diary was more than a management tool that they used as they learned to control Luke's asthma at home. It allowed the adults who cared for Luke to communicate clearly about his treatment, even though they worked different schedules. Luke's mom leaves for work at 6:00 A.M. and returns at 5:00 P.M. His dad works either from 3 P.M. to 3 A.M. or 11 P.M. to 7 A.M.. Luke's maternal grandmother, aunt, and cousin fill in taking care of him. They all use the asthma diary to understand Luke's changing condition and keep track of his medicine. Wendy says they could not function without it.

ASTHMA DIARY
SIGNS

For children under
five years of age
O - Before quick relief
X - After quick relief

See back for
instructions. Please
bring to each visit.

Triggers, Comments — Visit specialist — start prednisone — out late in cold — sneezing — congested — cough at breakfast — slight cough

Date: 3/31 · 4/1 · 4/2 · 4/3 · 4/4 · 4/5 · 4/6 · 4/7 · 4/8

SIGNS

Signs	3/31	4/1	4/2	4/3	4/4	4/5	4/6	4/7	4/8
Cough	1 / 2	1 / 1	1 / 2 / 2	1 / 2 / 2	2 / 1 / 1	0	0	0	0
Wheeze	0 0 / 0	0 0 0 0	1 1 0 0	0 0 0 0	0 0 0 0	0 0 0 0	0	0	0
Chest skin	0 0 0	0 0 0 0	0 0 0 0	0 0 0 0	0 0 0 0	0 0 0 0	0	0	0
Breathing faster	1 1 1 0	1 0 1 0	1 0 0 0	1 0 0 0	1 1 0 0	0 0	0	1	0
TOTAL:	2 2 4 1	2 1 2 1	4 2 2 1	2 1 2 1	3 3 2 2	1 1 1 0	0	1	0

ZONES

Zone	Score
Green Zone	0, 1
High Yellow Zone	2, 3, 4, 5
Low Yellow Zone	6, 7, 8
Red Zone	9

MEDICINES

* 2 AMP 2x Cromolyn	√√	√√	√√	√√	√√	√√	√√	√√	√√
* Inhaled steroid									
* albuterol 0.25 cc into cromolyn — Quick relief	√√	√√	√√	√√	√√	√√	√√	√√	√√
* 4 cc (12 mg) Oral steroid			√	√	√	√	√	√	√

DAILY

	3/31	4/1	4/2	4/3	4/4	4/5	4/6	4/7	4/8
Activity	0	1	1	0	1	0	0	0	0
Sleep	0	1	0	0	1	0	0	0	0

SIGNS

◆ Cough in past 5 minutes
None 0
Less than 1 per minute 1
1 - 4 per minute. 2
More than 4 per minute 3

◆ Wheeze
None 0
End of exhale 1
Throughout exhale 3
Inhale and exhale 5

◆ Sucking in chest skin
None 0
Barely noticeable 1
Obvious 3
Severe 5

◆ Breathing faster
None 0
Slight increase 1
Up to 100% increase 2
Over 100% increase 3

DAILY ROUTINE

◆ Activity
Fully active 0
Runs less 1
Plays quietly 2
Sleeps during day 3

◆ Sleep
Fine 0
Slight wheeze or cough 1
Awake 2 - 3 times because
of wheeze or cough 2
Awake most of the night 3

* Fill in the brand name of your medicine, dose, and number of times per day you take it.

Figure 43. Asthma Signs Diary After Luke's Consultation

How to Choose a Diary

There are more than twenty diaries available from various companies, organizations, and publications. Which one should you use? An effective diary should be easy to use and analyze and include instructions that are clear. Most importantly, the diary should help guide your treatment. I recommend that you use a diary that has the following attributes:

- *Visual Display of Peak Flow or Asthma Signs:* Peak flow monitoring is an essential component of asthma learning and management for people 5 years of age and older.

Signs scores guide treatment in younger children. A graphic display allows you to see trends at a glance and to understand zones. (A display of numbers in a column or list is much harder to interpret.)

- *A Place to Record Asthma Medicines:* Asthma medicines are an important part of treatment, and your diary should have a space to record the type, brand name, dose, and frequency of each one that you need. But is this enough? I don't think so.

A diary should have space for you to record each dose of medicine you take every day. With this record, you will be less likely to skip or repeat a dose by mistake. You will also be more likely to notice how your medicines affect peak flow, signs, symptoms, and asthma control. Seeing these connections in your diary will help you understand how your asthma medicines work.

- *A Place to Record Signs and Symptoms:* A diary should have a designated space to record scores for asthma signs and symptoms.

- *A Place to Record Comments:* Comments increase the helpfulness of a diary by allowing you to identify new triggers and see how a combination of triggers adds up to cause trouble. The diary should give you space to write any additional information each day that you think is important about your asthma.

- *Shows the Connections:* A good asthma diary should show you how the pieces of the asthma puzzle fit together, since understanding these connections is part of achieving excellent asthma control. This means that all of the information from one day should be recorded in a single column or row.

- *Color:* For many years in my practice I used a black-and-white diary, like the examples displayed in this book. I like to keep things simple, and I didn't think adding colors would improve the diary.

Then I noticed that many of my patients had colored in the green, yellow and red zones on the diaries they brought to their visits. They said that color helped them pay better attention to the boundaries between the zones. When scores dropped even slightly into the yellow zone, they noticed right away. A score in the brightly colored red zone urgently communicated the need for treatment. After I produced a three-color diary, my patients used it more frequently because it was easier to interpret.

In Summary

A comprehensive asthma diary can help you understand asthma and, as a result, manage it more effectively. The diary provides an ongoing record of fluctuations in peak flow rates, asthma medicines, suspected triggers, and your signs and symptoms. It will help you identify triggers that provoke an episode, learn when to start and when to reduce medicines, remember to take medicines regularly, and to see trends in your peak flow and asthma signs scores. At the doctor's office, the diary will help you accurately recall events since the last visit. It will both improve communication with your doctor and give him a wealth of clinical information to use in guiding treatment and addressing your progress.

Once you achieve excellent control of your asthma, you can gradually decrease the frequency of diary entries. Some patients keep a diary only when they have signs or symptoms, enter a threatening environment, make a change in medicine routine, or encounter a trigger. All of my patients keep a diary for the week prior to their appointment. The diary is one of the most powerful tools you can use to manage your asthma.

Chapter Seven

Asthma Treatment

You must work closely with a competent doctor to control your asthma safely and effectively. Ask your doctor to give you an individualized written plan to guide your asthma treatment.

Asthma treatment is much more effective today than it was even ten years ago because we have new medicines, new inhalation devices, new monitoring devices and educational aids, and a fuller understanding of the asthma process in the lungs. Each of these advances can help you achieve better control of your asthma. But using new asthma management tools effectively requires that you gain more knowledge, acquire new skills, and monitor your asthma more closely than was necessary before.

If you had seen a pediatrician, family practitioner or internist in the office or in the emergency room for an asthma episode before 1979, you probably would have been given a shot of adrenaline and a prescription for theophylline to take at home. No monitoring. No learning. Preventive management was often limited to reducing triggers, and many doctors did not even discuss this subject. It was quite possible that you would be back in the emergency room with your next episode.

By the 1980s, treatment had improved greatly. Many doctors were using inhaled beta$_2$-agonist medicines instead of adrenaline shots to relieve asthma episodes. Allergists and pulmonologists were routinely prescribing cromolyn and inhaled steroids to prevent asthma episodes.

In 1991, the National Heart, Lung and Blood Institute published the first *Expert Panel Report: Guidelines for the Diagnosis and Management of Asthma,* prepared by a panel of national asthma experts. A second set of *Guidelines* was published in 1997 to update the original document. These reports, which summarize information that has appeared in thousands of scientific articles, describe the care currently recommended for most patients with asthma. They were produced to provide guidance for health professionals who care for patients with asthma.

Not all experts agree with every part of the *Guidelines,* and individual patients may require a different approach. However, the *Guidelines* are the best and most comprehensive resource available today for the treatment of asthma. The overall approach to asthma treatment which you will read about in this chapter is consistent with the expert opinion found there. If your doctor recommends treatment that varies from the *Guidelines,* ask her to explain her reasoning so you can understand why your treatment differs.

Asthma treatment calls for more than simply taking the right asthma medicine. It starts with proper expectations, by you and by your doctor. As you learn about the basics of asthma and the medicines used to treat it, you build the foundation for effective treatment. When you identify and learn to avoid your asthma triggers, you can reduce the occurrence of episodes and the need for medicine.

Monitoring peak flow scores and asthma signs guides you in changing your medicine routine during an episode and teaches you more about asthma, triggers, and medicines. Asthma medicines help reduce inflammation in your airways, prevent symptoms, and relieve episodes that do occur. Your doctor helps you integrate these principles of treatment into a written asthma treatment plan that you can use at home to guide you to excellent asthma control.

The first half of this chapter discusses the principles of asthma treatment, relevant to people of all ages. Almost all asthma patients will benefit from using the zone system to guide their asthma management. For adults, teenagers, and children ages 5 years and older, peak flow scores provide the basis for the treatment zones. For children under 5, the four signs of asthma determine the zones. For this reason, the second half of the chapter is divided into two parts: one for adults, teenagers, and children ages 5 and older, the other for young children. When you reach that point, you may want to read only the section that ap-

plies to your situation. For both age groups, I provide examples based on actual patients. Your treatment plan should be individualized by your doctor.

You have already read about many pieces of the asthma puzzle. This chapter places those pieces in proper relationship to one another. Use this chapter to review and apply what you already know, and to learn where new information fits into the puzzle you are solving.

■

Two Treatment Stories

Maria Brown, age 39
First visit in the 1990s

Maria spent much of her childhood with runny noses, frequent colds, and multiple diagnoses of pneumonia and bronchitis. She often missed school during the winter. Strenuous exercise always seemed more difficult for her than for her friends, so she chose more sedentary activities. During this time, she lived in a house with five cats, five siblings, and two parents, both of whom smoked. Many of her relatives had "hay fever," and three had asthma.

Diagnosed with asthma at the age of 27, Maria started taking theophylline twice a day. Her allergist determined that she was allergic to dust, cats, various pollens, and grasses, but Maria didn't make any changes in her home environment. Her asthma symptoms worsened, waking her up at night and lasting a long time after each cold.

A respiratory specialist recommended environmental changes and prescribed several more medicines: albuterol, an inhaled steroid, a nasal steroid, an antihistamine, and a decongestant, in addition to the theophylline. Maria took all of these until she became pregnant, when she dropped all of them except for theophylline. She continued to have between twelve and fifteen asthma episodes a year, but she never required treatment in the emergency room.

Maria initially came to see me because her son was having trouble with his asthma. Our discussions about Lewis led her to make the changes in her home environment that she had deferred, as well as to come in for a consultation for herself. She wrote this account prior to her first consultation.

■

On your advice, we have made major changes in the house. We now have no pets (except fish). My mattress, box spring and pillows all have allergy covers. I am still aware of having many sinus headaches and infections. I wheeze and have a tight throat and watery eyes if I am in the presence of cats, dogs, cigarette smoke, and some grasses. I always take albuterol prior to aerobic exercise.

Since I have stopped living with cats, my symptoms have decreased significantly at home. I still react acutely when I come into contact with them. My present treatment includes environmental measures, an inhaled steroid, theophylline, and albuterol as needed, as well as inhaled nasal cromolyn and an antihistamine. In the year before I saw you with Lewis, whenever I had a cold, coughing awakened me at night. I had a tight chest, wheezing, coughing, and felt miserable every fall and winter. I have had no emergency visits to the hospital or doctor in the past twelve months.

■

At her first visit, I observed that Maria had poor technique in using the metered dose inhaler (MDI). She inhaled quickly and held her breath for about four seconds, instead of inhaling for three to five seconds and holding for five to ten seconds. She had never used a holding chamber and was probably getting less than half of the benefit from the inhaled steroid she was taking. After instruction, she used the MDI with holding chamber properly.

At a follow-up visit four months later, Maria was very satisfied with her ability to control her asthma. She attributed her improvement to the use of a holding chamber, which she demonstrated perfectly, and to making further changes in her environment. Two months later she stopped taking the inhaled steroid and reduced her theophylline dose by 50 percent.

Two years after her initial visit, Maria described her improvement.

■

Since last year my asthma control has been excellent, in that I have had very few symptoms and have been able to run and kayak regularly. My primary triggers are still upper respiratory infections and exercise. I use albuterol during respiratory infections and prior to exercise. I have not needed to use prednisone.

■

Nancy Grossman, age 46
First visit in the 1990s

Nancy's goals for her first asthma consultation were to prepare for a trip to Poland and to develop a plan to manage her asthma on a regular basis. She had her first episode of difficult breathing in her early twenties when she moved into a new apartment. A few years later, two weeks after the sudden traumatic death of her significant other, she had a second episode of difficult breathing, much worse than the first. Because she couldn't breathe while standing, she had to crawl down the steps to a taxi to take her to the emergency room. She then moved to the Northwest to attend chiropractic school, not aware that she had an asthma condition, and started having many asthma episodes each year. At this time, she was diagnosed with asthma. Here is the story that she brought to her first visit with me, almost 20 years later.

■

During that first year in the Northwest, I had about eight "attacks" that knocked all the strength out of me. Because I had no management plan, and because I didn't want to take any drugs, I did homeopathic remedies and vitamins once I started getting sick. Then, as I got worse and worse, I waited, sort of hoping I would get well by the alternative treatments I was doing. During this time, in addition to homeopathy and vitamins, I also utilized acupuncture care, chiropractic care, polarity therapy, herbs, and anything else that seemed would help.

Only once did I go to the ER, though I was bad enough to go several other times. The one time I went, my blood gases were pretty low, and they said I was in respiratory distress. In fact, I was so far gone that the drugs didn't kick in immediately and after spending all night in the ER with seemingly no relief, I checked myself out against doctor's orders and went home to deal with my asthma. Because no medical doctor taught me how to deal with my asthma I used holistic therapies to treat an attack. In hindsight they were not helpful in an acute situation. By the time I finally would take the drugs I was so far gone that it would take a few days to get some relief.

During those days of struggle, I would be down on all fours, trying hard to breathe, not able to lie down, not able to sleep, not able to eat, barely able to crawl out of bed to go to the bathroom, wheezing away, waiting for the next

four hours to pass so that I could take some more medicine. And finally, finally, it would kick in and after a few days of sheer agony and struggle, I would start to feel some relief. This cycle continued during my four years of chiropractic school.

After chiropractic school, I moved to Boston in 1981. I had serious asthma problems several times and had to miss work for as much as two weeks on three occasions between 1983 and 1994. In addition to these episodes I had two others, which I cut short by taking prednisone, something I don't like to do. Traditionally, the fall has been my worst time, specifically the change from summer to autumn. During this time, I usually take albuterol as needed. The rest of the year, I have been basically drug-free unless I've had an acute episode.

In May 1994, you and I had a curbside consultation. You introduced me to the concept of peak flow monitoring and the idea of using drugs early in an episode, instead of only in serious situations. A year later, I began a regimen of albuterol up to 2 puffs four times a day, when needed. What's different this year is that although I have not been close to an "attack," I also have not been able to get off albuterol for months now, which concerns me. Normally, by winter I am able to stop all drugs. This year, I haven't had very many days that I have been drug-free since September.

After reading your asthma book and writing this narrative, I can recognize my relationship to asthma more clearly. To me, taking drugs — any drugs, any amount — seems like I'm not okay. For years, I have tried many, many programs and therapies to avoid taking drugs and healing this condition for good. I do believe the holistic work I've done has diminished the severity of my illness. What I now realize is that I may (probably will) have asthma all my life. Learning how to deal with it effectively and with gratitude that drugs can help me is an important new step that began last year when I started using the peak flow meter.

As for going to Poland, I have no control over the environment. People who have no breathing problems tell me how hard it was for them in Poland and how everyone smokes and there's tons of industrial waste and pollution and that I should think carefully about going. So I have been concerned about doing this trip. I am eager for some plan both to get me through this trip with ease, and also to help me in my concerns of living here, an area that aggravates my asthmatic condition.

■

After a thorough history, physical exam, and a pulmonary function test (spirometry), Nancy and I discussed asthma, asthma medicines, asthma learning, environmental measures, and monitoring. I recommended that she take prednisone (an oral steroid) for the next seven days, an inhaled steroid for the long term, and albuterol before each dose of the inhaled steroid for the first month of treatment.

At her next visit a month later, Nancy explained that she had decided not to take the prednisone but had been taking the inhaled steroid daily, and that her peak flow score had climbed ten percent. Because of phlegm and coughing, she had gone to see her primary care physician. He had recommended that she add salmeterol (a long-acting beta$_2$-agonist medicine) to her daily routine. The next day her peak flow scores reached the green zone and stayed there.

A few months later she traveled to Poland. She continued taking the inhaled steroid and salmeterol every day for the two months before and then during her trip. She had absolutely no asthma difficulties during her three weeks of travel.

Two years after her initial visit, Nancy told me her asthma control is excellent. Since she knows when to treat her asthma symptoms and when to call for help, her anxiety about asthma has decreased greatly, and she checks her peak flow scores only when she isn't feeling well. Nancy uses albuterol before exercising when she has a cold. She treats episodes with albuterol and adds an inhaled steroid if symptoms don't clear up promptly. She has taken no oral steroids and made only one visit to the doctor for asthma. Because Nancy has only occasional symptoms and can run three miles or use the Stairmaster for thirty minutes without asthma symptoms, she does not take a daily controller medicine. She is very satisfied with her ability to control her asthma.

■

Proper asthma treatment greatly improved the lives of both Maria and Nancy. They were able to become more active, almost free from symptoms, and live with greater peace of mind. And both were able to substantially reduce the amount of asthma medicine they needed by avoiding asthma triggers, learning the proper technique for inhaling medicine, treating symptoms early, and following a written Home Treatment Plan. Because of a combination of diligence and good luck, at present neither of them has to take a controller medicine daily.

Unlike Maria and Nancy, most people with asthma who take a controller medicine will need to continue treatment to maintain excellent control. You certainly can reduce your need for asthma medicine by avoiding your asthma triggers and treating asthma episodes early. However, if you have symptoms more than twice a week (unrelated to strenuous exercise), you need to take controller medicine each day to control inflammation in your airways and protect you from symptoms and episodes.

Effective Asthma Treatment

You have read the phrase "excellent asthma control" many times in this book. Do you know what excellent control feels like? Many of my patients experience it after taking oral steroids for seven days, learning to inhale controller and quick relief medicine properly, and reducing triggers in their environment. They then can sleep through the night, breathe without wheezing, stop coughing, and have more energy for exercise. People who didn't think they were slowed down by their asthma realize that they feel much better than they have in a long time. Some people become aware that they had asthma symptoms only after their symptoms have vanished. All of these people have taken the first giant step toward effective asthma treatment: they have realized just how good they can feel.

When your asthma is under excellent control, you should be able to do whatever you want to do. That means exercising as hard and as long as you choose, not missing any activities, and rarely staying home from work or school because of asthma. You should not cough at night or need a quick relief medicine more than twice a week to clear your symptoms. You should rarely need an emergency visit to the doctor or hospital, and your peak flow scores should be in the green zone. The treatment plan that helps you achieve this control should include a medicine routine that produces minimal or no adverse effects.

THE STEP-DOWN APPROACH TO EXCELLENT ASTHMA CONTROL

All of my patients follow a step-down routine, starting at their first asthma visit. This routine calls for intensive treatment and reducing triggers from the outset, to clear airways, resolve symptoms and fulfill high expectations rapidly. Once these goals have been accomplished, medicine doses are carefully and gradually reduced (stepped down) to the minimum amount needed to maintain excellent control.

Many people come to see me after living for months or years with asthma symptoms. They want to take control of their asthma as quickly as possible. The step-down routine eliminates or reduces their symptoms greatly within two weeks and shows them that their asthma can be controlled.

If your doctor follows the 1997 *Guidelines*, you can expect her to guide you through the following steps to excellent asthma control:

1. Realize that your asthma control can be excellent.
2. Learn about asthma, medicines, peak flow, and treatment.
3. Monitor peak flow scores and record them in a peak flow diary.
4. Reduce triggers in your environment.
5. Establish and follow an intensive medication routine to rapidly clear your airways and therefore reduce symptoms.
6. Achieve excellent control for two to three months with this routine.

Then:

7. Gradually step down your medicines to the minimum dose needed to maintain excellent control.
8. Continue to monitor peak flow periodically to evaluate your ongoing routine.

I expect almost all of my patients with mild or moderate persistent asthma to begin feeling better within two weeks after their first visit. If they follow an effective plan, they can expect to achieve excellent symptom control in one to three months. Three or four visits with your regular doctor should be enough to take most or all of these steps toward excellent control. You should start to feel better in two weeks and continue to improve from then on. If you are not making good progress toward asthma control within two weeks, it makes sense to look for complicating factors, such as rhinitis, sinusitis, or environmental triggers at home or at work.

This time frame sets out general expectations to help you and your doctor judge whether your progress is satisfactory. It is based on a treatment approach in which almost all of my patients take an oral steroid during the first seven days of treatment. This clears up airway inflammation and symptoms very quickly. If you and your doctor follow a different approach, it may take longer before you can expect to feel free of almost all asthma symptoms and to blow peak flow scores consistently in the green zone.

STEPS TOWARD EXCELLENT ASTHMA CONTROL

Learning About Asthma

Asthma is not a simple condition. It involves complex reactions in the lungs which vary from morning to afternoon, day to day, season to season, and person to person.

Even the best asthma specialist cannot develop an optimal plan unless you collect and provide information on your day-to-day condition. With this information and your doctor's guidance, you can contribute to the development of a written treatment plan and adjust medicines according to the plan. As a result, you will feel confident that you can handle most asthma episodes at home and that you know when to seek a doctor's help.

If you do not have a clear understanding of asthma, it will be difficult to know when you need to change treatment, to judge what action to take, and to communicate well with your doctor. It is likely that you will experience unnecessary asthma symptoms and take too much or too little medicine.

Learning about your asthma is not a luxury. It is just as important as taking the proper medicines in the proper doses. People who want an appointment with me read this book before they come in for their first office visit. From the first consultation, we begin building a relationship based on knowledge and communication. I send them my typewritten office notes (four to six pages) after each visit to document the details of our conversation. Once their asthma is under good control, they return to the care of their primary care doctor, who handles the rare emergencies that occur. I adjust the treatment plan as needed in visits at three- to twelve-month intervals.

Reducing Triggers in the Environment

The purpose of making environmental changes is to reduce the burden of asthma on you, not to create an additional burden. Asthma is a condition in which the airways are easily inflamed and hyperresponsive (overreactive) to various triggers in the environment. Cat dander, pollen, smoke, exercise, dust, or many other allergens or irritants may trigger your asthma. When a trigger enters your lungs, it can set off a reaction that leads to inflammation, bronchoconstriction, and increased production of mucus, all of which narrow the airways. If that trigger is present in your bedroom, car, school, or workplace, it may be aggravating your asthma continuously. Removing the trigger from places you commonly use can make a huge difference.

The impact of making a change in your environment may not be as dramatic as when you start to take the proper asthma medicine with the proper technique, but the effect will be substantial and long-lasting. During the twenty-five years I practiced general pediatrics, I was impressed with how much my patients improved with proper medicines. I did not appreciate the importance of improving a patient's environment. But about ten years ago, an experience with my teenage son enlightened me.

We moved into our wall-to-wall-carpeted house when David was 8 years old. He was diagnosed with asthma a year later, and he started taking several medicines. David took his asthma treatment seriously, learned about asthma, followed his medicine routine closely, and was fully active in sports all through high school. His skin tests for allergies were negative. When he went off to college, he lived in a dorm room that had no rugs on the floors. He felt better when he was away. When he returned home during school vacations, he noticed an increase in his occasional asthma symptoms. This happened several times before I realized the need to take the carpeting out of David's bedroom. Since the carpet has been removed, David has had fewer asthma complaints when he stays in his old bedroom.

I have repeatedly seen the importance of environmental measures in treating asthma. I try to help my patients make informed decisions about making changes in the places they live and work. Some triggers are easy and inexpensive to remove, while others may require time, effort, and money to eliminate. And before you can remove triggers, you need to identify them, which can be done with the help of an asthma diary.

When your peak flow scores drop or asthma signs scores increase, record the possible triggers that you have encountered. Watch for a pattern that correlates a drop in peak flow score with exposure to a particular trigger. If the trigger is easily removed, such as a moldy carpet in the basement family room, the course of action is clear. If removal of a trigger de-mands more energy, consider your asthma severity and the ease, cost, and effectiveness of the environmental measure. Below are some general guidelines I offer to my patients.

Suggested Environmental Control Measures

If you have mild intermittent or mild persistent asthma, strongly consider:

- not allowing smoking in the house or car
- keeping humidity in the house between 25 and 50 percent
- keeping the cat (if you are allergic to it) out of the bedroom
- bathing the cat once a week
- wearing a mask in cold weather or around known irritants or allergens
- burning your wood stove hot (to reduce smoke)
- encasing mattresses and pillows in allergen-proof covers

If you have moderate or severe persistent asthma, strongly consider these environmental controls as well:

- removing carpets, especially from the bedroom
- purchasing nonleaking vacuum cleaner bags to reduce dust
- installing a filter on the furnace heating vents, air conditioners, and windows (in pollen season)
- purchasing a HEPA air filter for the bedroom
- having a friend or neighbor adopt your cat

If you know that you have allergies, you may also want to consider specific environmental controls to reduce your exposure to those substances. Environmental measures and approximate cost and labor involved in implementing them are discussed in Chapter 2, "The Basics of Asthma."

Some environmental changes make an enormous difference. I recently spoke with the mother of Abigail, an 11-year-old girl whom I first saw four years ago. She came in then because her daughter was having four to six colds a year which triggered asthma symptoms each time. These symptoms had kept her home from school. After our asthma consultation, Abigail's mother stopped smoking. Abigail now has the same number of colds but no longer misses school because of them.

Monitoring Your Asthma

Monitoring peak flow scores and asthma signs scores gives you the information you need to decide about environmental measures and medicines. It is very difficult to figure out and follow an effective treatment plan without daily monitoring.

Once you achieve excellent asthma control, you can monitor less often. But whether you monitor once a week or once a month, you can always do it more often if the need arises. A change in season, your location, or the severity of your asthma may make your treatment plan less effective. With daily monitoring, you and your doctor can quickly figure out what is going on and adjust your plan.

Asthma Medicines

The goal of taking a controller medicine daily for persistent asthma is to keep you in the green zone all the time. An effective medicine routine treats the inflammation of asthma in addition to its symptoms. Until recently, doctors did not understand that inflammation is a more basic and important aspect of asthma than bronchoconstriction. The first NHLBI *Guidelines on the Diagnosis and Management of Asthma*

(1991) made it clear that asthma is mainly a disease of inflammation in which the airways are hyperresponsive, and that daily medicines are needed to treat the inflammation. In 1997, the updated *Guidelines* explained that preventing inflammation can reduce the possibility of long-term damage to the airways.

The two types of asthma medicine are controllers and quick relief medicines. Inhaled steroids, taken daily, are the mainstay of medicine treatment for persistent asthma. They prevent and reduce inflammation in the airways, making you less vulnerable to triggers and episodes. In the case of mild asthma, another daily controller medicine can sometimes be substituted for the inhaled steroid. In cases of moderate or severe asthma, other controllers may be added to daily treatment with an inhaled steroid to improve asthma control or reduce a high dose of inhaled steroid. In some cases of severe asthma, an oral steroid is taken long-term as a controller medicine.

Quick relief medicines are taken as needed to relieve symptoms or prevent symptoms with exercise. Doctors use the term "p.r.n." to mean "as needed." Ask your doctor what as needed means for you. It varies from patient to patient.

You may need a quick relief medicine daily before strenuous exercise. You should not need a quick relief medicine more than twice a week (unrelated to strenuous exercise) to relieve asthma symptoms. If you do, it most likely means that your controller medicine is not doing its job. It may be that you are not inhaling your medicine properly and thus not receiving full benefit from it. Ask your doctor to check your technique. It is also possible that the dose of your controller medicines needs to be adjusted. Reducing triggers can reduce symptoms and the need for a quick relief medicine.

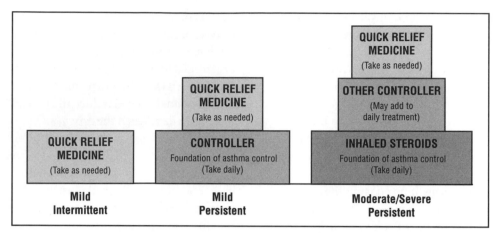

Figure 44. Types of Medicine Taken Based on Asthma Severity. Controller medicines are the foundation of treatment for everyone with persistent asthma.

CONCERNS ABOUT TAKING MEDICINE From many years of talking with patients and parents, I know that people have concerns about the medicines they take. Some people worry about adverse effects. Others are concerned that they might become dependent on or addicted to a medicine. Many parents find the idea of giving medicine to their child each day overwhelming, another commitment in an already busy life.

The best way to address these concerns is to learn how good you can feel using an effective treatment plan. I encourage my patients to try the medicine routine and environmental changes I recommend so they can see how much they benefit. They monitor their condition by keeping a daily asthma diary. After they have achieved and maintained excellent control for a month or two, they are in a good position to decide whether they want to continue with the plan or modify it in some way.

My patients provide me with specific information about their asthma. I supply them with general information about asthma and each medicine they are taking. They read about the adverse effects that can occur, and they learn

how often they do. We discuss whether a particular adverse effect is medically important or simply a nuisance.

I tell my patients how long it should take before a medicine starts to work. It may be one minute (albuterol), six to twelve hours (oral steroids), three days (nedocromil), a week (inhaled steroids), or several weeks (cromolyn). I prefer giving specific information to using vague terms like "promptly," "in a short time," or "in a few days."

My patients want facts that help them learn about asthma medicine and assess their progress toward asthma control. They use my estimates as reference points for their own observation. They find it helpful to know that they should start to feel improvement from taking inhaled albuterol in a few minutes and that it will reach its full effect in fifteen minutes.

Given this knowledge, my patients will not wait for thirty minutes hoping to feel better before they make their next move. If they don't start to improve, they will follow the next step of their treatment plan or call for help. Likewise, they know that an oral steroid, when taken early in an asthma episode, begins to take effect in six to twelve hours. Taken late, the effect is much delayed. Because they understand that peak flow or asthma signs scores usually start to improve two or three days after starting an oral steroid, they can ask their primary care physician to reassess their situation if the improvement does not occur.

When improvement does not occur as predicted, you and your doctor should look for an additional problem. Perhaps the dose is too low or the medicine is being taken incorrectly. Triggers in your environment may be overpowering the helpful effects of medicine. You may have another health condition that is aggravating your asthma or be taking medicine that makes your asthma worse. When you have proper expectations of how good you can feel and how long it should take to get better, you can make informed judgments about what is going on with your health. Good information enables you to take an active role in your asthma treatment.

My patient Molly is a good example. Her parents, who live in New York, brought her to see me when she was two years old (in the 1980s). They were concerned because Molly had been treated in the emergency room for asthma three times in the preceding four months. She seemed fine after each episode and then, three weeks later, suddenly developed asthma symptoms with horrible coughing, wheezing, retractions, and a high respiratory rate. After receiving adrenaline shots, oral steroids, and theophylline in the emergency room, Molly would recover within a week and be fine until the next episode. Because her parents didn't notice any asthma symptoms between episodes, they were reluctant to give her a daily controller medicine. They had tried giving cromolyn by compressor driven nebulizer a few times, but it had not made much difference. They gave her albuterol syrup three or four times a day when needed.

On hearing Molly's story, I thought her airways were probably inflamed between as well as during episodes and that she needed daily treatment with a controller medicine. The cromolyn probably had not helped for two reasons. Molly's doctor probably had not cleared her airways by giving an oral steroid for seven days when starting treatment. In addition, Molly's parents did not give cromolyn long enough to see a benefit. However, I did not want to encourage them to start giving cromolyn daily unless they were convinced it was necessary.

I taught Molly's parents how to observe and assess the four signs of asthma. They agreed to record their observations in an Asthma Signs Diary for one week. When I received the diary, it showed that Molly had coughed every day since the visit. Although this had not interfered with her activity, it had disrupted her sleep. Her parents had always thought of Molly as their "coughing kid" and had never connected the coughing to her asthma.

Over the phone, we discussed that chronic cough is the most common sign of uncontrolled asthma, and that a daily cough meant that Molly's airways were continuously inflamed. These airways were vulnerable to asthma triggers and explained her frequent asthma episodes. The Asthma Signs Diary showed me and Molly's parents that her asthma was persistent, not intermittent.

Based on their own observations and recordkeeping, Molly's parents realized that she might benefit from daily treatment with a controller medicine. They agreed to try a treatment plan giving cromolyn and albuterol by compressor driven nebulizer twice per day, and using prednisolone (an oral steroid) for the first seven days of treatment.

Two months later they came to see me for a follow-up visit. Molly was sleeping well through the night and had not experienced any more asthma episodes. We agreed that they would continue to monitor her signs so we could assess whether to reduce her daily use of albuterol and cromolyn in the future.

SETTING UP AN INITIAL MEDICINE PLAN

The initial plan you work out with your doctor should clear your airways and asthma symptoms quickly. To accomplish this, almost all my patients take an oral steroid for seven days, in addition to their other asthma medicines. This one-week treatment usually causes a remarkable improvement in symptoms and often brings peak flow scores into the green zone.

A few patients prefer to take a moderate to high dose of an inhaled steroid for 30 days to clear their airways, instead of taking an oral steroid. After they have cleared their airways, they continue to take an inhaled steroid daily. If they have mild persistent asthma, I may recommend that they change over to cromolyn or nedocromil instead of inhaled steroids as their controller medicine.

An effective medicine plan should keep your peak flow scores in the green zone almost all the time. If symptoms reappear or peak flow scores drop, you and your doctor know that your medicine dose is too low. If your peak flow scores stay in the green zone and symptoms do not occur, your doctor may be able to reduce your dose safely by 20 to 25 percent in two or three months. Even the best medicine plan won't prevent every asthma episode. However, if you have asthma symptoms more than twice a week, you may not be taking enough medicine. If you never have asthma symptoms, even when you have a cold, you may be taking too much medicine. Keeping a daily record in your asthma diary will help you and your doctor reduce your medicine to the lowest effective dose.

UNDERSTANDING THE ASTHMA TREATMENT ZONES: A REVIEW

Over the course of three visits, I help my patients learn how to adjust medicines and under what circumstances to do so. They learn about the zone system, what to expect in each zone, and how the zones can reliably guide asthma treatment.

The Green Zone

In the green zone, you should feel great, be fully active, and be able to go to work or school every day. When you are in this zone, your airways are almost always clear of inflammation, bronchoconstriction, and excess mucus. Contact with a minor asthma trigger will probably not cause you any trouble. Contact with a major trigger may cause some symptoms, but they should pass quickly with prompt treatment. If you are living consistently in the green zone, your asthma is under excellent control.

The High Yellow Zone

If you are living in the high yellow zone, you are probably having symptoms a few times a week, and your activity is close to normal. Your airways are slightly inflamed, constricted, or both. They may be producing somewhat more mucus as well.

In the high yellow zone your airways are more vulnerable to asthma triggers than they are in the green zone. Contact with a trigger, even a minor one, is more likely to provoke an asthma episode or worsen your symptoms. I advise my patients to change their medicine routine when their peak flow or asthma signs scores fall into the high yellow zone. If they act promptly, they usually will return to the green zone quickly and can soon stop taking the extra medicine.

A few of my patients choose not to take additional medicine immediately upon entering the high yellow zone. They are satisfied with their level of activity and prefer occasional minor asthma symptoms to taking medicine. If their symptoms worsen, they start taking additional medicines to treat the episode. They have learned a lot about asthma and monitoring their airways, and they know how to achieve excellent control by following the medication plan I recommend. After they have worked with the plan, I am happy to discuss their preferences for less-than-excellent control.

The Low Yellow Zone

In the low yellow zone, your airways are narrowed by constricted muscles and the swelling caused by increased inflammation. Excessive mucus production can narrow your airways further. If bronchoconstriction is the main cause of your problem, an inhaled quick relief medicine can often bring you back into the high yellow zone by relaxing airway muscles. If inflammation is the main problem, you will usually need to take an oral steroid to reduce the inflammation and clear up the episode. Close observation of your peak flow scores or your child's total signs scores will guide you in what medicines to take.

The Red Zone

If your asthma is well controlled, you will rarely end up in the red zone. In this zone, your airflow is reduced by 50 percent or more. This is serious. You must take action right away. A common routine is to immediately take an inhaled beta$_2$-agonist medicine (albuterol) by holding chamber or nebulizer. If your peak flow scores improve rapidly, reach the low yellow zone, and stay there for four hours, you can take an oral steroid and continue to treat the episode at home. However, if your peak flow scores are stuck in the red zone after taking a beta$_2$-agonist, take an oral steroid and *go to the doctor or emergency room right away.*

TAKE THE RED ZONE SERIOUSLY   It is impossible to predict the outcome of your red zone situation, so you should not try to handle the problem at home. You are always safest going for medical help once you know that you are stuck in the red zone.

Several of my patients had been living with peak flow scores in the red zone for months by the time I first saw them. They had become used to their symptoms and didn't worry about them. Some did not even realize that they were wheezing even though I could hear the wheezes from across the room. Living in the red zone is dangerous because your airways are continually inflamed and narrowed. Contact with a single trigger may cause many of your airways to close completely. It is not safe to continue living in this condition.

If you cannot blow hard enough to move the marker on the peak flow meter, you are at risk for respiratory failure and need medical help right away. The inability to blow indicates that your respiratory muscles are probably exhausted. Take a minute to determine whether the low peak flow score really indicates a severe problem or was due to incorrect technique or poor effort. If there is any doubt, get intensive treatment as fast as possible.

You should not waste time checking your peak flow if you have bluish lips or nail beds, are breathing hunched over, have trouble saying a sentence, or have severe retractions. These are all signs of an asthma episode that is extremely serious and requires immediate medical help at a hospital. *Go to the emergency room or call an ambulance immediately.*

In most cases, an emergency room is best equipped to provide the care you need for a serious episode. Hospital staff can monitor peak flow and asthma signs frequently, administer high doses of inhaled quick relief medicines along with oxygen, and give live-saving respiratory support (intubation) if needed. Very few doctors are specially trained and equipped to handle a problem of this severity in their offices. Clarify with your doctor ahead of time where you should go if an emergency arises. If you are unsure, go to the emergency room.

The Home Treatment Plan Based on Peak Flow

The written Home Treatment Plan provides a step-wise approach to the use of medicines for each zone of asthma episode severity (see Figure 45). The 1997 *Guidelines* state that all patients with asthma should be given a clear, written plan that covers daily asthma treatment and emergency care.

The Home Treatment Plan I developed for my patients is based on peak flow scores and covers both of these situations. A blank copy of this single page form is included at the back of the book. Doctors around the country use it to guide their patients' asthma management, and you may reproduce the plan for your doctor to use. Your doctor will modify this outline to conform with her practice routine and your individual situation. Consider bringing a blank plan to your next asthma visit.

The Home Treatment Plan describes asthma treatment in each zone based on peak flow scores. The green zone plan instructs you to take a controller medicine daily and pretreat before exercise, if necessary. When your peak flow scores drop into the high yellow zone, add the medicines indicated in that zone. If your peak flow scores drop into the low yellow zone,

continue the high yellow zone medicines and add low yellow zone treatment. Scores in the red zone call for accurate and rapid judgment of your condition, which may indicate the need for emergency treatment. Red zone scores require that your doctor reevaluate your asthma plan after the emergency has passed. In all zones, continue to take your daily green zone medicines.

Treatment plans vary somewhat from person to person, but the general approach to treatment in each zone is similar for most patients with persistent asthma. John, whom you met in the last chapter, has moderate persistent asthma, so he takes two controller medicines daily (an inhaled steroid and theophylline). John is 6 feet tall and weights about 200 pounds, so his dose of theophylline is larger than that needed by many people. Your doctor will work out an individualized plan with you based on the overall severity of your asthma, your size, and your usual response to treatment.

John's asthma diary showed that he was having asthma symptoms daily before he came in for his first visit (see Figure 36). Because his airways were inflamed, he could only blow a peak flow score of 540. After a week of treatment with prednisone, he was able to blow 640. This number became the basis for establishing his peak flow zones (see Table 43). You or your doctor can calculate the limits of your peak flow zones or copy them from Table 38 on page 156.

THE GREEN ZONE PLAN

In the green zone, you should have no symptoms and be fully active. Your treatment plan will tell you what medicines to take before vigorous exercise or contact with an unavoidable allergen. The green zone plan lists your daily medicines, including what brand of medi-

For Adults, Teens and Children Age 5 and Over
PEAK FLOW BASED HOME TREATMENT PLAN
Do not guess. Call the doctor if you have any questions about this plan.

Name: _____ Date: _____ Best Peak Flow: _____

Green Zone

GREEN ZONE: peak flow between _____ and _____.
- **Normal activity.**
  - ❑ Quick relief medicine _____ : 1 or 2 puffs 15 minutes before exercise.
  - ❑ Nedocromil or cromolyn _____ : 2 puffs before contact with cat or other allergens.
- **Medicine to be taken every day:**
  - ❑ Inhaled steroid _____ : ____ puffs by holding chamber ____ times a day.
  - ❑ Other controller medicine _____ : _____ .
  - ❑ Quick relief medicine _____ : ____ puffs before taking inhaled controller medicine
    for the first month.

High Yellow Zone

HIGH YELLOW ZONE: peak flow between _____ and _____.
- **Eliminate triggers and change medicines. No strenuous exercise.**
- **Medicines to be taken:**
  - ❑ Quick relief medicine: ____ puffs ____ to ____ times in 24 hours. Continue until peak flow is in the
    Green Zone for 2 days.
  - ❑ Double dose of inhaled steroids to ____ puffs ____ times per day. Continue until peak flow is in the
    Green Zone for as long as it was in the Yellow Zone.
  - ❑ Continue other controller medicines as instructed in the Green Zone.

Low Yellow Zone

LOW YELLOW ZONE: peak flow between _____ and _____.
- ✓ Take 4 puffs of quick relief medicine.
- ✓ **Check your peak flow again 10 minutes after inhaling quick relief medicine.**

  If your score has increased into the High Yellow Zone, follow the High Yellow Zone plan and continue to
  check peak flow every 1 to 2 hours.

  If your score is still in the Low Yellow Zone, or falls back into the Low Yellow Zone in less than 4 hours,
  follow the Low Yellow Zone plan (below):
  - ❑ Continue treatment with High Yellow Zone medicines as above.
  - ❑ Add oral steroid* ____ mg immediately. Continue daily until peak flow scores are in the Green Zone for
    at least 24 hours.
  - ❑ Please call the office before starting oral steroid.

  * If your condition does not improve within 2 days after starting oral steroid, or if peak flow does not reach
    the Green Zone within 7 days of treatment, see your doctor.

Red Zone

RED ZONE: peak flow score less than _____.
- ✓ Take 4 puffs of quick relief medicine.
- ✓ Take oral steroid ____ mg immediately.
- ✓ **Check your peak flow again 10 minutes after inhaling quick relief medicine.**
  - If your peak flow score has increased into the Low Yellow Zone, follow the Low Yellow Zone plan and
    continue to check peak flow every 1 to 2 hours.
  - If your peak flow score is still in the Red Zone, or falls back into the Red Zone within 4 hours, visit your
    doctor or **GO TO THE EMERGENCY ROOM NOW.**

Figure 45. Peak Flow Based Home Treatment Plan

Table 43. John's Asthma Treatment Zones Based on Peak Flow

Zone	Percent of Personal Best	Scores
green	80–100%	510–640
high yellow	65–80%	415–510
low yellow	50–65%	320–415
red	less than 50%	less than 320

cine, how many puffs or tablets to take at a time, and how many times per day to take it. The brand name is important because different brands of the same medicine may contain a different dose in each puff or tablet. I prescribe daily controller medicines to be taken only once or twice a day, so there is no need to bring them to work or school.

When John's peak flow scores are between 510 and 640, he is in the green zone. He should be having hardly any asthma symptoms. In this zone, John takes inhaled albuterol before exercise or contact with an allergen (see Figure 46). During his first month of treatment, John also takes the albuterol before he takes his inhaled steroid (flunisolide). The albuterol helps open up his airways, which may be constricted, and allows the inhaled steroid to reach cells deep in his lungs. John takes six puffs of the inhaled steroid daily (3 puffs, twice a day). He also takes 800 mg of theophylline daily (one 400 mg tablet, twice a day). After the first month, John will continue to take the inhaled steroid and theophylline, but will take albuterol only if he needs it before strenuous exercise or contact with an allergen.

THE HIGH YELLOW ZONE PLAN

Peak flow scores in the high yellow zone indicate that you are having an asthma episode of mild severity. If you start the high yellow zone plan right when your scores drop, you can often prevent the episode from becoming worse. In this zone, you eliminate triggers, avoid strenuous exercise, and add medicines. My patients double the usual dose of their inhaled steroid, still taking it twice a day. This increased dose helps fight the inflammation that is worsening in their airways. If they act promptly, they can often avoid the need to take an oral steroid. In addition, they add two puffs of albuterol, three to six times per day, while they are in the high yellow zone. If they need to take albuterol more than six times in twenty-four hours, they start to follow the low yellow zone plan.

John's high yellow zone falls between peak flow scores of 415 and 510. When John's score dips into the high yellow zone, he starts to take albuterol 3 to 6 times per day, depending on how often he needs it to relieve symptoms (see Figure 47). He doubles his inhaled steroid dose to 12 puffs per day, 6 in the morning and 6 in the evening. The written plan instructs him to continue taking this double dose until his peak flow scores have been in the green zone for as many days as they were in the high yellow zone. This ensures that the increased inflammation is under control.

Figure 48 shows that John was in the high yellow zone for three days. He continued taking 12 puffs of inhaled steroids until his peak flow was in the green zone for three more days in a row. John took a quick relief medicine several times a day until his peak flow scores were in the green zone for two days.

For Adults, Teens and Children Age 5 and Over
PEAK FLOW BASED HOME TREATMENT PLAN
Do not guess. Call the doctor if you have any questions about this plan.

Name: _John Mott_   Date: _____   Best Peak Flow: _640_

GREEN ZONE: peak flow between __510__ and __640__ .

Green Zone

- **Normal activity.**
  - ☑ Quick relief medicine __albuterol__ : 1 or 2 puffs 15 minutes before exercise.
  - ☐ Nedocromil or cromolyn _____: 2 puffs before contact with cat or other allergens.
- **Medicine to be taken every day:**
  - ☑ Inhaled steroid __flunisolide__ : __3__ puffs by holding chamber __2__ times a day.
  - ☑ Other controller medicine __theophylline__ : _400 mg tablet 2 times/day_ .
  - ☑ Quick relief medicine __albuterol__ : __2__ puffs before taking inhaled controller medicine
    for the first month.

HIGH YELLOW ZONE: peak flow between _____ and _____ .

High Yellow Zone

- **Eliminate triggers and change medicines. No strenuous exercise.**
- **Medicines to be taken:**
  - ☐ Quick relief medicine: _____ puffs _____ to _____ times in 24 hours. Continue until peak flow is in the
    Green Zone for 2 days.
  - ☐ Double dose of inhaled steroids to _____ puffs _____ times per day. Continue until peak flow is in the
    Green Zone for as long as it was in the Yellow Zone.
  - ☐ Continue other controller medicines as instructed in the Green Zone.

LOW YELLOW ZONE: peak flow between _____ and _____ .

Low Yellow Zone

- ✓ Take 4 puffs of quick relief medicine.
- ✓ Check your peak flow again 10 minutes after inhaling quick relief medicine.

  If your score has increased into the High Yellow Zone, follow the High Yellow Zone plan and continue to
  check peak flow every 1 to 2 hours.

  If your score is still in the Low Yellow Zone, or falls back into the Low Yellow Zone in less than 4 hours,
  follow the Low Yellow Zone plan (below):
  - ☐ Continue treatment with High Yellow Zone medicines as above.
  - ☐ Add oral steroid* _____ mg immediately. Continue daily until peak flow scores are in the Green Zone for
    at least 24 hours.
  - ☐ Please call the office before starting oral steroid.

  * If your condition does not improve within 2 days after starting oral steroid, or if peak flow does not reach
     the Green Zone within 7 days of treatment, see your doctor.

RED ZONE: peak flow score less than _____ .

Red Zone

- ✓ Take 4 puffs of quick relief medicine.
- ✓ Take oral steroid _____ mg immediately.
- ✓ Check your peak flow again 10 minutes after inhaling quick relief medicine.
  - • If your peak flow score has increased into the Low Yellow Zone, follow the Low Yellow Zone plan and
    continue to check peak flow every 1 to 2 hours.
  - • If your peak flow score is still in the Red Zone, or falls back into the Red Zone within 4 hours, visit your
    doctor or **GO TO THE EMERGENCY ROOM NOW**.

Figure 46. Peak Flow Based Home Treatment Plan: Green Zone

Asthma Treatment

For Adults, Teens and Children Age 5 and Over
PEAK FLOW BASED HOME TREATMENT PLAN
Do not guess. Call the doctor if you have any questions about this plan.

Name: _John Mott_   Date: _____   Best Peak Flow: _640_

Green Zone

GREEN ZONE: peak flow between ___510___ and ___640___.
- **Normal activity.**
  - ☑ Quick relief medicine _albuterol_ : 1 or 2 puffs 15 minutes before exercise.
  - ☐ Nedocromil or cromolyn _____: 2 puffs before contact with cat or other allergens.
- **Medicine to be taken every day:**
  - ☑ Inhaled steroid _flunisolide_ : _3_ puffs by holding chamber _2_ times a day.
  - ☑ Other controller medicine _theophylline_ : _400 mg tablet 2 times/day_ .
  - ☑ Quick relief medicine _albuterol_ : _2_ puffs before taking inhaled controller medicine for the first month.

High Yellow Zone

HIGH YELLOW ZONE: peak flow between ___415___ and ___510___.
- **Eliminate triggers and change medicines. No strenuous exercise.**
- **Medicines to be taken:**
  - ☑ Quick relief medicine: _2_ puffs _3_ to _6_ times in 24 hours. Continue until peak flow is in the Green Zone for 2 days.
  - ☑ Double dose of inhaled steroids to _6_ puffs _2_ times per day. Continue until peak flow is in the Green Zone for as long as it was in the Yellow Zone.
  - ☑ Continue other controller medicines as instructed in the Green Zone.

Low Yellow Zone

LOW YELLOW ZONE: peak flow between _____ and _____.
- ✓ Take 4 puffs of quick relief medicine.
- ✓ Check your peak flow again 10 minutes after inhaling quick relief medicine.

  If your score has increased into the High Yellow Zone, follow the High Yellow Zone plan and continue to check peak flow every 1 to 2 hours.

  If your score is still in the Low Yellow Zone, or falls back into the Low Yellow Zone in less than 4 hours, follow the Low Yellow Zone plan (below):
  - ☐ Continue treatment with High Yellow Zone medicines as above.
  - ☐ Add oral steroid* ____ mg immediately. Continue daily until peak flow scores are in the Green Zone for at least 24 hours.
  - ☐ Please call the office before starting oral steroid.

  * If your condition does not improve within 2 days after starting oral steroid, or if peak flow does not reach the Green Zone within 7 days of treatment, see your doctor.

Red Zone

RED ZONE: peak flow score less than _____.
- ✓ Take 4 puffs of quick relief medicine.
- ✓ Take oral steroid ____ mg immediately.
- ✓ Check your peak flow again 10 minutes after inhaling quick relief medicine.
  - • If your peak flow score has increased into the Low Yellow Zone, follow the Low Yellow Zone plan and continue to check peak flow every 1 to 2 hours.
  - • If your peak flow score is still in the Red Zone, or falls back into the Red Zone within 4 hours, visit your doctor or **GO TO THE EMERGENCY ROOM NOW**.

Figure 47. Peak Flow Based Home Treatment Plan: High Yellow Zone

Dr. Tom Plaut's Asthma Guide for People of All Ages

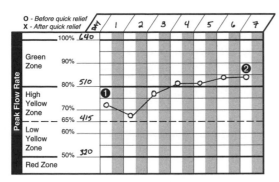

Figure 48. John Adjusts His Medicine Routine During a Mild Asthma Episode (High Yellow Zone).

1. John doubles the usual daily dose of his inhaled steroid and starts taking a quick relief medicine.
2. John returns to his usual dose of inhaled steroid after his peak flow scores are in the green zone for as many days as they have been in the high yellow zone (three full days).

THE LOW YELLOW ZONE PLAN

The low yellow zone differs dramatically from the high yellow zone. A peak flow score in the low yellow zone indicates an asthma episode of moderate severity. Prompt and adequate treatment often can prevent the episode from worsening and lead to improvement in a few days. Delayed or inadequate treatment can lead to a longer or more serious episode for which emergency treatment may be necessary.

In the low yellow zone, you usually need to take an oral steroid promptly to reduce inflammation and speed recovery. The 1997 *Guidelines* recommend that patients have an oral steroid available at home to treat a moderate or severe asthma episode. If your doctor prefers not to prescribe enough oral steroids for complete treatment of an episode, make sure that you at least have a two-day supply on hand to start treatment in an emergency. If your doctor wants you to call the office before starting an oral steroid, she can write that request as part

of your low yellow zone routine. Prompt treatment with an oral steroid will almost always reduce the total dose you need to take, because it shortens the duration of episode.

However, it does not make sense to take an oral steroid unless you need it. You can judge whether you do by observing how well you respond to a quick relief medicine (albuterol). If your peak flow score clears the low yellow zone within ten minutes after inhaling albuterol and stays clear for four hours after that, you don't need to take an oral steroid at that point. If you are stuck in the low yellow zone, you have significant airway inflammation and need to take an oral steroid to stop the episode from worsening. John, like my other patients, follows the routine described below to decide how to handle a low yellow zone episode (see Figure 49).

Clearing the Low Yellow Zone

When John blows a peak flow score in his low yellow zone (320 to 415), he takes 4 puffs of inhaled albuterol immediately. The medicine works quickly to relax tightened airway muscles. He checks his peak flow score again in ten minutes to find out if it has improved. If his score has reached the high yellow zone and stays there for the next four hours, he has cleared the low yellow zone (see Figure 50). He does not need to take an oral steroid at this time and can follow his high yellow zone plan. However, John continues to check his peak flow score every few hours to make sure he stays out of the low yellow zone. He can take a dose of quick relief medicine every four hours to help him stay in the high yellow zone.

In a situation like this one, John's extra peak flow monitoring and recording tells him he doesn't need to take an oral steroid. But, even though John has cleared the low yellow zone for now, he must continue to monitor his condition several times a day. The episode may worsen and require more intensive treatment.

For Adults, Teens and Children Age 5 and Over
PEAK FLOW BASED HOME TREATMENT PLAN
Do not guess. Call the doctor if you have any questions about this plan.

Name: John Mott   Date: _____   Best Peak Flow: 640

GREEN ZONE: peak flow between __510__ and __640__ .

- **Normal activity.**
  - ☑ Quick relief medicine __albuterol__ : 1 or 2 puffs 15 minutes before exercise.
  - ❑ Nedocromil or cromolyn _____ : 2 puffs before contact with cat or other allergens.
- **Medicine to be taken every day:**
  - ☑ Inhaled steroid __Flunisolide__ : __3__ puffs by holding chamber __2__ times a day.
  - ☑ Other controller medicine __theophylline__ : __400 mg tablet 2 times/day__ .
  - ☑ Quick relief medicine __albuterol__ : __2__ puffs before taking inhaled controller medicine for the first month.

HIGH YELLOW ZONE: peak flow between __415__ and __510__ .

- **Eliminate triggers and change medicines. No strenuous exercise.**
- **Medicines to be taken:**
  - ☑ Quick relief medicine: __2__ puffs __3__ to __6__ times in 24 hours. Continue until peak flow is in the Green Zone for 2 days.
  - ☑ Double dose of inhaled steroids to __6__ puffs __2__ times per day. Continue until peak flow is in the Green Zone for as long as it was in the Yellow Zone.
  - ☑ Continue other controller medicines as instructed in the Green Zone.

LOW YELLOW ZONE: peak flow between __320__ and __415__ .

✓ Take 4 puffs of quick relief medicine.

✓ Check your peak flow again 10 minutes after inhaling quick relief medicine.

If your score has increased into the High Yellow Zone, follow the High Yellow Zone plan and continue to check peak flow every 1 to 2 hours.

If your score is still in the Low Yellow Zone, or falls back into the Low Yellow Zone in less than 4 hours, follow the Low Yellow Zone plan (below):

☑ Continue treatment with High Yellow Zone medicines as above.

☑ Add oral steroid*__40__ mg immediately. Continue daily until peak flow scores are in the Green Zone for at least 24 hours.

❑ Please call the office before starting oral steroid.

* If your condition does not improve within 2 days after starting oral steroid, or if peak flow does not reach the Green Zone within 7 days of treatment, see your doctor.

RED ZONE: peak flow score less than _____ .

✓ Take 4 puffs of quick relief medicine.

✓ Take oral steroid _____ mg immediately.

✓ Check your peak flow again 10 minutes after inhaling quick relief medicine.

- If your peak flow score has increased into the Low Yellow Zone, follow the Low Yellow Zone plan and continue to check peak flow every 1 to 2 hours.
- If your peak flow score is still in the Red Zone, or falls back into the Red Zone within 4 hours, visit your doctor or **GO TO THE EMERGENCY ROOM NOW**.

Figure 49. Peak Flow Based Home Treatment Plan: Low Yellow Zone

Dr. Tom Plaut's Asthma Guide for People of All Ages

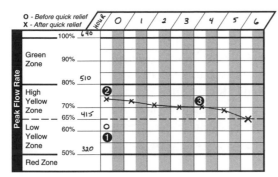 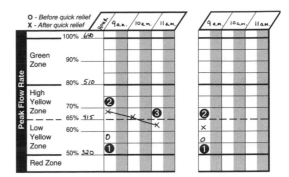

Figure 50. Clearing the Low Yellow Zone.

1. John blows a peak flow score in the low yellow zone, so he takes 4 puffs of albuterol.

2. Ten minutes later, John checks his peak flow again and sees that it has improved into the high yellow zone. He continues to check peak flow every one or two hours.

3. John's peak flow scores stay in the high yellow zone for at least four hours. He has cleared the low yellow zone.

Figure 51. Stuck in the Low Yellow Zone.

Here are two scenarios in which John needs an oral steroid.

In the left panel:

1. John blows a peak flow score in the low yellow zone, so he inhales 4 puffs of albuterol.

2. He checks his peak flow in ten minutes and finds that his score has reached the high yellow zone. He continues to check peak flow every hour.

3. Two hours later, John's peak flow is back in the low yellow zone. He is stuck.

In the right panel:

1. John blows a peak flow score in the low yellow zone, so he inhales 4 puffs of albuterol.

2. He checks his peak flow in ten minutes and finds that he is still in the low yellow zone. He is stuck.

Whenever John's peak flow scores drop into the low yellow zone, he follows this routine to determine his treatment.

Stuck in the Low Yellow Zone

Sometimes, John will have to use an oral steroid. When he is having an episode of moderate severity, his peak flow score may not reach the high yellow zone after he inhales albuterol, or it may fall back into the low yellow zone in less than four hours (see Figure 51). In either scenario, he is stuck in the low yellow zone and should follow the low yellow zone instructions in his plan.

In this case, John knows that he needs an oral steroid to take care of the episode. The oral steroid rapidly reduces airway inflammation and production of mucus. When John starts taking an oral steroid promptly, he usually needs it for only a few days to clear up the episode. He sometimes needs to miss work when he is stuck in the low yellow zone.

John's oral steroid dose of 40 mg is written in the low yellow zone plan. John starts the oral steroid immediately when he realizes that he is stuck in the low yellow zone. He then continues to take it each morning. He also continues the double dose of inhaled steroid and takes albuterol three to six times a day as needed, according to his high yellow zone plan.

John will continue to take an oral steroid each morning until his peak flow scores blown before taking albuterol have stayed in the green zone for at least twenty-four hours. The peak flow diary in Figure 52 guides him in stopping the oral steroid, even as it helped him decide when to start it.

If John does not begin to improve two days after taking an oral steroid, or fails to reach the

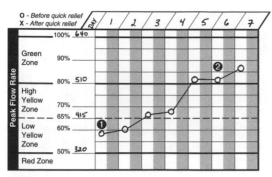

Figure 52. When to Stop Taking an Oral Steroid.

1. John starts taking an oral steroid because his peak flow score is stuck in the low yellow zone.

2. John stops taking an oral steroid on Day 6, after his peak flow scores have been in the green zone for twenty-four hours.

green zone after seven days, the treatment plan instructs him to see his doctor. His lack of improvement often indicates that something else, such as sinusitis or a trigger, is complicating his asthma. This complication must be resolved before his asthma treatment will be fully effective.

THE RED ZONE PLAN

If you are stuck in the red zone, you need medical help right away. "Stuck" means that your peak flow score fails to improve for at least four hours after you inhale a quick relief medicine. In this situation, there is no room for wishing or hoping things will get better on their own.

Do not try to handle a red zone episode by yourself. Emergency situations are usually a sign that your asthma treatment plan is not working properly. After your red zone emergency has been treated by your doctor or the emergency room, review your treatment plan with your regular doctor or asthma specialist. If your doctor thinks that your current plan is satisfactory, it may be time to find a new doctor.

Clearing the Red Zone

John takes four puffs of albuterol immediately after he blows a peak flow score in the red zone (less than 320). He checks his peak flow again in ten minutes. If his peak flow score increases into the low yellow zone and stays there for at least four hours, John has cleared the red zone. He can follow the low yellow zone plan, taking 40 mg of prednisone. He checks his peak flow score every hour or two to make sure he stays clear of the red zone.

Stuck in the Red Zone

In the case of a severe asthma episode, John's peak flow score may not climb out of the red zone within ten minutes after inhaling albuterol, or his score may drop back into the red zone in less than four hours. In either case, he is stuck in the red zone.

This is a serious problem. A phone call to the doctor is *not* enough. His red zone plan instructs him to take 40 mg of an oral steroid immediately and go to the doctor or the emergency room right away, certainly within an hour (see Figure 53). He can take additional albuterol while waiting for the ambulance or on the way to the hospital.

If you are unable to move the marker on the peak flow meter, your problem is even more serious. You must do the following immediately and simultaneously:

- Start taking a quick relief medicine by MDI or nebulizer.
- Call 911 and take an oral steroid.
- Take the quick relief medicine again on the way to the hospital.

USING THE HOME TREATMENT PLAN WITH THE PEAK FLOW DIARY

The Home Treatment Plan based on peak flow scores works best if used in conjunction with the Asthma Peak Flow Diary. The diary

For Adults, Teens and Children Age 5 and Over
PEAK FLOW BASED HOME TREATMENT PLAN
Do not guess. Call the doctor if you have any questions about this plan.

Name: _John Mott_   Date: _____   Best Peak Flow: _640_

GREEN ZONE: peak flow between _510_ and _640_ .

Green Zone

- **Normal activity.**
  - ☑ Quick relief medicine _albuterol_ : 1 or 2 puffs 15 minutes before exercise.
  - ☐ Nedocromil or cromolyn _____: 2 puffs before contact with cat or other allergens.
- **Medicine to be taken every day:**
  - ☑ Inhaled steroid _flunisolide_ : _3_ puffs by holding chamber _2_ times a day.
  - ☑ Other controller medicine _theophylline_ : _400 mg tablet 2 times/day_ .
  - ☑ Quick relief medicine _albuterol_ : _2_ puffs before taking inhaled controller medicine for the first month.

HIGH YELLOW ZONE: peak flow between _415_ and _510_ .

High Yellow Zone

- **Eliminate triggers and change medicines. No strenuous exercise.**
- **Medicines to be taken:**
  - ☑ Quick relief medicine: _2_ puffs _3_ to _6_ times in 24 hours. Continue until peak flow is in the Green Zone for 2 days.
  - ☑ Double dose of inhaled steroids to _6_ puffs _2_ times per day. Continue until peak flow is in the Green Zone for as long as it was in the Yellow Zone.
  - ☑ Continue other controller medicines as instructed in the Green Zone.

LOW YELLOW ZONE: peak flow between _320_ and _415_ .

Low Yellow Zone

- ✓ **Take 4 puffs of quick relief medicine.**
- ✓ **Check your peak flow again 10 minutes after inhaling quick relief medicine.**

  If your score has increased into the High Yellow Zone, follow the High Yellow Zone plan and continue to check peak flow every 1 to 2 hours.

  If your score is still in the Low Yellow Zone, or falls back into the Low Yellow Zone in less than 4 hours, follow the Low Yellow Zone plan (below):
  - ☑ Continue treatment with High Yellow Zone medicines as above.
  - ☑ Add oral steroid* _40_ mg immediately. Continue daily until peak flow scores are in the Green Zone for at least 24 hours.
  - ☐ Please call the office before starting oral steroid.

  * If your condition does not improve within 2 days after starting oral steroid, or if peak flow does not reach the Green Zone within 7 days of treatment, see your doctor.

RED ZONE: peak flow score less than _320_ .

Red Zone

- ✓ **Take 4 puffs of quick relief medicine.**
- ✓ **Take oral steroid _40_ mg immediately.**
- ✓ **Check your peak flow again 10 minutes after inhaling quick relief medicine.**
  - If your peak flow score has increased into the Low Yellow Zone, follow the Low Yellow Zone plan and continue to check peak flow every 1 to 2 hours.
  - If your peak flow score is still in the Red Zone, or falls back into the Red Zone within 4 hours, visit your doctor or **GO TO THE EMERGENCY ROOM NOW.**

Figure 53. Peak Flow Based Home Treatment Plan: Red Zone. This treatment plan was designed for my patient, John Mott. Your doctor must individualize a plan for you.

Asthma Treatment

provides the detailed information you need to make good judgments in following your plan.

Your diary displays trends in your peak flow scores and enables you to start additional treatment at the first sign of symptoms. This reduces the likelihood that you will need an oral steroid. The diary shows you whether you have cleared a zone or are stuck there. As your airways respond to treatment, the trend of improvement will be displayed in your diary, a reassuring sign that you are adjusting treatment properly. If you don't see an improvement and don't know what to do next, you will know to call or see your doctor for guidance.

A diary also helps you decide when to stop taking additional medicine. Once your scores have returned to the green zone for a specified amount of time, you can return to your usual medicine routine with confidence. To get full benefit from using the Home Treatment Plan, keep an asthma diary every day, at least until you have achieved excellent asthma control for several months. At that point, you can decide how often you need to make diary entries.

Keeping a diary and following a Home Treatment Plan takes a lot of work at first. But once you have learned how to keep a diary and to follow your treatment plan, the job becomes easier. My patients find that the improvement in their asthma control and peace of mind are well worth the time and effort they spend. As they become more experienced, the benefit continues and the burden lessens.

I have found that peak flow scores provide consistent, reliable, and early warning of asthma trouble, so these scores form the basis of my treatment plans. However, I tell my patients to watch their asthma signs and symptoms closely as well. A peak flow meter does not measure changes of airflow in the small airways. If they are inflamed, you may have symptoms even though your peak flow is normal.

If you regularly experience symptoms while your peak flow scores are in the green zone, your zone boundaries are not properly set. Treatment with an oral steroid for a week or with a moderate dose of an inhaled steroid for a month can clear inflamed airways. This usually will lead to an increase in your personal best score. If it doesn't, a green zone of 20 percent is too wide for you. The lower boundary of the green zone should be adjusted to 85 to 90 percent of your personal best, as I did with my patient Elizabeth.

Elizabeth has never blown a peak flow score below the green zone. Yet when she gets a cold in the winter, she notices a wheeze on expiration, tight chest, and prolonged cough. Albuterol brings relief from these symptoms, and a low dose of inhaled steroid taken daily keeps her symptoms from dragging on after the cold. To make her treatment plan more sensitive, we raised the lower boundary of her green zone to 90 percent. She rarely notices symptoms in this revised green zone and adjusts treatment earlier when her peak flow scores drop.

Your treatment plan should be written on a single sheet of paper and clearly identify the treatment zones. The yellow zone should be divided into high and low parts because scores in each zone call for different treatment. The plan should use peak flow scores to establish the zones and include both daily and emergency plans. The plan should flow smoothly from one zone to another, covering all possible asthma situations. It should guide you in discontinuing medicines you have added during an asthma episode. Finally, it should direct you to call the doctor's office if you have questions.

Treatment For Children Under 5 Years of Age

For more than twenty years, cromolyn has been the main controller medicine used for young children with mild or moderate persistent asthma. The most effective way to give this medicine is by compressor driven or ultrasonic nebulizer. Inhaled steroids became available for use by holding chamber with mask in 1990 and by nebulizer in 1999, and they can now be used as controller medicines for young children.

Young children with persistent asthma (symptoms more than twice a week) need to take a daily controller medicine to avoid asthma episodes, to live fully active lives, and to prevent long-term damage to the lungs. They need to take additional medicines when asthma episodes occur.

Providing good asthma care at home for children can seem like a daunting task at first. It requires that you have knowledge and skill in monitoring your child for the four signs of asthma (cough, wheeze, retractions, and breathing faster), assessing his asthma condition, and then following the proper medicine routine based on your observations. It takes time and practice for parents and other caregivers to become competent and confident in providing this care.

The Home Treatment Plan Based on Asthma Signs

A written Home Treatment Plan based on asthma signs is an essential tool for managing your child's asthma at home (see Figure 54). Parents of almost all of my patients under 5 use the plan you will see here. (A blank copy that you may reproduce for your doctor to use is included in the back of the book.) When filled out by your doctor, this plan gives you clear, stepwise instructions on what medicine to give your child.

If the course of action is not clear, you can present your observations to the doctor and get good advice over the phone or in person. The general approach outlined in the signs based treatment plan, combined with environmental measures, helps almost all children with mild or moderate persistent asthma, and many with severe asthma, achieve excellent asthma control. Here I will illustrate how Luke DeLaura's parents used the signs based plan to bring his asthma under excellent control.

When children are too young to blow reliable peak flow scores, the four signs of asthma provide the best indicators of their asthma condition. The four signs are scored individually based on severity or frequency. Table 44 reviews the scoring for each sign. By recording the signs scores in an Asthma Signs Diary, you can more easily calculate the total score and classify the episode by zone. The zone then guides you in adding and adjusting medicines promptly.

The Signs Based Home Treatment Plan is based on zones, identical to those found in the Asthma Signs Diary. The green zone plan tells you what medicine to give your child each day. When your child's total signs score drops into the high yellow zone, the plan instructs you to give additional medicines and limit exercise. A total signs score in the low yellow zone calls for careful assessment. If the score does not reach the high yellow zone within 10 minutes after treatment with inhaled quick relief medicine (and does not stay there for four hours), the plan calls for an oral steroid to be given daily for a short period of time.

If your child has an asthma signs score in the red zone which does not improve with quick relief medicine, it is time to go for help from your doctor or an emergency room. In each zone, the treatment plan clearly states when to start and when to stop giving additional medicine. The Asthma Signs Diary enables you to judge whether your child is improving with treatment. You should con-

For Children Under Age 5
SIGNS BASED HOME TREATMENT PLAN
Do not guess. Call the doctor if you have any questions about this plan.

Name: _____ Date: _____

GREEN ZONE: absolutely no cough, wheeze, breathing faster or sucking in of the chest skin.
 	
• **Normal activity.**
• **Medicine to be taken every day:**
   ❑ Cromolyn _____ : _____ ampules _____ times a day.
   ❑ Inhaled steroid _____ : _____ puffs _____ times a day by holding chamber with mask.
   ❑ Quick relief medicine _____ : 0. _____ cc by compressor-driven nebulizer with each cromolyn dose for the first month OR give _____ puffs from MDI by holding chamber with mask before each inhaled steroid dose for the first month.
	Treatment Plan based on total score of all 4 signs:
	
	Cough in past 5 minutes
	None 0
	Less than 1 per minute 1
	1 - 4 per minute 2
	More than 4 per minute 3
	
	Wheeze
	None 0
	End of exhale 1
	Throughout exhale 3
	Inhale and exhale 5

HIGH YELLOW ZONE: total asthma signs score 1 to 4 measured before inhaling quick relief medicine.
 	
• **Eliminate triggers and add medicines. No strenuous exercise.**
• **Medicine to be taken:**
   ❑ Cromolyn: as above.
   ❑ Double dose of inhaled steroid to _____ puffs _____ times a day. Continue until signs score is in the Green Zone as long as it was in the High Yellow Zone.
   ❑ Quick relief medicine 0. _____ cc by compressor-driven nebulizer with each cromolyn dose OR give _____ puffs from MDI by holding chamber with mask before each inhaled steroid dose. Give _____ to _____ times in 24 hours.*
   Continue until signs score is _____ for 2 days.
   * If you need to give more than 6 treatments of quick relief medicine in 24 hours, start the Low Yellow Zone plan.
	Sucking in the chest skin
	None 0
	Barely noticeable 1
	Obvious 3
	Severe 5
	
	Breathing faster
	None 0
	Up to 50% increase 1
	Up to 100% increase 2
	Over 100% increase 3

LOW YELLOW ZONE: total asthma signs score 5 to 8.

✓ Give 0._____ cc of quick relief medicine by compressor-driven nebulizer OR give _____ puffs from MDI by holding chamber with mask.

✓ Check your child's total signs score again 10 minutes after giving quick relief medicine.

If your child's total score has improved into the High Yellow Zone, follow the High Yellow Zone plan and continue to check signs every 1 to 2 hours.

If your child's total score is still in the Low Yellow Zone, or falls back into the Low Yellow Zone in less than 4 hours, continue with High Yellow Zone treatment and:

❑ Give oral steroid† _____ mg, _____ cc immediately. Continue once daily until total signs score is _____ for at least 24 hours.

❑ Please call the office before starting oral steroid.

† If your child's condition does not improve within 2 days after starting oral steroid, or does not reach the Green Zone within 7 days of treatment, see your doctor.

RED ZONE: total asthma signs score 9 or more.

✓ Give 0._____ cc of quick relief medicine by compressor-driven nebulizer OR give _____ puffs from MDI by holding chamber with mask.

✓ Give oral steroid _____ mg, _____ cc immediately.

✓ Check your child's total asthma signs score again 10 minutes after giving quick relief medicine.

If your child's total score has improved into the Low Yellow Zone, follow the Low Yellow Zone plan and continue to check signs every 1 to 2 hours.

If your child's total score is still in the Red Zone, or falls back into the Red Zone in less than 4 hours, visit your doctor **OR GO TO THE EMERGENCY ROOM NOW.**

Figure 54. Signs Based Home Treatment Plan

Table 44. Scoring the Four Signs of Asthma

Cough		*Breathing Faster*	
None	0	None	0
Less than 1 per minute	1	Up to 50% increase	1
1–4 per minute	2	50–100% increase (double)	2
More than 4 per minute	3	More than 100% increase	3
Wheeze		*Sucking in the Chest Skin*	
None	0	None	0
Exhale only	1	Barely noticeable	1
Throughout entire exhale	3	Obvious	3
Both inhale and exhale	5	Severe	5

Some signs are scored from 0–3, while others are scored from 0–5. The total score of these four signs determines the zone that guides treatment (see Table 45). The Signs Based Home Treatment Plan displays this scoring system.

tinue to give your child his daily controller medicines in every zone.

In the last chapter, you met 7-month-old Luke during his first asthma visit. His Asthma Signs Diary showed that he had been in the yellow zone and had daily asthma symptoms during the preceding week. His parents were giving him cromolyn by compressor driven nebulizer twice a day. Cromolyn is an excellent medicine for young children and prevents most asthma symptoms and episodes, but it did not seem to be helping Luke. I suggested that Wendy give him an oral steroid for seven days, along with cromolyn and albuterol by compressor driven nebulizer each day. Once the oral steroid cleared Luke's airways of inflammation, the cromolyn effectively prevented most of his asthma symptoms.

During the visit, I developed a written plan that outlined Luke's daily treatment and what actions to take if an asthma episode did occur. His parents learned what medicines to add and how long to give them in each treatment zone. Here I present the plan that enabled Luke to achieve and maintain excellent asthma control. Your doctor can create a similar, individualized plan consistent with the 1997 *Guidelines*.

THE GREEN ZONE PLAN

Luke is in the green zone when he has no signs of asthma (a score of 0). His mother gives him 2 ampules of cromolyn by nebulizer in the morning and 2 in the afternoon or evening (see Figure 55). For the first month of treatment, she also adds 0.25 cc of albuterol to the cromolyn in the nebulizer cup. The quick relief medicine she has added helps open Luke's airways, allowing the cromolyn to reach deep into his lungs.

A standard nebulizer cup loses about half the medicine dose during a treatment. A year and a half after the initial visit, Wendy switched to a medicine-retaining cup to give Luke his medicine. Since this cup loses almost no medicine, I was able to reduce Luke's cromolyn dose to 1 ampule in the morning and 1 ampule in the afternoon or evening without decreasing its effect. (See page 126 for a discussion of nebulizer cups).

THE HIGH YELLOW ZONE PLAN

A total signs score of 1 to 4 places your child in the high yellow zone, meaning that a mild asthma episode is under way. Here you

For Children Under Age 5
SIGNS BASED HOME TREATMENT PLAN
Do not guess. Call the doctor if you have any questions about this plan.

Name: _Luke Delaura_   Date: _____

Green Zone

GREEN ZONE: absolutely no cough, wheeze, breathing faster or sucking in of the chest skin.

- **Normal activity.**
- **Medicine to be taken every day:**
  - ☑ Cromolyn _____ : __2__ ampules __2__ times a day.
  - ☐ Inhaled steroid _____ : _____ puffs _____ times a day by holding chamber with mask.
  - ☑ Quick relief medicine __Albuterol__ : 0. _25_ cc by compressor-driven nebulizer with each cromolyn dose for the first month OR give _____ puffs from MDI by holding chamber with mask before each inhaled steroid dose for the first month.

High Yellow Zone

HIGH YELLOW ZONE: total asthma signs score 1 to 4 measured before inhaling quick relief medicine.

- **Eliminate triggers and add medicines. No strenuous exercise.**
- **Medicine to be taken:**
  - ☐ Cromolyn: as above.
  - ☐ Double dose of inhaled steroid to _____ puffs _____ times a day. Continue until signs score is in the Green Zone as long as it was in the High Yellow Zone.
  - ☐ Quick relief medicine 0. _____ cc by compressor-driven nebulizer with each cromolyn dose OR give _____ puffs from MDI by holding chamber with mask before each inhaled steroid dose. Give _____ to _____ times in 24 hours.* Continue until signs score is _____ for 2 days.
  - * If you need to give more than 6 treatments of quick relief medicine in 24 hours, start the Low Yellow Zone plan.

Treatment Plan based on total score of all 4 signs:

Cough in past 5 minutes
None 0
Less than 1 per minute 1
1 - 4 per minute 2
More than 4 per minute 3

Wheeze
None 0
End of exhale 1
Throughout exhale 3
Inhale and exhale 5

Sucking in the chest skin
None 0
Barely noticeable 1
Obvious 3
Severe 5

Breathing faster
None 0
Up to 50% increase 1
Up to 100% increase 2
Over 100% increase 3

Low Yellow Zone

LOW YELLOW ZONE: total asthma signs score 5 to 8.

✓ **Give 0.____cc of quick relief medicine by compressor-driven nebulizer OR give _____ puffs from MDI by holding chamber with mask.**

✓ **Check your child's total signs score again 10 minutes after giving quick relief medicine.**

If your child's total score has improved into the High Yellow Zone, follow the High Yellow Zone plan and continue to check signs every 1 to 2 hours.

If your child's total score is still in the Low Yellow Zone, or falls back into the Low Yellow Zone in less than 4 hours, continue with High Yellow Zone treatment and:

- ☐ Give oral steroid† _____ mg, _____ cc immediately. Continue once daily until total signs score is _____ for at least 24 hours.
- ☐ Please call the office before starting oral steroid.

† If your child's condition does not improve within 2 days after starting oral steroid, or does not reach the Green Zone within 7 days of treatment, see your doctor.

Red Zone

RED ZONE: total asthma signs score 9 or more.

✓ **Give 0.____ cc of quick relief medicine by compressor-driven nebulizer OR give _____ puffs from MDI by holding chamber with mask.**

✓ **Give oral steroid _____mg, _____ cc immediately.**

✓ **Check your child's total asthma signs score again 10 minutes after giving quick relief medicine.**

If your child's total score has improved into the Low Yellow Zone, follow the Low Yellow Zone plan and continue to check signs every 1 to 2 hours.

If your child's total score is still in the Red Zone, or falls back into the Red Zone in less than 4 hours, visit your doctor **OR GO TO THE EMERGENCY ROOM NOW.**

Figure 55. Signs Based Home Treatment Plan: Green Zone

Table 45. Assigning a Zone to the Total Score of Asthma Signs

Zone	Total Score of Asthma Signs	Episode Severity
green	0	no episode
high yellow	1–4	mild episode
low yellow	5–8	moderate episode
red	9 or more	severe episode

should help your child avoid asthma triggers and strenuous activity and give albuterol to help clear the episode quickly. The albuterol can be added to cromolyn solution or given by itself every four hours, up to six times in twenty-four hours. If your child needs the albuterol treatments more often than every four hours to control symptoms, start to follow the low yellow zone plan or consult your doctor.

Albuterol is a bronchodilator that will open your child's airways by relaxing constricted airway muscles, allowing the cromolyn to keep working. In the case of a mild episode, additional albuterol may be the only treatment that your child needs to help him back into the green zone. You can stop the albuterol treatment after your child has a signs score of 0 or 1 for forty-eight hours. Sometimes, the inflammation in the airways continues to worsen, and the total score of asthma signs drops into the low yellow zone, calling for a different treatment.

THE LOW YELLOW ZONE PLAN

A total signs score from 5 to 8 falls in the low yellow zone and warns you that a moderate asthma episode is in progress. In the low yellow zone, your child should avoid strenuous exercise and other triggers that might cause the episode to worsen. Treated promptly, the episode may clear up within a few days to a week. In the case of strong or multiple asthma triggers, the episode may worsen even though you followed the treatment plan exactly.

The treatment plan in the low yellow zone instructs you to give an oral steroid to your child under some circumstances. Parents are often reluctant to do this, especially the first time. Certainly, you want to give an oral steroid only if your child needs it. The low yellow zone plan calls for an oral steroid only if your child is stuck in that zone after taking albuterol.

Using an oral steroid for seven days or less, once or twice in a year, rarely causes serious adverse effects. If you delay starting treatment with an oral steroid when your child needs it, the episode may become more severe. It may then require more prolonged treatment with an oral steroid at home or in the hospital.

If you understand asthma and monitor your child's signs accurately, you will know when to use an oral steroid and also when it is safe not to use it. If your doctor wants you to notify the office before starting an oral steroid at home, she can write this step as part of the low yellow zone routine (see Figure 59).

Clearing the Low Yellow Zone

When you observe that your child has a total score of asthma signs in the low yellow zone (score of 5 to 8), give inhaled albuterol by nebulizer or holding chamber with mask. The medicine will often relieve symptoms and reduce asthma signs. Five to ten minutes after the treatment, score your child's signs again. Did they reach the high yellow zone (score of 1 to 4)? If so, follow the high yellow zone plan and

For Children Under Age 5
SIGNS BASED HOME TREATMENT PLAN
Do not guess. Call the doctor if you have any questions about this plan.

Name: _LUKE DELAURA_   Date:

Green Zone	**GREEN ZONE: absolutely no cough, wheeze, breathing faster or sucking in of the chest skin.**

- **Normal activity.**
- **Medicine to be taken every day:**
  - ☑ Cromolyn _____ : __2__ ampules __2__ times a day.
  - ❑ Inhaled steroid _____ : _____ puffs _____ times a day by holding chamber with mask.
  - ☑ Quick relief medicine __Albuterol__ : 0. __25__ cc by compressor-driven nebulizer with each cromolyn dose for the first month OR give _____ puffs from MDI by holding chamber with mask before each inhaled steroid dose for the first month.

HIGH YELLOW ZONE: total asthma signs score 1 to 4 measured before inhaling quick relief medicine.

- **Eliminate triggers and add medicines. No strenuous exercise.**
- **Medicine to be taken:**
  - ☑ Cromolyn: as above.
  - ❑ Double dose of inhaled steroid to _____ puffs _____ times a day. Continue until signs score is in the Green Zone as long as it was in the High Yellow Zone.
  - ☑ Quick relief medicine 0. __25__ cc by compressor-driven nebulizer with each cromolyn dose OR give _____ puffs from MDI by holding chamber with mask before each inhaled steroid dose. Give __3__ to __6__ times in 24 hours.* Continue until signs score is __0 or 1__ for 2 days.
    - * If you need to give more than 6 treatments of quick relief medicine in 24 hours, start the Low Yellow Zone plan.

Treatment Plan based on total score of all 4 signs:

Cough in past 5 minutes
None 0
Less than 1 per minute 1
1 - 4 per minute 2
More than 4 per minute 3

Wheeze
None 0
End of exhale 1
Throughout exhale 3
Inhale and exhale 5

Sucking in the chest skin
None 0
Barely noticeable 1
Obvious 3
Severe 5

Breathing faster
None 0
Up to 50% increase 1
Up to 100% increase 2
Over 100% increase 3

LOW YELLOW ZONE: total asthma signs score 5 to 8.

- ✓ Give 0.____cc of quick relief medicine by compressor-driven nebulizer OR give _____ puffs from MDI by holding chamber with mask.
- ✓ **Check your child's total signs score again 10 minutes after giving quick relief medicine.**

  If your child's total score has improved into the High Yellow Zone, follow the High Yellow Zone plan and continue to check signs every 1 to 2 hours.

  If your child's total score is still in the Low Yellow Zone, or falls back into the Low Yellow Zone in less than 4 hours, continue with High Yellow Zone treatment and:

  - ❑ Give oral steroid† _____ mg, _____ cc immediately. Continue once daily until total signs score is _____ for at least 24 hours.
  - ❑ Please call the office before starting oral steroid.

  - † If your child's condition does not improve within 2 days after starting oral steroid, or does not reach the Green Zone within 7 days of treatment, see your doctor.

RED ZONE: total asthma signs score 9 or more.

- ✓ Give 0.____ cc of quick relief medicine by compressor-driven nebulizer OR give _____ puffs from MDI by holding chamber with mask.
- ✓ Give oral steroid _____mg, _____ cc immediately.
- ✓ **Check your child's total asthma signs score again 10 minutes after giving quick relief medicine.**

  If your child's total score has improved into the Low Yellow Zone, follow the Low Yellow Zone plan and continue to check signs every 1 to 2 hours.

  If your child's total score is still in the Red Zone, or falls back into the Red Zone in less than 4 hours, visit your doctor **OR GO TO THE EMERGENCY ROOM NOW.**

Figure 56. Signs Based Home Treatment Plan: High Yellow Zone

keep monitoring asthma signs every hour or two.

If your child's total score of asthma signs stays in the high yellow zone for four hours after treatment with inhaled albuterol, your child has cleared the low yellow zone (see Figure 57). As long as your child stays out of the low yellow zone for at least four hours after each albuterol dose, you don't need to give an oral steroid. If your child worsens before four hours have passed, recheck the signs score to see if an oral steroid is needed.

Stuck in the Low Yellow Zone

If your child's signs score does not improve into the high yellow zone after receiving albuterol, he is stuck in the low yellow zone. Similarly, your child is stuck if he improves but then drops back into the low yellow zone in less than four hours (see Figure 58).

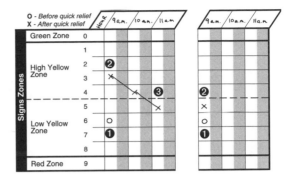

Figure 58. Stuck in the Low Yellow Zone.
Here are two scenarios in which Luke needs an oral steroid.

In the left panel:
1. Luke's parents score his asthma signs and realize that he is in the low yellow zone, so they give him 0.25 cc of albuterol by nebulizer.
2. They check his total score of asthma signs again and find that it has reached the high yellow zone. They continue to observe him.
3. In three hours, Luke's total score of asthma signs is back in the low yellow zone. He is stuck.

In the right panel:
1. Luke's parents score his asthma signs in the low yellow zone, so they give him 0.25 cc of albuterol by nebulizer.
2. They check his total score of asthma signs again and find that he is still in the low yellow zone. He is stuck.

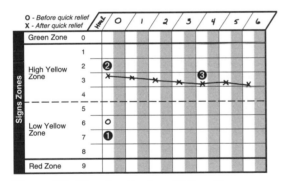

Figure 57. Clearing the Low Yellow Zone.
1. Luke's parents score his asthma signs in the low yellow zone, so they give him 0.25 cc of albuterol by nebulizer.
2. After the albuterol treatment, Luke's parents score his asthma signs again. Luke is now in the high yellow zone, so he does not need to take an oral steroid. His parents continue to check his asthma signs every one to two hours.
3. Luke's total score of asthma signs stays in the high yellow zone for at least four hours.

In either circumstance, you should start giving an oral steroid. By starting the medicine promptly, you are helping to stop the increasing inflammation in the airways. Your child's condition should begin to stabilize six to twelve hours after starting treatment with an oral steroid and begin to improve within two or three days. Continue to give treatments with inhaled albuterol as outlined in the high yellow zone plan, not more often than every four hours. Call your doctor if the beneficial effect of albuterol does not last for four hours or if your child does not improve in two days.

For Children Under Age 5
SIGNS BASED HOME TREATMENT PLAN
Do not guess. Call the doctor if you have any questions about this plan.

Name: LUKE DELAURA   Date:

GREEN ZONE: absolutely no cough, wheeze, breathing faster or sucking in of the chest skin.
 	
 • **Normal activity.**
 • **Medicine to be taken every day:**
     ☑ Cromolyn _____ : __2__ ampules __2__ times a day.
     ☐ Inhaled steroid _____ : _____ puffs _____ times a day by holding chamber with mask.
     ☑ Quick relief medicine __Albuterol__ : 0.__25__ cc by compressor-driven nebulizer with each cromolyn dose for the first month OR give _____ puffs from MDI by holding chamber with mask before each inhaled steroid dose for the first month.
	Treatment Plan based on total score of all 4 signs:
	
	 Cough in past 5 minutes
	 None 0
	 Less than 1 per minute 1
	 1 - 4 per minute 2
	 More than 4 per minute 3

HIGH YELLOW ZONE: total asthma signs score 1 to 4 measured before inhaling quick relief medicine.

• **Eliminate triggers and add medicines. No strenuous exercise.**

• **Medicine to be taken:**
    ☑ Cromolyn: as above.
    ☐ Double dose of inhaled steroid to _____ puffs _____ times a day. Continue until signs score is in the Green Zone as long as it was in the High Yellow Zone.
    ☑ Quick relief medicine 0. __25__ cc by compressor-driven nebulizer with each cromolyn dose OR give _____ puffs from MDI by holding chamber with mask before each inhaled steroid dose. Give __3__ to __6__ times in 24 hours.*
    Continue until signs score is __0 or 1__ for 2 days.
    * If you need to give more than 6 treatments of quick relief medicine in 24 hours, start the Low Yellow Zone plan.

Wheeze   None 0   End of exhale 1   Throughout exhale 3   Inhale and exhale 5   **Sucking in the chest skin**   None 0   Barely noticeable 1   Obvious 3   Severe 5   **Breathing faster**   None 0   Up to 50% increase 1   Up to 100% increase 2   Over 100% increase 3

LOW YELLOW ZONE: total asthma signs score 5 to 8.

✓ Give 0.__25__ cc of quick relief medicine by compressor-driven nebulizer OR give _____ puffs from MDI by holding chamber with mask.

✓ Check your child's total signs score again 10 minutes after giving quick relief medicine.

If your child's total score has improved into the High Yellow Zone, follow the High Yellow Zone plan and continue to check signs every 1 to 2 hours.

If your child's total score is still in the Low Yellow Zone, or falls back into the Low Yellow Zone in less than 4 hours, continue with High Yellow Zone treatment and:

☑ Give oral steroid† __15__ mg, __5__ cc immediately. Continue once daily until total signs score is __0 or 1__ for at least 24 hours.

☐ Please call the office before starting oral steroid.

† If your child's condition does not improve within 2 days after starting oral steroid, or does not reach the Green Zone within 7 days of treatment, see your doctor.

RED ZONE: total asthma signs score 9 or more.

✓ Give 0.____ cc of quick relief medicine by compressor-driven nebulizer OR give _____ puffs from MDI by holding chamber with mask.

✓ Give oral steroid _____mg, _____ cc immediately.

✓ Check your child's total asthma signs score again 10 minutes after giving quick relief medicine.

If your child's total score has improved into the Low Yellow Zone, follow the Low Yellow Zone plan and continue to check signs every 1 to 2 hours.

If your child's total score is still in the Red Zone, or falls back into the Red Zone in less than 4 hours, visit your doctor **OR GO TO THE EMERGENCY ROOM NOW.**

Figure 59. Signs Based Home Treatment Plan: Low Yellow Zone

For Children Under Age 5
SIGNS BASED HOME TREATMENT PLAN
Do not guess. Call the doctor if you have any questions about this plan.

Name: LUKE DELAURA   Date:

	Treatment Plan based on total score of all 4 signs:

GREEN ZONE: absolutely no cough, wheeze, breathing faster or sucking in of the chest skin.

- **Normal activity.**
- **Medicine to be taken every day:**
  - ☑ Cromolyn _____ : __2__ ampules __2__ times a day.
  - ❏ Inhaled steroid _____ : _____ puffs _____ times a day by holding chamber with mask.
  - ☑ Quick relief medicine __Albuterol__ : 0. __25__ cc by compressor-driven nebulizer with each cromolyn dose for the first month OR give _____ puffs from MDI by holding chamber with mask before each inhaled steroid dose for the first month.

Cough in past 5 minutes
None 0
Less than 1 per minute 1
1 - 4 per minute 2
More than 4 per minute 3

HIGH YELLOW ZONE: total asthma signs score 1 to 4 measured before inhaling quick relief medicine.

- **Eliminate triggers and add medicines. No strenuous exercise.**
- **Medicine to be taken:**
  - ☑ Cromolyn: as above.
  - ❏ Double dose of inhaled steroid to _____ puffs _____ times a day. Continue until signs score is in the Green Zone as long as it was in the High Yellow Zone.
  - ☑ Quick relief medicine 0. __25__ cc by compressor-driven nebulizer with each cromolyn dose OR give _____ puffs from MDI by holding chamber with mask before each inhaled steroid dose. Give __3__ to __6__ times in 24 hours.*
    Continue until signs score is _0 or 1_ for 2 days.
  - * If you need to give more than 6 treatments of quick relief medicine in 24 hours, start the Low Yellow Zone plan.

Wheeze
None 0
End of exhale 1
Throughout exhale 3
Inhale and exhale 5

Sucking in the chest skin
None 0
Barely noticeable............... 1
Obvious 3
Severe 5

Breathing faster
None 0
Up to 50% increase 1
Up to 100% increase 2
Over 100% increase 3

LOW YELLOW ZONE: total asthma signs score 5 to 8.

- ✓ Give 0.__25__ cc of quick relief medicine by compressor-driven nebulizer OR give _____ puffs from MDI by holding chamber with mask.
- ✓ **Check your child's total signs score again 10 minutes after giving quick relief medicine.**
  If your child's total score has improved into the High Yellow Zone, follow the High Yellow Zone plan and continue to check signs every 1 to 2 hours.
  If your child's total score is still in the Low Yellow Zone, or falls back into the Low Yellow Zone in less than 4 hours, continue with High Yellow Zone treatment and:
  - ☑ Give oral steroid† __15__ mg, __5__ cc immediately. Continue once daily until total signs score is _0 or 1_ for at least 24 hours.
  - ❏ Please call the office before starting oral steroid.
  - † If your child's condition does not improve within 2 days after starting oral steroid, or does not reach the Green Zone within 7 days of treatment, see your doctor.

RED ZONE: total asthma signs score 9 or more.

- ✓ Give 0. __25__ cc of quick relief medicine by compressor-driven nebulizer OR give _____ puffs from MDI by holding chamber with mask.
- ✓ Give oral steroid __15__ mg, __5__ cc immediately.
- ✓ **Check your child's total asthma signs score again 10 minutes after giving quick relief medicine.**
  If your child's total score has improved into the Low Yellow Zone, follow the Low Yellow Zone plan and continue to check signs every 1 to 2 hours.
  If your child's total score is still in the Red Zone, or falls back into the Red Zone in less than 4 hours, visit your doctor **OR GO TO THE EMERGENCY ROOM NOW.**

Figure 60. Signs Based Home Treatment Plan: Red Zone. This treatment plan was designed for my patient Luke DeLaura. Your child's doctor must individualize a plan for your child.

Once your child has had a signs score of 0, 1 or 2 for twenty-four hours, you can stop giving the oral steroid. Ask your doctor to decide which score to use in judging when to stop an oral steroid and to write it into the low yellow zone plan.

THE RED ZONE PLAN

A signs score of 9 or greater alerts you that your child is having a severe asthma episode. When your child is stuck in the red zone, you should not try to handle the situation at home. You need to give albuterol and an oral steroid immediately and score your child's signs again a few minutes later. If your child's total score of asthma signs improves into the low yellow zone (8 or less), and the improvement holds for at least four hours, you should follow the low yellow zone plan. Continue to monitor asthma signs, every one to two hours, to make sure his condition remains stable.

If your child's score is stuck in the red zone, go to the doctor or emergency room right away. "Stuck" means that your child's total score of asthma signs remains in the red zone after treatment with albuterol. Your child is also stuck in the red zone if the signs score clears into the low yellow zone but then drops back into the red zone in less than four hours. In this situation, a phone call to the doctor is *not* enough. Give a dose of an oral steroid and go to your doctor's office or the emergency room, or call the ambulance immediately. Give additional albuterol while waiting for the ambulance or in transit to the doctor, if giving the medicine causes no delay.

Wendy gives Luke 0.25 cc of albuterol as soon as she observes that his signs scores are in the red zone (see Figure 60). If Luke clears out of the red zone into the low yellow zone, his mother gives 15 mg of prednisolone (an oral steroid) and follows the low yellow zone plan.

She monitors Luke's asthma signs closely, scoring them every one to two hours.

If Luke is stuck in the red zone, Wendy gives 15 mg of an oral steroid and goes to the emergency room. She knows that Luke may need oxygen and administration of inhaled albuterol in large doses that are not safe to give at home. In a critical situation, he may need a respiratory support system to breathe for him.

Signs Based Treatment Plan for Young Children Taking Inhaled Steroids

Treating young children with daily inhaled steroids is a relatively new approach. It has only been possible since the development of the holding chamber with mask, and more recently the availability of an inhaled steroid solution for use in a compressor driven or ultrasonic nebulizer. As you already know, inhaled steroids are the most effective controller medicine available. They work by preventing inflammation and reducing inflammation that may already be under way. Because inhaled steroids (unlike cromolyn) can reduce inflammation, they are sometimes effective in treating an asthma episode. By doubling your child's usual daily dose of an inhaled steroid in the early stage of an episode, you can often avoid the need to give an oral steroid.

When my patient Shoshana was 3½ years old, her parents found that cromolyn did not adequately prevent her asthma symptoms and episodes. Her primary care doctor substituted a low dose of an inhaled steroid for the cromolyn. Her parents delivered the medicine by a holding chamber with mask and brought Shoshana's asthma under excellent control. Figure 61 shows the treatment plan they follow to keep Shoshana, now 6½, healthy and fully active.

For Children Under Age 5
SIGNS BASED HOME TREATMENT PLAN
Do not guess. Call the doctor if you have any questions about this plan.

Name: Shoshana   Date:

GREEN ZONE: absolutely no cough, wheeze, breathing faster or sucking in of the chest skin.
- **Normal activity.**
- **Medicine to be taken every day:**
  - ☐ Cromolyn _____ : _____ ampules _____ times a day.
  - ☑ Inhaled steroid _flunisolide_ : _2_ puffs _1_ times a day by holding chamber with mask.
  - ☑ Quick relief medicine _albuterol_ : 0. _____ cc by compressor-driven nebulizer with each cromolyn dose for the first month OR give _2_ puffs from MDI by holding chamber with mask before each inhaled steroid dose for the first month.

HIGH YELLOW ZONE: total asthma signs score 1 to 4 measured before inhaling quick relief medicine.
- **Eliminate triggers and add medicines. No strenuous exercise.**
- **Medicine to be taken:**
  - ☐ Cromolyn: as above.
  - ☑ Double dose of inhaled steroid to _4_ puffs _1_ times a day. Continue until signs score is in the Green Zone as long as it was in the High Yellow Zone.
  - ☑ Quick relief medicine 0. _____ cc by compressor-driven nebulizer with each cromolyn dose OR give _2_ puffs from MDI by holding chamber with mask before each inhaled steroid dose. Give _3_ to _6_ times in 24 hours.* Continue until signs score is _0 or 1_ for 2 days.
  - * If you need to give more than 6 treatments of quick relief medicine in 24 hours, start the Low Yellow Zone plan.

LOW YELLOW ZONE: total asthma signs score 5 to 8.
- ✓ **Give 0._____ cc of quick relief medicine by compressor-driven nebulizer OR give _2_ puffs from MDI by holding chamber with mask.**
- ✓ **Check your child's total signs score again 10 minutes after giving quick relief medicine.**

  If your child's total score has improved into the High Yellow Zone, follow the High Yellow Zone plan and continue to check signs every 1 to 2 hours.

  If your child's total score is still in the Low Yellow Zone, or falls back into the Low Yellow Zone in less than 4 hours, continue with High Yellow Zone treatment and:
  - ☑ Give oral steroid† _15_ mg, _5_ cc immediately. Continue once daily until total signs score is _0 or 1_ for at least 24 hours.
  - ☐ Please call the office before starting oral steroid.
  - † If your child's condition does not improve within 2 days after starting oral steroid, or does not reach the Green Zone within 7 days of treatment, see your doctor.

RED ZONE: total asthma signs score 9 or more.
- ✓ **Give 0._____ cc of quick relief medicine by compressor-driven nebulizer OR give _4_ puffs from MDI by holding chamber with mask.**
- ✓ **Give oral steroid _15_ mg, _5_ cc immediately.**
- ✓ **Check your child's total asthma signs score again 10 minutes after giving quick relief medicine.**

  If your child's total score has improved into the Low Yellow Zone, follow the Low Yellow Zone plan and continue to check signs every 1 to 2 hours.

  If your child's total score is still in the Red Zone, or falls back into the Red Zone in less than 4 hours, visit your doctor **OR GO TO THE EMERGENCY ROOM NOW.**

Treatment Plan based on total score of all 4 signs:

Cough in past 5 minutes
None 0
Less than 1 per minute 1
1 - 4 per minute 2
More than 4 per minute 3

Wheeze
None 0
End of exhale 1
Throughout exhale 3
Inhale and exhale 5

Sucking in the chest skin
None 0
Barely noticeable 1
Obvious 3
Severe 5

Breathing faster
None 0
Up to 50% increase 1
Up to 100% increase 2
Over 100% increase 3

Figure 61. Signs Based Home Treatment Plan: Inhaled Steroid. This treatment plan was designed for my patient Shoshana Moriarty. Your child's doctor must individualize a plan for your child.

SHOSHANA'S TREATMENT PLAN

When Shoshana is in the green zone, her parents give her a single dose of two puffs of inhaled steroid by holding chamber with mask between 3:00 P.M. and 5:00 P.M. For the first month of treatment, Shoshana also received two puffs of albuterol by holding chamber with mask before her inhaled steroid dose. The albuterol was given to make sure that her airways were open, allowing the inhaled steroid to reach deep into her lungs and do its job.

In the high yellow zone (score of 1 to 4), Shoshana's parents double her dose of inhaled steroid to 4 puffs, still giving it once a day in the afternoon. They also give Shoshana 2 puffs of inhaled albuterol by holding chamber with mask, 3 to 6 times per day.

In the low yellow zone (a score of 5 to 8), Shoshana's parents figure out whether she can clear the low yellow zone or is stuck there. If Shoshana clears the low yellow zone, they follow the high yellow zone plan. If Shoshana's total score of asthma signs does not improve into the high yellow zone after inhaling albuterol, or drops back into the low yellow zone in less than four hours, her parents start treating her with 15 mg of an oral steroid daily.

A total signs score in the red zone (9 or higher) calls for immediate action. Shoshana receives 4 puffs of albuterol by holding chamber with mask and 15 mg of an oral steroid. If she is stuck in the red zone, her parents take her to the pediatrician or the emergency room. This scenario is very unlikely because they have worked out an effective treatment plan.

Once your doctor has worked out a Home Treatment Plan for your child, it can be followed by other family members, noncustodial parents, caregivers, parents of the child's friends, school nurses, and other doctors. This ensures that a child receives consistent treatment in any setting, from any adult. The Home Treatment Plan helps parents feel more comfortable and confident when they leave their child under someone else's care.

USING THE SIGNS BASED HOME TREATMENT PLAN WITH THE ASTHMA SIGNS DIARY

The Home Treatment Plan works best if used alongside the Asthma Signs Diary. The diary helps you score your child's asthma signs and track how the signs change. It tips you off early about trends in asthma signs so you can start additional treatment at the first sign of symptoms. A diary also helps you figure out when to stop giving additional medicine. Once your child's asthma signs scores have returned to the green zone for a specified amount of time, you can return to the usual medicine routine with confidence.

Keeping a diary and following a Home Treatment Plan takes a lot of work, but once you have learned to score signs, record them in a diary, and follow the Home Treatment Plan, the job becomes easier. Parents usually find that the improvement in asthma control and the peace of mind they earn from keeping a diary is well worth the time and effort. And as they become more experienced, the benefit continues and the burden lessens. To get full benefit from using the Home Treatment Plan, keep an asthma diary every day at least until your child has achieved excellent asthma control. After that point, you can decide how often you need to make diary entries.

In Summary

The key to effective treatment is a written plan developed by your doctor. This is based on the treatment zones defined by your peak flow scores or asthma signs score. Each zone includes day-to-day routines and special steps for asthma episodes. Your written plan will give you clear instructions about when to start and stop additional medicines and how to judge when emergency care is needed.

Initially, I recommend a treatment plan that usually clears the airways rapidly and eliminates asthma symptoms. If it does not produce good results, I modify it. After my patients gain excellent control over their asthma, I reduce their medicine dose gradually to the lowest effective amount. Eliminating and avoiding triggers helps them keep medicine to a minimum. A review of the plan every three to twelve months allows us to adjust it to maintain excellent asthma control at the lowest possible dose of medicine.

Chapter Eight

Working With Your Doctors

You must work closely with a competent doctor to control your asthma safely and effectively. That doctor will give you written instructions, teach you to use your devices, measure air flow at each visit, and treat you in a manner consistent with the 1997 NHLBI *Guidelines*.

I believe you can achieve excellent asthma control only when you and your doctor actively share with each other complementary knowledge, skills, attitudes, and behaviors. A good doctor brings a breadth of experience and medical knowledge to the collaboration. You bring the daily observations, insights, and growing understanding of your own asthma situation. It takes both of you to build and carry out a successful asthma management plan.

Your doctor needs to have comprehensive knowledge of asthma and the medicines used to treat it. He must recognize that you want to be the primary manager of asthma once you acquire the skills and knowledge you need. He must support you as you learn, and he must also be readily accessible to answer your questions.

If you want to be a major manager of your asthma, you have to work, too. By reading this book, you have begun the process of building your knowledge and exploring your attitudes about asthma care. With the support and guidance of your doctor, you can become skilled in measuring and monitoring peak flow, observing the signs and symptoms of asthma, and using devices to deliver medicines.

Once you and your doctor have worked out an asthma management plan, you can make that plan effective by following its guidelines and continuing to observe how well it is working. Most asthma problems will be temporary, and you will be able to manage them at home. However, even after you have acquired extensive knowledge about your asthma, treating it still requires collaboration with your doctor. There may be some situations that you cannot or should not handle at home. Don't guess. Stay within the boundaries of your written plan.

Taking care of asthma is a shared responsibility. In the early stages of your learning, it is only safe to take on a small portion of that responsibility. As you grow in knowledge, skills, confidence, and experience, you will be able to take on more. A good doctor will help you judge your ability to manage asthma and transfer responsibility to you in an appropriate and timely way. In my experience, patients and parents move through five general stages as they learn to care for asthma at home. As they became more advanced through learning and experience, they are ready to take on more of the responsibility (see Figure 62).

The approach I describe in this chapter is based on my experience and is followed by many asthma specialists. It works well for patients who want to take control of their asthma and to prevent or manage most of their episodes. Once you have high expectations for asthma control, you can make sure that you get the care you want. The following stories illustrate how two mothers found doctors that they could work with.

■

My New Doctor Listens
Cathleen Henning, Florida
Written in the 1980s

The day I read your book was truly a day of awakening for me. I realized that it was totally unnecessary for Douglas, my son, to be receiving a shot of adrenaline as the only conclusion to each and every asthma attack he had. My 3-year-old child was taking 400 mg of theophylline a day and bouncing off the walls from its effects. We made seemingly endless trips to the six different on-call pediatricians to enable him to breathe normally.

The pediatricians were treating the asthma episodically and telling me to consult the allergist if I needed anything further. The allergist told me to take Douglas to the pediatricians for rou-tine treatments. By the time I found your book, I was ready to move to Phoenix, the beaches, or to get an M.D. degree so that I could treat him myself! The day I arrived at the allergist's office, your book in hand, asking to discuss whether Douglas would benefit from cromolyn, I was treated as a necessary evil who had to be dealt with and forgotten. The allergist gave us a prescription for cromolyn, but when I asked him about a particular holding chamber, he told me he'd never heard of it, that he didn't want to see your book, and that there was no need for me to be asking about albuterol, steroids, or any other medications.

A well-informed mother was a threat to this man. Yet, somehow, I no longer cared. I trusted my new knowledge enough to know that I wanted to play an active role in Douglas' care. My next choice of allergist would be one who respected my knowledge of my child's needs as well as my knowledge of asthma, and my desire to prevent the attacks rather than treat them episodically.

At our first visit with the new allergist, he asked me to review Douglas's medical history and treatment. He asked questions and listened to my answers and opinions. He immediately demonstrated and prescribed the holding chamber I had asked about. I asked for an inhaler to replace the albuterol liquid that made Douglas irritable and sleepless during the attacks; he agreed.

I told the allergist that cromolyn had maintained Douglas without an attack for the previous five months, and he agreed that we should continue with it and use theophylline only as needed. When I asked him if he would be interested in reading *Children with Asthma: A Manual for Parents,* and explained your concept of teaching parents to manage asthma at home, he borrowed the book, read it, ordered his own copy, and now recommends it to parents. Finally, when

STAGES IN PATIENT ABILITY TO MANAGE ASTHMA

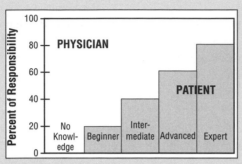

Figure 62. Shared Responsibility

No Knowledge:
- Cannot recognize an asthma episode.
- Knows nothing about asthma medicines.

Beginner:
- Can recognize an asthma episode but cannot judge the severity.
- Needs help in deciding when to start medicine.
- Cannot communicate clearly with doctor over the phone.

Intermediate:
- Can handle an episode well with doctor's help.
- Knows how to judge the severity of an episode, how to use a peak flow meter and when to start treatment.
- Can communicate clearly with doctor over the phone using an asthma diary to describe progress.
- Has made some changes in the environment to reduce triggers.

Advanced:
- Has good knowledge of asthma signs, triggers and medicines.
- Is skilled in analyzing peak flow scores and symptoms and starting/stopping medicines.
- Has made major changes in the environment.
- Can handle most episodes safely at home without consulting the doctor.

Expert:
- Has full knowledge of asthma signs, triggers and medicines needed for asthma care.
- Can accurately assess an episode and knows when to call or go for help.
- Can handle almost all episodes without consulting the doctor.
- Understands the course and pattern of asthma episodes.
- Is able to analyze episodes and, using this information, can discuss possibilities for improving treatment.
- Still needs the doctor when stuck in the red zone and to review treatment at three to twelve month intervals.

I expressed an interest in starting a support group, he provided me with literature from the Allergy and Asthma Foundation of America and now provides referrals to our group.

I left that first visit with a written plan for treatment that I knew would work for my son, and a tremendous sense of relief. What a difference it made to have the support and confidence of a doctor who was more concerned with my child's well-being than with his own insecurities about who was going to control my child's care.

In the last ten months, through the use of a well-established plan of preventive maintenance and early intervention, we have had only two episodes that actually reached "attack" proportions. Only once did I need to call the doctor, at which point we decided on an increased dose of medication. That was it. It worked. No expensive and painful trip to the emergency room. NO SHOT! Douglas is nearly five now, playing soccer, swimming — a normal healthy child with occasional episodes of asthma, and I can't even remember his last shot of adrenaline.

■

I Can Talk With My Doctor
Kristine Uravich, Idaho
Written in the 1980s

Julie had been coughing for three months following a suspected case of pneumonia in January. She was only 2½ then and could not describe how she was feeling. She looked healthy and her growth continued to be good. But she coughed all the time. She stayed awake at night, propped high on bed pillows and engulfed in the vapor of a cool mist machine. She coughed so hard that tiny blood vessels broke in her cheeks. Our doctor prescribed what seemed to be gallons of metaproterenol syrup, and later what he described as a "powerful drug" (slow-release theophylline) to help open her airways.

Our family doctor gave me lots of explanations: it's a lung irritation, maybe she's allergic to your dog, her lungs were temporarily damaged by the infections. We took her to an allergist for skin patch tests, got rid of our long-time family dog and tried to free our home of house dust. But, she was still "sick." Late one afternoon in April, during a particularly hard cold, I crawled into Julie's bed to try and help her sleep. Her breathing was labored and fast. I became frightened. Maybe she would stop breathing. Maybe she would die!

Our family doctor was out of town, so I called the allergist in a town 40 miles from home. After a brief exam in his office, the doctor handed me a prescription. "What's wrong with her?" I wanted to know. The reply was so matter-of-fact that I was stunned: She was having an asthma attack. I had never heard the word "asthma" used in association with my daughter's health. That's when I began to learn about asthma. That's when I decided that the day-in/day-out medical care for this child was in my hands. I had to find out about symptoms, medications, and treatment so I could ask intelligent questions during doctor visits. I would be my child's advocate in the doctor's office.

Through an article on asthma in *American Baby* magazine, I learned about *Children With Asthma: A Manual for Parents.* I read it through the day it arrived in the mail and went to the doctor's office with a barrage of questions. Our family doctor was at first surprised by some of them. He had assumed that I would prefer to give theophylline at breakfast and supper rather than every twelve hours as recommended. I think he should have asked me. He didn't realize that I would gladly inconvenience myself to help my child to breathe better.

When I inquired about the advantages that I would gain by delivering medicine for Julie with a compressor driven nebulizer, he told me he thought it was too expensive and too complicated for me to manage. After some discussion, he agreed to let me make the decision. Then things began to go our way. We purchased a compressor driven nebulizer for use at home. It is simple to operate and was paid for primarily by our insurance coverage. We got a firm grip on asthma through a good medication routine.

Most importantly, I've learned that professional medical treatment is a service that requires intelligent consideration by the patient as a consumer.

In order to deal effectively with my physician, I must be informed. I need to be able to describe symptoms in terms the doctor understands and know the whys and hows of medicines so we can use them properly and effectively. Using my physician as a consultant I have accepted the responsibility of managing Julie's asthma until she is old enough to take it on herself.

How to Choose a Doctor

A doctor's particular specialty is not as important as his interest in asthma. It takes time and effort for a doctor to stay up-to-date in diagnosis and treatment, although the 1997 NHLBI *Guidelines* have made that job easier. If you have mild intermittent or mild persistent asthma, you may be able to achieve excellent control working with a good primary care physician (pediatrician, family practitioner, or internist). If you do not achieve excellent control, or if you have moderate persistent asthma, periodic consultation with an asthma specialist will be helpful in almost all cases (see "Seeking a Consultation," this chapter). Once you have worked out a good plan with a specialist, you can follow this plan with your primary care physician and see the consultant occasionally for review. If you have severe persistent asthma, you should be treated by an asthma specialist.

To judge whether your regular doctor will be able to help you achieve excellent control, you need to consider several issues:

- Does the doctor follow currently recommended treatment?

- Can the doctor communicate to you what you need to know to manage asthma?
- Does the doctor listen well enough to learn about your specific asthma situation?
- Does the doctor want to help you to learn to manage your asthma at home?

I will discuss each of these points to help you make an informed decision about whether your current physician has the qualities that will help you to gain control of your asthma.

CURRENT APPROACH TO ASTHMA CARE

Use the following criteria to assess whether your doctor is up-to-date in his approach to asthma care. A competent asthma doctor:

- *Gives you written instructions.* This means that your doctor provides you with a written home treatment plan that you can understand. The plan should clearly list all of your asthma medicines and doses, when and how to take them, and when to add or stop taking additional doses. The plan should be based on peak flow or signs scores and the zone system.
- *Teaches and monitors your use of devices.* The office staff or the doctor should teach you how to use each prescribed device (inhaler, holding chamber, nebulizer, peak flow meter) and observe you as you use each one. Even after your technique is perfect it will need to be checked at office visits.
- *Measures your peak flow or FEV_1 at each visit.* At an office visit, your doctor can get important information about your airways by checking your peak flow score with a peak flow meter or your forced expiratory volume (FEV_1) with a spirometer.

This airflow information is essential to monitor your progress and adjust your treatment.

- *Approaches asthma treatment in a manner consistent with the* Expert Panel Report 2: Guidelines for the Diagnosis and Management of Asthma, *published in 1997.* The *Guidelines* are the most comprehensive guide to effective asthma care currently available. Your doctor and the office staff should be familiar with this document, or with the more readable version, *Practical Guide for the Diagnosis and Management of Asthma.* Treatment consistent with its recommendations will almost always lead to good results.

Not all experts agree on every part of the *Guidelines.* A good doctor may suggest treatment that differs from the *Guidelines* and will be able to explain clearly why he recommends that approach for you. I suggest that you purchase the *Practical Guide* and become familiar with its key points (see Resource Section).

If your doctor meets the four criteria discussed here, he is up-to-date on asthma treatment and can help you take control of your asthma and live a fully active life. However, consider these additional factors before making your final decision.

ATTITUDE TOWARD HOME MANAGEMENT

Now you need to decide how well the doctor's attitude toward home management fits with yours. Please remember, no matter how good the doctor, you have the primary responsibility for your care. A good doctor will teach you how to provide this care within certain well-defined limits. He will help you learn the skills you need to manage asthma at home and help you judge how much you can handle as you become more skilled.

Home management of asthma depends on your ability to observe, score, record, and assign a zone to peak flow scores and the signs of asthma. Your observations guide the actions that you take based on your written plan. Effective home management also depends on your ability to take the medicines you need properly and promptly. It is your doctor's job, and yours, to make sure that you understand your asthma medicines and how to take them.

ATTITUDE TOWARD THE PATIENT'S CONTRIBUTION

A doctor needs detailed information from you to develop the most effective treatment plan. Both his medical knowledge and your individual knowledge are necessary to reach the goal of asthma control. You need to write an account of your life experience with asthma similar to the stories (from the 1990s) in Chapter 1. Your doctor needs to read it. Does he supplement this information by careful questioning? Does he analyze the information you have collected in your asthma diary? Does he want to know about the environment you live and work in? As your doctor conducts an asthma visit, it will become clear how much he values your input.

COMMUNICATION

A doctor may know everything there is to know about asthma. However, that knowledge won't do you any good unless the doctor can communicate the important information to you.

Doctors vary widely in their ability to communicate, just as patients do. If you feel that you are getting the information you need from your doctor, his communication style is probably compatible with yours. Patients often find that communication with their doctor improves greatly after they read this book. If you leave the office confused or frustrated, you might benefit from working with a doctor who can communicate more clearly with you.

How Often Should You See Your Doctor for Asthma?

Once you have chosen a doctor, it may take several months for you to achieve excellent control of your asthma.

I believe a preliminary plan for the management of mild or moderate asthma can be worked out during the first consultation visit with your primary care physician. If you have mild intermittent asthma, you will find it helpful to review your plan after you manage the next episode. If you have mild or moderate persistent asthma, a second visit with your doctor should take place one to two weeks after the first, and a third visit in one month, to adjust your treatment and provide additional asthma education. Once you have achieved excellent asthma control, you probably will be able to maintain it with review visits spaced three to twelve months apart. Patients with severe persistent asthma may need to be seen more often.

Until you have learned to manage asthma with the proper treatment plan, your doctor may need to see you once a month or more often to fine-tune your treatment. An unscheduled urgent care visit does not substitute for a planned asthma review.

Achieving Excellent Asthma Control

When your asthma is under excellent control, you:

- can exercise as hard and as long as you want.
- need urgent care for asthma once a year or less.
- are not hospitalized for asthma.
- miss school or work one day per year or less.
- have minimal side effects from treatment.
- take the lowest effective dose of asthma medicines.

You should start to feel better in two weeks after starting treatment. If you have mild or moderate persistent asthma, your symptoms should occur no more than two days a week after one to three months of effective treatment. It may take three to six months for your doctor to "step down" your medicine dose to the minimum amount you need to maintain excellent asthma control. If you have severe persistent asthma, the process will take longer. If you are not making progress within this general time frame, it is time to seek a consultation with an asthma specialist.

After you achieve asthma control, the frequency of review visits depends on the severity of your asthma and how it is affecting your life. If you have mild intermittent or persistent asthma and you rarely miss school or work be-

Table 46. Time Required to Achieve Excellent Asthma Control

Asthma Severity	Feel Improvement	Symptoms: ≤ 2 times/week	Lowest Medicine Dose
mild persistent	1–2 weeks	1–2 months	2–3 months
moderate persistent	1–2 weeks	2–3 months	3–6 months
severe persistent	1–2 weeks	2–6 months	4–6 months

cause of symptoms, a review visit once a year should suffice. During the visit, your doctor will review your treatment plan and techniques for using your medicine devices and peak flow meter. He may also teach you about recent improvements in asthma care.

If you miss work or school more than one day a year, or you limit your activity or wake up at night because of asthma, your doctor needs to adjust your treatment plan. You should have a thorough review at least every six months. If you have been hospitalized or received emergency care in the office or the emergency room during the past month, it may require several visits until you are able to reestablish excellent control. Remember, "excellent control" means you have no more than one urgent visit to the doctor's office or the emergency room in a year.

Seeking a Consultation

Even when patients and parents have had a good experience and work well with their doctor, they may want a second opinion from an asthma specialist on some prescribed course of action or to get a fuller understanding of their situation.

This is accepted medical practice, and you should not feel at all uncomfortable in asking for it. Involve your regular doctor in the process by asking that he provide a clinical summary and suggest a consultant. A competent physician will not be insulted by this request. In fact, he will want to be involved in recommending a consultant who would be particularly skilled to help with your care. Some patients prefer to make all the consultation arrangements on their own.

I recommend that you seek a consultation if:

- you limit your activity or miss school or work more than one day per year because

of asthma, in spite of reviewing the situation with your regular doctor.
- your doctor suggests that you limit activities because of asthma.
- you have to go to the doctor's office or emergency room for urgent care more than once a year.
- you have recently been hospitalized for asthma.
- you have nighttime symptoms (cough or wheeze) that wake you up one night a week or daytime symptoms more than twice per week, despite reviewing the situation with your regular doctor.

In addition, the NHLBI *Guidelines* recommend that a primary care physician refer a patient to an asthma specialist if the patient:

- has had a life-threatening asthma episode.
- has complicating factors, such as sinusitis, severe rhinitis, COPD, and others.
- needs more education and guidance than is currently being provided.
- requires an oral steroid long-term or a high dose of an inhaled steroid to control asthma, or has received more than two short-term treatments with an oral steroid in the past year.
- is younger than 3 years of age and has moderate or severe persistent asthma.
- needs additional diagnostic tests, such as allergy skin testing.
- is being considered for immunotherapy (allergy shots).
- requires confirmation of a history of occupational or environmental causes that provoke or contribute to asthma.
- has signs or symptoms that are not typical of asthma.

FINDING A GOOD ASTHMA SPECIALIST

Almost all asthma specialists are allergists or pulmonologists (lung specialists). A well-trained and experienced allergist will have a comprehensive knowledge of asthma, asthma treatment, and the significant role that allergens play. Pulmonologists are particularly good at defining structural problems in the lungs and in the rest of the respiratory tract. However, not every doctor who is board-certified in allergy or pulmonology will be able to provide asthma care that is optimal for you.

Some investigation on your part will help you find an asthma specialist who will meet your needs. Start with a call to your local hospital, and ask the secretary of the medical staff to recommend someone who matches all of the criteria of a good asthma doctor described earlier in this chapter.

If no one from the first hospital matches these criteria, try another hospital. You may have to travel as far as one hundred miles to find someone qualified to provide the care that you need. Since you will rarely have an asthma emergency after you work out an effective plan with a consultant, that doctor does not have to be local. Occasional urgent problems will be handled by your regular doctor or the emergency room staff.

PREPARING FOR AN ASTHMA CONSULTATION

I will describe how I conduct an asthma consultation and illustrate this with a patient's story. I have high expectations of my patients, and they have high expectations of me. I expect every patient to do considerable preparation before the first visit. Were you to want an appointment with me, I would ask you to do the following:

- Read this book from cover to cover.
- Write your asthma story.
- Fill out an asthma questionnaire.
- Keep a daily Asthma Peak Flow Diary for the week before your appointment.

Consider preparing for your consultation with any asthma specialist in the same way. By reading this book, you are beginning to build the understanding you need to take an active role in managing your asthma. As a result, you come to the visit with informed questions and can use your time highlighting and analyzing important information instead of covering basic facts. This makes your first visit much more interactive and productive.

The asthma narrative is your written personal story, including your observations, experiences, feelings, fears, and goals. I have found that you can give more thought to your asthma history if you have the opportunity to consider it at home. There you have access to your medical records and calendars, which can help you write an accurate account. The writing requires you to review, organize, and analyze a substantial amount of information before coming to the office. In writing your story, you can get perspective on your experience and emphasize what you think is important. After your doctor reads the narrative, he can ask questions to clarify or add to it.

The stories you read in the first chapter of this book are all narratives written by my patients. As you saw from those stories, people know a great deal about their asthma from observing their own lives. One unexpected benefit of the narrative has been that patients learn about their asthma while writing about it. Most people have never taken a good look at their complete asthma story. When they do, they see patterns that had previously escaped their notice. They may identify triggers, see that symptoms are limited to a single season, or find that a change in their environment was beneficial or caused symptoms. They can also see under what circumstances an episode got out of hand and how they might have avoided that situation.

Writing down these observations and making some sense of them is the crucial first step in taking control of your asthma. Patients usually read my book before they write their stories and use their new understanding as a foundation for writing their narrative. They gain power over their asthma as they increase their knowledge of it.

By completing a two-page questionnaire, you state your goals for the visit and write any specific questions you have. You also provide details about your asthma, including triggers, early clues, episodes, missed work or school, emergency room or hospital visits, medicines, asthma education, and the environment in your home.

I require patients to complete the questionnaire and return it, along with their asthma story, before I will schedule an appointment. I also ask them to record peak flow scores and symptoms in an Asthma Peak Flow Diary for a week before their visit. Parents of a young child use the Asthma Signs Diary instead.

The previsit routine underscores my interest in working interactively with patients. Before the visit I read all the material you send. Sometimes I call to clarify questions raised in the narrative or questionnaire. When we meet, I will already know a great deal about you and your asthma.

This preparation saves time in the visit and vastly improves our results. We can spend valuable visit time analyzing information instead of trying to gather and organize it. In this way, I can learn a great deal about your asthma that I might never have found out, or not found out until a later visit.

A VISIT OVERVIEW

A consultation is a cooperative enterprise. If you compile information before your visit, you will be confident and clear about your communication, rather than struggling to dredge up facts on the spot. I spend about half of the initial visit reviewing historical facts. First we discuss your goals for the visit. After that, we discuss your narrative and questionnaire in detail. Learning takes place as I ask about the details of your story and demonstrate the changes that occur in the airways during an asthma episode. It continues as we analyze the trends in peak flow and asthma signs in your asthma diary and see how they are affected by triggers and medicines.

During the physical examination, I check your height, weight, blood pressure, ears, nose, throat, sinuses, heart, and lungs. I remark on any signs of asthma that are present, and I explain how to assess them. I observe how you use the peak flow meter and then provide feedback and coaching. Since most patients do not take inhaled medicine in a fully effective manner, I review and correct your technique for the inhalation device you are using. Then I observe while you use the device by yourself, to make sure you have learned well enough to continue using it properly at home.

At this point in the visit, I usually have a basic understanding of your asthma situation. We spend the rest of the visit working out a preliminary treatment plan and discussing how you will implement it. I suggest a step-down approach to asthma care which calls for starting treatment with enough medicine and environmental changes to clear up your current asthma symptoms rapidly. I send a typed copy of my office notes in a few days so you can review them and discuss them with your family.

During the second visit, one to four weeks later, I review your account of events since the preceding visit, as well as your diary. I make suggestions for further education, environmental changes, and monitoring of peak flow and asthma signs. I adjust medicine doses and review routines for zones based management. I send my notes to you and to your primary care physician.

After this review, you can handle most asthma problems at home. Your primary care physician is able to provide emergency care in the rare event that it is needed. He checks to make sure that your asthma control continues to be excellent and refills prescriptions during your regular visits to the office. I usually see you again in one month and then at three- to twelve-month intervals. Patients who travel a great distance make a single visit of several hours to clarify their status and work out a plan. Fine-tuning can be done by mail, fax, and phone or with another asthma specialist closer to their home.

The initial medicine routine usually calls for a dose higher than you will need once you have reduced triggers and cleared your current asthma symptoms. After you have achieved asthma control and sustained it for two or three months, we step down to a lower dose of medicine. If your peak flow scores drop slightly or symptoms reappear, we know that the reduced dose is too low and must be increased to the previous step. If the peak flow remains stable for two or three months after a reduction in medicine dose, we may be able to reduce the dose further.

Karen Warren's Asthma Visits

Karen's asthma narrative appears in the first chapter of this book. She first came to see me in 1993 as a 22-year-old college senior. She had been struggling with asthma for the previous twelve years. For months her symptoms had limited her activity every day and awakened her every night. I saw her several times during her last month of college. By graduation she had learned to control her asthma and was fully active.

Before I can help any patient work out an effective asthma plan, I must learn and understand a great deal about her asthma. The asthma narrative Karen sent to me before her visit told a story of asthma that had been out of control for years. She frequently took medicine to treat asthma symptoms but had never been given a plan to prevent them. She had been seen for emergency care many times. I was convinced that Karen could achieve excellent asthma control by making some simple changes in her medicine routine and her environment. Here are the steps that we followed at her first visit.

In her questionnaire, Karen stated, "I would like to learn how to use the various asthma devices properly — so I can best benefit from their use. In addition, I would like to feel that there can be an end to this restless-night, achy-chest, twelve-year pain in the butt!"

Since she was 10, Karen has had frequent episodes of asthma. In the past twelve months she has missed twelve days of college classes due to asthma. Her asthma triggers include respiratory infections, pollutants, cold air, exercise, and allergens.

Karen knows the three changes that occur in the airways during an episode (see page 36) and the major signs of asthma. Currently, she takes albuterol and knows the action of this medicine. During the college year, Karen spends most of her time in a smoke-free room.

Karen has read *Children With Asthma: A Manual for Parents* and kept an Asthma Peak Flow Diary every day for the two weeks before her visit. Prior to this visit, she has been instructed in the use of a nebulizer but has not consulted a doctor other than her regular physician about asthma. Aside from her asthma, she is in excellent health.

Her physical exam includes various measurements and review of her metered dose inhaler (MDI) technique. Karen inhales medicine for two seconds and then holds her breath for two seconds. After I instruct her, her technique is perfect: she inhales the medicine for five seconds and holds her breath for ten seconds. I also instruct her in the use of a holding chamber with her MDI. Now Karen knows how to take her medicine properly. We will review her technique at each follow-up visit.

ASSESSMENT OF KAREN'S ASTHMA

This 22-year-old college senior has severe persistent asthma. She is athletic but at present is unable to participate in sports because of her asthma symptoms. Karen would like to run when she wants to run and would like to bike when she wants to bike. At present, she drives to classes to avoid wheezing.

At this point, I have a good sense of Karen's asthma. Now we can develop a preliminary treatment plan. I prescribe prednisone for seven days to clear up the inflammation that Karen has had in her airways for months. In addition, I prescribe albuterol for the first month and cromolyn daily for the long term.

Karen will follow this plan when she leaves the office after her first visit. She will continue to check her peak flow scores, signs, and symptoms and record them in the asthma diary. This monitoring will allow us to judge how well the plan is working. When she comes back a week later, we will discuss asthma and her specific management plan in detail.

At the end of our first visit, I fill out a Home Treatment Plan to give step-by-step instructions on what medicines Karen will take in each of her asthma treatment zones. While I fill out the plan for the chart, she fills out her own copy and we discuss any questions that come up. She leaves the office with a completed plan and her questions answered.

Karen is doing much better when she returns. She can sleep through the night for the first time in three weeks. She is walking without wheezing or coughing for the first time in six months. She has taken a three-hour self-defense class and did not wheeze. A one-hour hike did not trigger symptoms as it had four months ago. She has stopped driving to her distant classes because she can now walk there without any problem.

During the second visit, Karen and I discuss the many ways she can control her asthma, including reducing triggers, increasing her understanding of asthma and asthma medicines, monitoring peak flow, and taking controller medicine. Karen and I discuss what might be done to reduce the triggers she is encountering in her dorm room. I recommend that she encase her mattress to keep out dust mites, buy a humidity gauge, and keep the humidity between 25 and 50 percent to decrease the growth of dust mites and mold. I also suggest that she buy a HEPA air cleaner to reduce airborne dust, pollutants, and other triggers in her room. We make no changes in her medicine plan except to discontinue the use of prednisone.

Karen has previously had allergy testing that did not identify any allergic triggers. I think she would benefit from looking for additional asthma triggers in her environment. She agrees to do this by recording possible triggers in her peak flow diary. Karen will continue to monitor peak flow twice a day. I also recommend that she read *One Minute Asthma: What You Need to Know* and watch an asthma videotape. For some patients I also recommend *Asthma Update* (a newsletter), the NHLBI *Practical Guide to the Diagnosis and Management of*

Asthma, Children's Allergies, or *The Asthma Self Help Book.*

A week after her second visit, Karen is back in my office because she was wheezing following a three-hour welding class. Her peak flow diary shows she has experienced trouble with welding class in the past, but usually improved the next day. This time, she did not recover after class and continued to get worse. We decide to substitute an inhaled steroid for cromolyn as her controller medicine. The inhaled steroid will reduce the inflammation in her airways more effectively. Karen's daily medicine plan will now be 8 puffs of an inhaled steroid, taken in two doses. The rest of her plan remains the same.

Later that month, Karen returns with her parents who are in town for graduation. I tell them we will continue to adjust her medicines to find the lowest dose that will prevent symptoms. Karen knows how to treat the occasional episode that may occur. She is moving to Vermont and will make contact with a primary care physician to review her treatment plan.

FOLLOW-UP ONE YEAR LATER

Karen has been doing great on 4 puffs of an inhaled steroid and 2 puffs of albuterol each day. She had no asthma episodes in the previous year. She is in terrific shape, very active, and works out on the Stairmaster for forty-five minutes at 80 percent of her cardiac capacity. Two months after this visit, Karen is able to reduce her inhaled steroid dose to 2 puffs daily. She continues to pretreat with albuterol before exercise.

LONG-TERM FOLLOW-UP

I spoke with Karen in 1998, five years after her initial visit. She has had little trouble with asthma over the past four years. She stopped taking her inhaled steroid in 1996. She is in excellent health and works out five days a week. Sometimes, when she works out particularly hard, she gets a tight chest and wheezy cough. However, she can prevent this by pretreating with albuterol before the workout. She also gets slightly wheezy with a cold. But overall, her asthma control has been excellent. She has not taken prednisone, visited an emergency room, been seen by an asthma doctor, nor missed a single day of work because of asthma in the past four years.

Asthma Visits for Young Children

When children under the age of 5 come in for an asthma consultation with their parents, I follow the same routine as I did with Karen. I always recommend that both parents come in, or one parent and another adult, so one parent can focus on the discussion. Since young children usually cannot blow peak flow properly, we concentrate on learning the four signs of asthma. The parents learn how to observe and score the signs, and we develop a Home Treatment Plan based on them. Parents also learn to use a holding chamber with mask or a nebulizer to deliver medicines to their child. The timetable for follow-up visits is the same as for adults.

In the Emergency Room and Hospital

If your asthma is under excellent control, it is unlikely that you will need to visit the emergency room. However, under some circumstances you should not hesitate to go for help. You need to go to the emergency room if you are very sick or your doctor is not prepared or available to take care of emergencies in the office. "Very sick" means that you can't move the marker on a peak flow meter, your peak flow is stuck in the red zone, or you have one of the emergency signs of asthma (see page 44).

Before the emergency room staff can treat an asthma episode, they must evaluate the seriousness of your breathing problem. This can be done by checking your peak flow and evaluating the four signs of asthma. Often, the oxygen level in your blood will also be measured. A nurse or other staff member should check your peak flow at the registration desk to decide if you are in the red zone and whether you should receive immediate treatment. When a patient is so sick that her nail beds or lips are bluish, she is unable to speak in sentences, or is breathing hunched over, she needs treatment immediately. There is no need to check the peak flow.

If the critical signs of asthma are absent, you still may need intensive treatment. Often a doctor cannot tell how seriously ill you are by performing only a standard physical examination. Your airflow must be checked by measuring peak flow or FEV_1 to assess your condition.

I was asked to review the record of a patient who died an hour after she entered the emergency room. Her doctor wrote that she had diffuse expiratory wheezes but was not in acute distress. He did not believe that she was having serious trouble, but he had not checked her peak flow. If he had, he might have realized that her respiratory muscles were exhausted, causing her asthma signs to look less serious. Immediate preparation to intubate her probably could have prevented her death.

The 1997 NHLBI *Guidelines* strongly recommend that emergency rooms assess a patient's airflow right away. It is not safe to be treated in an emergency room that fails to do this. Doctors must understand how sick you are to decide what level of treatment you need. The basic medicines they will use to treat you in the emergency room are similar to those that you use at home: inhaled quick relief medicine and an oral steroid. However, the doses and frequencies are usually increased, oxygen is often given, and additional medicines may be needed.

The doctor and nurses will continue to treat and observe you to see if you are improving until they feel you are out of danger. If your episode is moderate or severe, the staff must make sure your condition is stable before you are discharged by checking your peak flow and asthma signs thirty minutes after your last treatment. They should also review your medicines and treatment plan with you and recommend a follow-up visit. If your problem does not respond adequately to intensive treatment, you should be admitted to the hospital.

DISCHARGE FROM THE EMERGENCY ROOM

When you leave the Emergency Room, you must have a written home treatment plan that you understand. If you received a steroid by mouth or intravenously in the emergency room, you should continue to take it for three to ten days. You will also need to continue taking an inhaled quick relief medicine and an increased dose of your inhaled steroid. By monitoring peak flow scores or asthma signs after leaving the emergency room, you can tell whether you are improving or worsening. After you are discharged, arrange for a follow-up visit with your regular doctor or an asthma specialist.

ADMISSION TO THE HOSPITAL

Admission to the hospital is necessary if:

- essential observation and treatment cannot be provided at home, in the office, or in the emergency room.
- quick relief medicine given by nebulizer is needed frequently or continuously. (Since this treatment should be given with oxy-

gen and requires professional observation and laboratory tests, it cannot be done at home.)

- your breathing difficulty is worsening despite intensive treatment.

In addition to the state of your airways, other factors may affect a doctor's decision to hospitalize you. Physician coverage of the office may decline drastically at night or on weekends, making admission to the hospital prudent.

If the emergency room is working with insufficient nursing staff or lacks proper equipment, a patient may receive better care in the hospital. If you are not prepared to continue treating the episode at home after an emergency visit, a hospital stay may be necessary. This will depend on your knowledge of asthma and asthma medicines, your skill in using various devices (such as a nebulizer and the peak flow meter), and whether you know how to keep an asthma diary. It will also depend on your doctor's experience in consulting with a moderately ill asthma patient by phone. Your access to a telephone and transportation are also important factors.

When a doctor recommends admission to the hospital because you are having an asthma episode, you can discuss your ability to handle asthma at home but don't fight the admission. Spend your energy on getting better, and making sure that you know how to prevent another hospitalization in the future.

AVOIDING HOSPITALIZATIONS

Doctors cooperating in a national asthma project were asked to analyze the records of patients they admitted to the hospital. In almost every case, they felt the admission was necessary at the time the patient was seen. However, they believed that most admissions for asthma might have been avoided if the patient had a written plan, proper devices, and medicines to take in a timely fashion.

The hospital is a good place to learn about asthma by reading, watching videotapes, and discussing questions and concerns with nurses, respiratory therapists, and doctors. If you learn enough about asthma and its treatment while you're there, you will reduce the chance of an admission in the future.

In Summary

To achieve excellent control over your asthma, you need the guidance of a doctor whose knowledge is current and who accepts you as a partner in management. You should seek a consultation with an asthma specialist if you fail to achieve excellent control. For best results, prepare for the consultation by writing your asthma story and keeping an asthma diary.

Chapter Nine

Asthma at School

You must work closely with teachers, nurse, administration, and other parents to ensure that your school's policies and practices provide a safe environment for your child.

■

Monica's Asthma Attack
Monica Cyran
Written in the 1980s

It was Friday and ever since second period gym, I was having a hard time breathing, but I was too busy and too embarrassed to go and use my inhaler between classes. We only have three minutes to run to our lockers and get our books for next period. By the time fifth period English came, I realized I'd better get my inhaler or die on the spot. That's when I went to my teacher, to ask for a pass to my locker. Of course she said no. I had tried to get out of her classes before. She yelled at me and said I should go sit because I had tried to get out and visit my friends during first period lunch (this is normally true, but this time it was different).

I asked her a second time if I could go to my locker and get my inhaler. She said, "No" again. She was especially grouchy because there were so many people around her desk. By that time, if she didn't let me go, I was gonna go without her permission and worry about it later. Then I thought, she already hates me anyway, I'd better try one more time. So I screamed at her, "I have asthma." (It took just about everything I had to say this.) "I have to get my inhaler, I'm having an attack."

"Go, go, go ahead! I don't care what you do anyway!" she said. So I booked.

While running down three flights of stairs to get to the freshmen lockers in the basement (they make us start at the bottom), I thought I'd never make it there. I was having a hard time breathing. I know that sounds dramatic, but I felt lousy!

I got there and just really wanted that medicine in my lungs so I could feel better. I felt so dizzy. Just then the nurse's aide saw me and brought me to her office. She sat me down and I was so weak I fell down and I passed out. All that because I do not bother to carry my inhaler — I know I should. Also, I took my medicine carelessly. It's too late now to say what I should have done, but everyone says, you learn valuable lessons from dumb mistakes.

Monica is a typical teenager. She did not want her peers to know that she had asthma. So she did not give my note (written several months previously) to the school nurse. Thus, the school had no knowledge of her condition. After this episode, Monica's mother wrote a letter to the principal with my note attached which explained Monica's asthma and her periodic need to use an albuterol inhaler during school. The principal made sure that all the teachers were aware of Monica's asthma so they would be able to respond appropriately in the future.

Once a parent has notified the school that a child has asthma, the school should be prepared to collect the information it needs to care for that student.

The child's doctor provides a formal, written diagnosis of asthma and orders for medicine that is needed at school. In most states, parents and the doctor need to sign authorizations for medicine administration and emergency treatment. This documentation enables the school nurse, other school staff, and the student's parents and physician to protect the student's health. With a good plan in place, Monica's asthma symptoms due to exercise would be rare. Her teachers would know about her condition, and she would have fast and safe access to her medicines.

Like controlling asthma at home, effective asthma management at school involves more than just medicine. It requires an understanding of asthma and how the environment can cause airway inflammation and symptoms. It requires monitoring of peak flow and asthma signs and use of a written treatment plan to enable school staff to make appropriate and safe decisions. However, school is different from home. At school, many other people make decisions about your child's activities and the environment.

Schools vary in the appropriateness of their policies and commitment to health planning, the physical conditions in the school building, the accessibility of a certified school nurse, and the level of teacher knowledge about asthma. Evaluate your school's policies and practices by answering the questions in "How Asthma-Friendly Is Your School?" (see sidebar). Students also vary in the severity of their asthma and their specific needs. The goal of this chapter is to identify important aspects of asthma management at school. Doing so will help you work with the school staff and administrators to ensure a safe and healthy education for your child. I have included references to additional resources so you can go beyond this introduction if you choose (see Resource Section and Bibliography).

Health Planning

In some circumstances, you need only notify the school that your child has asthma to initiate an effective management plan. In other cases, a more formal and ongoing planning process may be necessary. School health professionals have developed a framework for health planning known as the Individualized Health Plan (IHP). An IHP is a written record of a school's comprehensive health management plan for meeting a particular child's special health needs. Creating an IHP involves a series of steps to identify those needs, develop strategies to meet them, and provide for scheduled evaluation of how well the plan is working. The

HOW ASTHMA-FRIENDLY IS YOUR SCHOOL?

1. Is your school free of tobacco smoke all of the time, including during school-sponsored events?
2. Does the school maintain good indoor air quality? Does it reduce or eliminate allergens and irritants that can make asthma worse?
3. Is there a school nurse in your school all day, every day? If not, is a nurse regularly available to the school to help write plans and give students with asthma guidance about medicines, physical education, and field trips?
4. May children take medicines at school as recommended by their doctor and parents? May children carry their own asthma medicines?
5. Does your school have an emergency plan for taking care of a child with a severe asthma episode? Does it state clearly what to do? Whom to call? When to call?
6. Does someone teach school staff about asthma, asthma management plans, and asthma medicines? Does someone teach all students about asthma and how to help a classmate who has it?
7. Do students with asthma have good options for fully and safely participating in physical education class and recess? (For example, do students have access to their medicines before exercise? Can they choose modified or alternate activities when medically necessary?)

If the answer to any question is no, a student may be facing obstacles to asthma control. Asthma that is out of control can hinder a student's attendance, participation, and learning. School staff, health professionals, and parents can work together to remove obstacles and to promote students' health and education.

Contact the organizations in the Resource Section for information about asthma and for ideas to help make school policies and practices more asthma-friendly. Federal and state laws exist to help children with asthma.

Adapted from the National Heart, Lung and Blood Institute, National Asthma Education and Prevention Project.

plan should specifically address the areas of medication, environmental safeguards, physical education, teacher and staff planning, and emergencies. An IHP enables the school nurse to manage a student's condition at school.

Before your child enters school, notify the administration in writing about your child's condition. Ask your child's doctor to send a formal letter giving the diagnosis of asthma, documenting medicine needs, and recommending environmental safeguards and guidelines for exercise and emergencies. Request a planning meeting with all school staff who play a role in your child's well-being.

The certified school nurse should coordinate the health management team. Another health professional in your local health department, or the school's consulting physician, may serve as the team coordinator if there is no school nurse. In addition to the school nurse, other participating staff might include the principal or director of student services, teachers, teacher's aides, and other professionals.

In this meeting, consider the physician's documentation, orders for medicine, and recommendations for asthma management. These factors need to be examined in the specific context of the school and the classrooms your child will attend. Give the school the written authorizations it will need to carry out your doctor's instructions. You will also need to sign forms allowing designated school staff to discuss confidential information about your child with your doctor.

Several resources include sample IHP forms that can guide your child's planning team by helping you ask important questions and providing a framework for answering them. Consult *The School Nurse's Source Book of Individualized Health Care Plans, Serving Students with Special*

Health Care Needs, Massachusetts Comprehensive School Health Manual, and *Guidelines for Serving Students with Special Health Care Needs.* In addition, check with your state's Department of Education and Department of Public Health for guidelines for developing an Individualized Health Plan. The NHLBI produces "Managing Asthma: A Guide for Schools," which offers guidelines for administrators, teachers, coaches, and students, although not within the specific framework of an IHP.

WHAT IF THERE IS NO SCHOOL NURSE?

The development and implementation of an asthma management plan depends heavily upon the licensed school nurse. However, many districts do not have full-time nurses, or else they have nurses who provide services to many students, sometimes in different buildings. In either case, students may rely inappropriately on other school personnel to administer medicines or assist with health tasks. Because asthma problems do arise when no school nurse is available, the school administration needs to plan for safe delegation of health tasks. State medical practice acts regulate procedures for safe delegation. Contact the school health unit of your state's Department of Public Health for a copy of the regulations that apply to schools. Simply delegating a health task to a person who is available or willing to perform a task, but not necessarily trained or certified, is not safe.

If you are concerned about the lack of nurse staffing at your child's school, make your concerns known in writing to school officials. A school nurse is essential to developing the asthma management plan, training school staff, and making sure the plan is effectively implemented.

 AN INDIVIDUALIZED HEALTH PLAN (IHP) PROVIDES FOR:

- opportunities for collaborative planning and problem-solving among staff and parents.
- medically timely and convenient access to medication at all times.
- the achievement of personal fitness goals and safe participation in physical education and sports, field trips, and other special events.
- environmental controls and safeguards (maintaining air quality, eliminating irritants, allergens, pesticides, and other toxic hazards).
- coordination of physical, social, emotional, and academic goals.
- staff training and peer sensitization.
- academic and social continuity during periods of disrupted attendance.
- individualized crisis and emergency management.

Goldberg, E., "Individual Health Plans: A Strategy for Achieving Educational Equity," 1997.

MEDICATION POLICY AND STUDENT NEEDS

Just like at home, at day care, at a friend's house, or on vacation, your child's medicine routine is guided by the Home Treatment Plan. Clear documentation and ongoing communication with your child's doctor will help the school follow the plan. You and your child's doctor will work out the medicine type, dose, and method and frequency of administration.

When you discuss your child's medicines, explore options about the timing and methods of treatment. For example, you usually will be able to schedule use of controller medicine outside of school hours. If your doctor determines that giving controller medicine at school is necessary, she should provide specific written instructions to the school nurse on techniques for giving medicine, as well as the dosage.

The Home Treatment Plan also provides instructions for the use of a quick relief medicine at school, based on your child's peak flow scores and the signs and symptoms of asthma. The need for quick relief medicine can be greatly reduced by an effective asthma management plan that emphasizes reducing asthma triggers, monitoring peak flow, and taking controller medicine daily for persistent asthma. However, your child may need to take a quick relief medicine during the school day. He may take albuterol before physical education class, sports practice or a competition. He may need a quick relief medicine if asthma symptoms start during the school day. During an asthma episode in the high yellow zone, use of a quick relief medicine every three to four hours may be part of the medicine plan. The written Home Treatment Plan directs a school nurse or her trained delegate to respond to your child's changing asthma needs at school.

According to a ruling by the U.S. Department of Education, Office of Civil Rights, schools are responsible for providing students with reliable access to their prescribed medicines. "Reliable" in this case means that the child can quickly, conveniently, and safely get to his medicine and that school staff is sufficiently knowledgeable about asthma to care for the child's health and safety.

ENVIRONMENTAL SAFEGUARDS

Eliminating and avoiding asthma triggers can protect the lungs from sources of inflammation and reduce the amount of medicine needed to keep asthma under control. Just like at home, triggers at school need to be identified; then the trigger can be removed or the situation modified to reduce exposure. Peak flow is a huge help in identifying triggers. When peak flow scores drop at school, or asthma signs appear, you know that your child's lungs are responding to a trigger.

Teachers and staff can be involved in identifying these triggers. Because schools are complex facilities, an environmental "walk-through" can help identify conditions that are sources of air quality problems. It is best if known or likely triggers are dealt with before students encounter them. Because asthma is a condition that is provoked and aggravated by environmental exposure, environmental safeguards should be written into the asthma management plan (or IHP).

Some activities or rooms in the school may cause special problems for children with asthma. Field trips may bring a student into contact with an unexpected trigger. Sometimes a one-time exposure to an asthma trigger can cause a problem. My patient Robby predicted that he would have trouble attending study hall in the wood shop. He was right. Unfortunately, his teacher did not know about asthma and did not listen to Robby's concern. After the incident, I wrote this letter on Robby's behalf to the vice principal:

My patient, Robby, started attending your school September 14. On the 16th he was assigned to a study hall in the wood shop. He told the teacher that this would cause him to have trouble with his asthma. The teacher didn't believe Robby and made no change. Robby was in the wood shop for one hour. In the following two weeks, he missed seven days of school due to asthma and associated problems. I had to double some of his medicines and add an additional one in order to bring his asthma under control. Please be advised that Robby should not be in the wood shop, the metal shop, or any other place where he is likely to be subjected to dirty air.

Although he is only 13, Robby is a good judge of his condition. If he says he should not take gym, the school staff should respect that. His mother and I will follow up to confirm that he's not just trying to avoid gym.* I look forward to working together with you to see that Robby gets the education he needs in an environment that will be safe for him. Please call me if you have any questions about this letter or if I can answer any general questions about asthma for you. I enclose two books which I hope you will put in the school library as a resource for your students and staff.

The planning tools available through the Individualized Health Plan process could have

anticipated the wood shop problem, avoided placing Robby in a risky environment, and informed teachers that Robby was a good judge of his asthma needs. Guidelines in the plan could have made sure that Robby's teachers had the information they needed to make appropriate decisions that help him stay healthy.

GUIDELINES FOR TEACHERS AND SCHOOL STAFF

Your child's teachers may have little or no experience with asthma. The Individualized Health Plan offers an opportunity to provide guidelines and training for them. An informative booklet, *One Minute Asthma: What You Need to Know,* can teach the basics of asthma and the medicines used to treat it in about thirty minutes. Make this resource part of staff training, including it in your child's asthma management plan. Teachers who have learned about asthma will plan classroom activities and choose materials so every child can participate safely.

Part of the documentation you and your child's doctor provide to the school should include guidelines for avoiding exposure to asthma triggers. Teachers can integrate these guidelines into their lesson planning. For example, they will know to avoid bringing a guinea pig or rabbit into the classroom because it can provoke inflammation and asthma symptoms. They will know to provide alternative recess activities during cold weather or pollen season. Teachers also need guidelines to plan field trips and other activities outside the school building and instruction in how to handle asthma-related emergencies that occur outside of school. Good planning and communication help put teachers in an informed and comfortable position, able to consider the needs of all their students.

---

*The asthma plan for your child should include instructions that define conditions when modification of exercise is necessary. This will avoid the need for your child to negotiate with the physical education teacher.

Some materials used in classroom activities are not healthy for any student and put students with asthma at special risk. *The Artist's Complete Health and Safety Guide* discusses classroom hazards created by the use of some of these products and identifies safe school supplies. Although the book focuses on art classrooms, many of the same products are used in regular classrooms as well. It is a good resource for schools to use in developing guidelines for safe use of materials, and it directs readers to additional resources.

PESTICIDES

Does your child's school use pesticides? When are they applied? Are physical education and other teachers informed? Do students use areas that have been sprayed recently? Are applications on school grounds clearly posted? Are parents notified about pesticide applications? What is the school policy about using pesticides inside the school to control mold, insects, or rodents?

Pesticides present special health hazards for children, whose small body sizes make them more vulnerable to toxic chemicals and whose activities may bring them into closer contact with areas where pesticides are used. Classrooms may be treated with pesticides, and playgrounds and sports fields may be treated with chemicals (including turf treatments like insecticides, fertilizer, lime, and other supplements) which can irritate the lungs. Integrated Pest Management (IPM) is an approach to building and landscape management that corrects and prevents conditions where pests can thrive. These practices can greatly reduce the need for chemicals, protect student and staff health, and often save money.

PEER EDUCATION

Having students with asthma in a class offers a learning opportunity for everyone. These children are learning life skills that are important to all students: self-monitoring, taking medicines safely, and communicating their needs. Health management skills are part of many comprehensive health curricula. In addition, learning about the lungs, triggers, and the asthma reaction is well-suited to a health curriculum and can be integrated into many subjects.

The National Heart, Lung and Blood Institute has produced an asthma curriculum, *Asthma Awareness*, for elementary students, and a short video for school staff (kindergarten through eighth grade), *Making A Difference: Asthma Management in the School.*

ABSENCES

Absences due to asthma should be rare when asthma is well controlled by a combination of environmental safeguards, effective medicines and inhalation techniques, peak flow monitoring, and prompt action when symptoms begin. However, many students with asthma do miss school, sometimes for several days, and even a short absence can be disruptive to a student's education. When absences occur, teachers and school staff can help by planning for ways to keep students informed and to help them stay connected to peers.

PHYSICAL EDUCATION AND EXERCISE

The goal of physical education is to help students build skills for lifelong fitness and health. Exercise commonly triggers asthma symptoms, but students with asthma should not avoid it. Physical education teachers may unintentionally limit students with asthma, or they may push them too hard and thereby put them at risk for an asthma episode. Students with asthma may limit themselves if an activity is not appropriate for them, if asthma triggers are present, or if the situation is not supportive. Well-informed and thoughtful teachers can help these students truly pursue their personal best and gain confidence about physical activity.

Good communication and planning can help your child have a positive and safe experience during physical education class. The pamphlet *Asthma & Physical Activity in the School: Making A Difference*, developed by the NHLBI, provides an excellent framework for this planning. Its "Safety Guidelines for Physical Education Teachers" state that safe physical activity depends on:

- activities that match a student's changing asthma status and take into account environmental conditions (outdoor temperature, presence of allergens, etc).
- proper use of medicines before exercise, if needed.
- prompt use of quick relief medicines when needed.
- reliable access to medicines during exercise.

A physical education teacher can adjust the type, pace, or intensity of an activity when a student's peak flow scores drop, symptoms are present, or the student expresses a need for reduced activity. Because exercise is a common trigger for people with asthma, physical education teachers and peers need to be able to recognize the early signs of an asthma episode and know what action to take, especially in the case of a serious asthma problem.

Students whose asthma is under excellent control should also be able to play any extracurricular sport they choose. Exercise is discussed extensively in Chapter 2, "The Basics of Asthma."

EMERGENCIES AT SCHOOL

Careful planning can reduce the risk of asthma emergencies. Even so, a detailed emergency plan should be in place as part of the overall asthma management plan (or IHP). The plan should define emergency situations and outline sequential action steps to be taken by designated staff members. Anyone who is responsible for your child during the school day needs instruction in how to identify an asthma emergency, because she may be the first responder if a problem occurs.

A peak flow score that is stuck in the child's red zone is an emergency. The red zone should be clearly identified in the Home Treatment Plan provided by your doctor. "Stuck" means that the peak flow score fails to improve into the low yellow zone within ten minutes after the child inhales 4 puffs of a quick relief medicine (see page 196). Once the nurse or certified staff delegate determines that the child is stuck in the red zone, the child must be taken to a medical facility (emergency room or doctor's office) without delay.

An *extreme asthma emergency* exists if a child can barely move the marker on the peak flow meter or if he shows any of the following signs:

- gray or bluish lips or fingernails
- difficulty talking or walking
- difficulty breathing, with any of the following:
  - chest and neck skin pulled in (retractions)

– breathing hunched over
– struggling to breathe

In the case of an extreme emergency, the child must be transferred to medical care within minutes. The step-by-step details of this transfer should all be spelled out in the emergency plan.

Teachers and school staff must be able to identify an emergency and know that it calls for immediate action. A good emergency plan will apply to all children with asthma and specify exactly what a teacher should do and who is responsible for carrying out each step of getting your child to medical care. The specific emergency plan itself will depend on the child's situation, the school, the personnel, the rescue service available, and many other factors.

Here are some questions to consider as you work with the school to develop the steps in an emergency plan:

- Who gives medicine if the nurse is not available?
- Where are medicines kept?
- How do teachers and staff communicate with the nurse, principal, and people outside the school? Does each classroom have an intercom? A telephone?
- Are teachers and other staff authorized to call for emergency service?
- What is the emergency phone procedure?
- Do teachers and other staff know the signs of an asthma emergency?
- Do staff members who may be responsible for your child all have a copy of the emergency plan and understand it? Where is the emergency plan posted?
- How should staff deal with emergencies that happen outside the classroom?
- How is a substitute teacher informed of the plan?

- Has the staff rehearsed a health emergency?
- Does the rescue team include an emergency medical technician (EMT)? Can team members administer oxygen? Do they carry epinephrine? Are they equipped to administer albuterol? How close are they? What happens if they are unavailable?
- If the student goes to the hospital in an ambulance, who accompanies the child?
- What are the procedures for contacting parents? What is done if parents cannot be reached?

Legal Aspects of Asthma at School

The rights of students with disabilities are defined under three federal laws: the Individuals with Disabilities Education Act (IDEA), Section 504 of the Rehabilitation Act of 1973, and the Americans with Disabilities Act (ADA) of 1990, as well as state statues and regulations. Federal rulings on specific cases continue to clarify what these laws mean for students with asthma. Your child does not have to be classified as "special needs" to qualify for accommodation or special planning, such as an Individualized Health Plan.

The three sections that follow were taken from the works of Ellie Goldberg, M. Ed., an educational rights specialist. References to her work appear in School Resources (see "Resource Section).

A SCHOOL'S DUTY TO CARE

Schools have a "duty to care" shared by all staff members. This duty arises because students are required to be at school, away from their usual sources of protection (parents). Schools have a duty to exercise "special care" for students known to have physical handicaps, injuries, or impairments. This duty may require administering medication, monitoring health status, providing specialized staffing or training to teachers, and protecting students from emotional distress caused by teasing, neglect, or abuse. Parents cannot waive a child's right to proper care nor release a school from its obligation to protect a student from harm.

COMPLAINT PROCEDURES

When efforts to work with school officials do not result in appropriate cooperation and supports for your child, you should exercise your due process rights. Federal laws require states to establish a system for working out parent-school disagreements, such as arbitration, mediation, and/or a hearing process. Both IDEA and Section 504 oblige schools to inform parents how to file complaints and seek remedies when they disagree with a school's decisions or practices.

Every school system should have a "parents' rights" document explaining its problem-resolution process and naming the person to contact to officially request consideration for a child's needs or to remedy a situation. If your school handbook or school office does not supply this information, call the district's director of pupil services, director of special education, or Section 504 coordinator. If you cannot find the appropriate official, call your state's Department of Education.

Schools sometimes assume that informal arrangements reduce their liability better than formal documentation of procedures, roles, and responsibilities. Many schools do not document accidents, injuries, and medication administration, mistakenly thinking that writing things down somehow exposes staff to liability that they might otherwise avoid. In fact, a school's best protection against liability is having an ongoing risk-management process that carefully records assigned tasks, responsible parties, and ensures that proper procedures are followed.

Indoor Air Quality

The U.S. Environmental Protection Agency has ranked indoor air pollution among the top five environmental health risks. Inadequate ventilation and poor maintenance can make the inside of buildings two to five times more polluted than the outdoors. Up to one hundred times the concentration of certain outdoor pollutants have been observed inside some buildings. Poor air quality in school can cause a wide range of health problems for occupants, especially for people with asthma.

People who have not been affected previously by allergies or asthma may become sensitized by chronic exposure to a substance or even by a single exposure. One approach to avoiding this problem is to create an indoor air quality team that works to promote safe practices, good maintenance, and control of pollutant sources, and promptly reports health symptoms, poor conditions, or hazards. Keeping in-house records of the nature, location, and timing of health symptoms in the school is a reliable and inexpensive way to identify air quality problems.

This section discusses the basics of indoor air quality so you can identify potential or existing problems and work to resolve them. It helps for schools to have some basic equipment for measuring parameters that affect air quality. The U.S. Environmental Protection Agency recommends measurement of air temperature, relative humidity, air movement, and volume of airflow. These measurements provide information more useful than sampling for specific pollutants, and cost much less. A carbon dioxide monitor also helps in situations where ventilation with outdoor air may be insufficient.

Throughout this section, I will direct you to resources that provide more detailed, technical, and authoritative information about this subject. Some circumstances call for expert consultation and advice. The resources and problem-solving tools I list here can help you figure out when the school should call in the experts and whom to call.

The Environment Plays a Key Role in Asthma

You are about to read a painful story written by the mother of a high school sophomore with asthma who attended an unhealthy school and was also exposed to major triggers at home and in her neighborhood. These environmental factors led to life-threatening asthma.

Although Tori is not my patient, I decided to include her mother's account here for several reasons. It demonstrates that even parents who are health professionals may have difficulty putting all of the pieces of the asthma puzzle together. It shows how an indoor air quality expert may misjudge the importance of environmental hazards and that careful attention to a student's story can help solve an indoor air quality mystery. It shows how a drop in peak flow scores can be a sign that indoor air is polluted. Finally, Tori's story illustrates the hazards from remodeling and construction and how they can cause long-standing asthma problems.

Although none of my patients has encountered difficulty of this magnitude, some of their experiences have been similar. Studying this story can teach you a lot about asthma.

■

Tori
Beckie Willis
January, 1998

Tori Lynn Willis was a normal, active, 15-year-old girl when she started her sophomore year at Poteau High School in 1995. She was on the honor roll, elected class president, played basketball, ran track, and got the part of Esmerelda in the musical play "Sleeping Beauty." Everything seemed to be going really well. Then suddenly, Tori started being really tired and sleeping a lot more than usual. She got a bad case of bronchitis after helping our neighbor, who has commercial chicken houses, pick up dead chickens after a heat wave killed thousands of them in a matter of hours. We also thought the bronchitis might have been due to some remodeling and repairs we were having done to replace a moldy carpet and ceiling because of a leaky fireplace. We have more knowledge of asthma than the average parents since Bill is a family practitioner and I am a pharmacist.

But Tori did not get better. She asked for an inhaler to use at school. She had used one occasionally in the 8th grade and 9th grade when she ran track in the spring, but had used it only two or three times even though she ran the two

mile. She told us she was having to use it "a lot." We told her that her symptoms were due to bronchitis and to take it easy in athletics for a few days. Then, her coach called and said she had passed out in the locker room when she went to get her inhaler. The coach said he did not want her "dying on him" and not to come back until she was completely well.

A day later Tori passed out at a pep assembly. She was just sitting there, but it was hot and there were a lot of people crammed in the assembly. She woke up quickly and a friend brought her home. Bill made an appointment for Tori to see a pulmonologist.

When Bill returned from the appointment, he was very upset. Tori's pulmonary function tests showed that her airflow was very low and her small airways were severely inflamed. She was treated with large doses of prednisone, inhaled steroids, an inhaled bronchodilator, and theophylline in addition to the antibiotics she was taking.

Tori was given a peak flow meter so we could tell how she was breathing. She did get somewhat better and insisted on returning to school, but each day she would call me by lunchtime and ask to come home. She was scared. She was afraid to go to sleep because she was afraid she wouldn't wake up. We kept a constant eye on her with help from her friends and the school. We could not break the severe inflammation of her lungs and things just kept getting worse no matter what we tried.

And we tried plenty. We had instructions about bedding, carpeting, air filters, washing hair, cleaning house, pets, fumes and odors and how to live a whole new way! We went to asthma education seminars and learned things we could do at home and how to efficiently use her inhalers and medicines.

We made an appointment with an asthma allergy specialist in Oklahoma City, four hours away. I would have gone to the moon if it would have helped my child! The asthma specialist did extensive testing and Tori showed up allergic to sixty-two of the sixty-five things for which he tested her. We got more instructions about mold and foods and vacuuming and avoidance of fumes and smoke. This meant more cleaning and treating and adjusting. But we did it all. He left her on the oral steroids for two months and then tapered for two more months. He increased her other medicine doses, added new medicines, and allergy injections. We carried an Epi-Pen for emergencies.

Tori was angry. She did not understand what was happening. She was also scared. So were we. We realized that if she were to be placed in a situation where there were fumes or smoke or even someone with a strong perfume that she could have an attack and if she did not have her medicines with her and use them quickly, she could die. We felt guilty and blamed ourselves for not catching her asthma more quickly but her doctors all said she probably compensated her way through the mild asthma because she was in such good shape. Then she got ill so quickly we just did not comprehend the severity of the inflammation due to all the dust and ammonia at the chicken farm, and all the dust and mold from remodeling we were doing in our home. (I remembered that for the first two years of Tori's life we had been remodeling an old farmhouse. I could not keep her out of all the mess since we continued to live there while we remodeled.)

Tori wanted to go to school. She went to her play practice and continued to try to run some in basketball. (They have to run a mile in a certain amount of time to qualify for the team). This had never been a problem, and now she couldn't even get a fourth of the way without her lips and nail beds turning blue. She kept pushing herself thinking that she just needed to

be in better shape. The coaches did not understand either. Once she kept going, because they kept telling her to "be tough." She ran until she passed out and had to have an epinephrine shot. She was having trouble singing in practice for the musical now too. There just wasn't enough air. And, every day she called me to come pick her up. She would be exhausted, and she just could not get through a whole day of school. By Wednesday she usually was home in bed with bronchitis again. She said she just couldn't breathe at school. She went to school and her peak flows would be 260, but by noon they would be 220 or 230. By Friday she would be down to 230 in the mornings and 190 to 150 in the afternoons. At 120 her lips and nail beds turned blue, and it got really scary. Several times the school called us because she had passed out.

Once at a dance she had to go to the restroom and kids had been smoking in there, and before she could get her jeans up and get out, she passed out. It embarrassed her to wake up with everyone standing around her and her gasping for breath. Several other times her friends would notice her turning blue, and they just drove her straight up to her dad's office. It was a nightmare and we couldn't figure out what to do. The doctors looked at the peak flow charts, but really couldn't believe the school was bad enough to cause the drops in peak flow. They did not really know her like we did and I'm sure they suspected that she wanted to come home or did not like school. But we knew Tori, and the teachers and kids knew Tori, and we all knew something was wrong at the school!

Then at the end of October, during the state teacher's meeting, while school was out, we saw some improvement. We were hopeful. She had improved her peak flows to up near 280 during those four days at home. But, Monday morning, back at school, she called and said she was getting really tight. I calmed her down and she took some more of her bronchodilator. At one o'clock she called me crying and scared. I picked her up. It was the same on Tuesday and Wednesday and on Thursday morning she was at 220 and I did not even send her to school.

We put a HEPA filter in chemistry class to help with the odors and fumes in there. She wore a mask. She said the only place she could breathe was the library. I told her that did not make sense because it was full of dusty books and it had carpet, but she said that was the only place she could breathe.

The teachers provided her with her assignments in the library when they could but she just was not getting any better. On Thursday and Friday, they brought her assignments to the house and sent a teacher out to help her. We decided to keep her home all the week of Thanksgiving. She got better. After she went back to school . . . same thing . . . peak flows dropped . . . she got sicker and sicker as the week went on. I kept her out of school except for special events or special lectures she needed to hear. She could go to ball games and watch, except when the school where we were playing had a new gym floor and the fumes from the varnish made us have to leave after just five minutes.

People started asking us what was the matter with Tori. What emotional conflicts was she having? Did she hate school? Were we having family problems? If she was too sick to go to school, why could she go to other activities in town?

Then I remembered my friend who is an RN had gone through this same thing three years before. They were building a new home and suddenly Danielle, her daughter who was a senior, got very sick. She also was active in everything, a good student, ballplayer, and loved school, but she ended up homebound too. It was the same scenario. Then, I remembered how people said they thought Danielle had emotional problems.

And I remembered that I had even asked my husband, who helped take care of her, "If she is too sick to go to school, how can she attend other functions and not be bothered?" Bill and I called Danielle and found out all the details of her illness. Much like Tori, she just suddenly got bad and she couldn't get well, especially not at school. There was something wrong at school.

Tori's pulmonologist commented that he had another patient from Poteau High School who was having similar problems, but not quite so severe. I knew we had to do something. I called the Environmental Protection Agency (EPA) in Washington. They told me to go through the Department of Labor (DOL) in Oklahoma. I kept getting the runaround. Finally, I found an engineering professor at Tulsa University who was an expert in air quality issues. He agreed to come and look at the school if I could get permission from the school board.

Well, I realized this was not going to be easy. Bill decided to run for school board and make indoor air quality one of his issues. He won. Now, we could get the school board's attention and the administration's attention. Ironically, one of the school board members, a lawyer, had a son who had just developed severe asthma (by the way, they were remodeling when this happened). A second member had a son in the same class as Tori whose asthma was worsening. A third had asthma and allergies and his children had allergies. A fourth member was a doctor whose kids have allergies and Bill was the fifth. Bill convinced them to ask the engineering professor to come and test the school.

By this time, we had decided to try Tori in another school even though both her doctors doubted this would be all that helpful. We felt it would because we knew from her peak flow charts that she always got worse during the school week. In addition, she had gone through Christmas vacation without having symptoms.

We moved Tori in with my mother in our hometown of Vian, about fifty miles away, and enrolled her in high school there. She had cousins, aunts and all her grandparents there and knew a lot of the kids through them. She came home weekends. We cried a lot. It wasn't easy, but she was going to school and functioning pretty well except for athletics, where she still had to take it really easy. By summer she was up to 320 on her peak flows and she was off the oral prednisone.

Bill used reports from the engineering professor to bring in a consultant from the Department of Labor. The consultant discounted all of the professor's findings except for mold on the ceilings and told them to repair that. Bill asked the consultant to run a carbon dioxide (CO_2) test to determine the indoor air quality. She said it wouldn't do any good because we just did not have adequate laws to enforce IAQ problems even if we found them. She said the CO_2 levels would have to be 5,000 ppm or above before they could require the school to do something and that she had never tested anything above a 2,000. Bill asked her again to run the test. She did so reluctantly and begrudgingly.

When the tests came back, the levels in the old part of the high school were at 5,000 in all areas except the library, which had been added and had a different air system. Since the school had no fresh air, all the pollutants like the mold and cleaning materials were concentrated and recycled. Because of the CO_2 reports and the pieces of the puzzle which we supplied, the school board voted to do major renovations and completely revamp the heating and ventilation systems.

In the meantime, Bill and I came up with some new facts. He remembered several patients who had asthma that had gotten worse during high school and better after they graduated. Two teachers told us they had to be moved from the old part to the new part of the high school because of allergies.

Tori is a senior at the Vian high school now. She is salutatorian (she only made one B and that was during the homebound period). She plays basketball and was the high point at the last game. We attribute her improvement to environmental measures, and to the addition of a new asthma medicine. She loves school and is learning to cope and live with asthma. She is a member of the American Lung Association, Allergy and Asthma Network/Mothers of Asthmatics, and anything that has to do with lungs. She gives talks to kids in school about smoking and asthma and keeps on keeping on! She even used asthma and lung diseases as her platform in the local Junior Miss pageant.

Health Problems Related to Indoor Air Quality

For a student or school staff member with asthma, poor air quality can cause an increase in the frequency or intensity of asthma symptoms. A school occupant who does not have asthma may experience problems as well. However, people may not recognize that their symptoms are caused by something in the air. When only a few individuals are affected, their symptoms may not be taken seriously. Even when symptoms are widespread, they may be non-specific and not easily linked to poor air quality. Symptoms commonly associated with poor indoor air quality include:

- coughing and shortness of breath
- sinus congestion and sneezing
- eye, nose, throat, and skin irritation
- headache, dizziness, nausea, and fatigue

Symptoms related to air quality often begin or intensify after a person has entered the school building and diminish or disappear entirely in the evening, over weekends, or during school vacations. Individual records that include peak flow scores, like a daily asthma diary, can reveal a pattern in symptoms that identifies air quality as the cause.

Schoolwide data collection of symptoms is an excellent way to track down indoor contaminants and ventilation problems. A health log should record the nature, time, and location of health symptoms. These records may reveal certain types of symptoms that are typically caused by specific contaminants. The pattern of symptoms in a building can identify a particular area or activities for closer investigation. For example, when health complaints are clumped in one or two classrooms, the office area, or the gym, the air handling system and activities in these areas may be at fault. However, health complaints that are spread out around the building may be due to a single source because a contaminant can be dispersed by airflow patterns or through a ventilation system.

Understanding Indoor Air Quality in Schools

The air quality inside a school building is the result of interactions among many factors: the site and climate, building structures and construction techniques (including any modifications), the mechanical systems in place to handle ventilation, and the activities of the occupants, including introduction of pollution sources. Good indoor air quality management requires control of pollution sources, introduction and circulation of sufficient outdoor air, and maintenance of an acceptable temperature and humidity.

Understanding these components is a challenging task. However, you and other concerned parents, staff, students, and administrators can learn what you need to know to participate in indoor air quality management and promote responsible practices. The U.S. Environmental Protection Agency has produced two excellent resources to help you: *Building Air Quality: A Guide for Building Owners and Facility Managers* and *Indoor Air Quality: Tools for Schools*. These documents are essential guides for learning about air quality, creating a proactive management team, and dealing with problems that arise. The information below is taken largely from these documents.

MECHANICAL AIR HANDLING SYSTEMS

The Heating, Ventilating and Air Conditioning (HVAC) system in a school includes boilers, furnaces, chillers, cooling towers, air handling units, exhaust fans, ductwork, and filters. If it is well designed and maintained and functioning properly, the system should control temperature and relative humidity in the building, distribute adequate amounts of outdoor air, and isolate and remove indoor pollutants through air pressure control, filtration, and exhaust fans.

However, the HVAC system in your child's school may not have been designed to perform all these functions, or lack of maintenance may have compromised its effectiveness. Depending on a building's age, design, modifications, changes in use, and quality of maintenance, the system may not perform its job to acceptable current standards.

Ventilation rates specified by building codes may have been much lower at the time your child's school was constructed than they are now. The energy crisis of the 1970s encouraged tight construction with low air exchange rates to save heating costs. In addition, "uni-vents" in individual rooms may have been turned off to reduce heat loss. The American Society of Heating, Refrigerating, and Air-Conditioning Engineers (ASHRAE) sets air exchange standards that are the basis for most building ventilation codes. The 1989 standard (Standard 62-1989) calls for the introduction of 15 to 20 cubic feet of fresh air per minute (CFM) for each person in an area served by the ventilation system. Many schools were constructed at a time when standards called for only 5 CFM, or one-third of present recommendations.

Current ventilation standards (15 to 20 CFM) do not take into account the need for dealing with certain kinds of indoor contaminants. Toxic airborne substances must be exhausted to the outside directly from the source. For example, a metal shop should have a local exhaust system in place to vent welding fumes away from students, out of the building, away from air-intake areas. The same applies to construction or remodeling work being done to the school building.

Unfortunately, not all harmful materials are easy to recognize as toxic airborne contaminants. Schools are filled with materials, furnishings, supplies, and activities that can create airborne hazards. Students or staff with asthma are particularly sensitive to these inhaled triggers and may become more sensitive if the exposure continues. Although individual concentrations of specific contaminants may be low, the combined effect of multiple pollutants may be much greater due to interactions among them. Therefore, achieving and maintaining good indoor air quality requires your school to remove sources of indoor contaminants from construction, furnishings, cleaning, and daily activities. No ventilation system is as effective as avoiding the hazard in the first place.

REMOVING SOURCES OF INDOOR POLLUTION

Many potential sources of indoor air pollution exist in a school. Table 47 identifies typical sources of indoor air pollutants but is not exhaustive. I will discuss several categories of contaminants here and refer you to the resources mentioned previously. Manufacturer's Safety Data Sheets (MSDSs) for individual products provide safety information and should be available from your school's vendors. Set up a committee of parents, staff, and other concerned citizens to establish purchasing criteria for supplies and materials used by the school district. This committee, or an indoor air quality team, can also make sure that storage, handling, use, and disposal conform with manufacturer recommendations.

CLEANING

Good housekeeping is part of good maintenance. Regular and thorough cleaning of the school reduces the amount of dust and other particles that can become airborne. In addition to causing trouble for people with asthma, dust, lint, and other particles can clog filters in the air-handling system and decrease their effectiveness. Schools can improve house cleaning by damp dusting, using high-efficiency vacuum cleaners, upgrading filters in ventilation systems, and changing filters frequently. Carpeting poses special difficulty, as it can harbor dust, moisture, dust mites, mold, or bacteria, as well as other allergens and irritants.

To avoid creating health problems, schools should not have carpeting at all. However, if your child's school does have carpeting, daily vacuuming using double-thickness vacuum bags can remove allergens and irritants without putting them into the air. Removal of carpeting can provide a safer school environment in the

Table 47. Typical Sources of Indoor Air Pollutants

Outside Sources
- Polluted Outdoor Air: pollen, dust, fungal spores, industrial emissions, vehicle emissions
- Nearby Sources: loading docks, odors from dumpsters, unsanitary debris, building exhausts near outdoor air intakes
- Underground Sources: radon, pesticides, leakage from underground storage tanks

Building Equipment
- HVAC Equipment: microbe growth in drip pans, ductwork, coils, and humidifiers; improper venting of combustion products; dust or debris in ductwork
- Non-HVAC Equipment: emissions from office equipment (volatile organic compounds, ozone); emissions from shops, labs, cleaning processes

Components/Furnishings
- Components: microbe growth on soiled or water-damaged materials, dry traps that allow the passage of sewer gas, materials containing volatile organic compounds, or damaged asbestos materials that produce particles (dust)
- Furnishings: emissions from new furnishings and floorings, microbe growth on or in soiled or water-damaged furnishings

Other Indoor Sources
- Science laboratories; vocational arts areas; copy/print areas; food prep areas; smoking lounges; cleaning materials; emissions from trash; pesticides; odors; volatile organic compounds from paint, caulk, and adhesives; occupants with communicable diseases; dry-erase markers and similar pens; insects and other pests; personal care products

Adapted from United States Environmental Protection Agency, *Indoor Air Quality: Tools for Schools,* 1995.

long term, but removal itself is hazardous. It should be done under strict guidelines for contaminant control. In addition, be alert to the need for more frequent air filter changes after carpet removal to keep small particles (previously trapped in the carpet) out of circulation.

Cleaning can introduce a range of chemical products into the school, products that may be sources of indoor air pollution. Solvent-based cleaners are hazardous. Fumes and vapors remain in the building long after cleaning is complete. Simply scheduling cleaning for after school does not mean that odors will be safely vented. Schools are multiuse facilities and are seldom empty of all occupants. In addition, unsafe cleaning materials pose a special risk to the persons using them.

Find out what materials are used for cleaning and how they are stored in your child's school. You should have access to labels and Manufacturer's Safety Data Sheets (MSDSs) for these materials. Select materials carefully and be aware that "natural" or "nontoxic" materials are not necessarily safe. Judge them by the same criteria you develop for any cleaning material. Some preliminary recommendations include:

- Avoid solvents and volatile organic compounds (VOCs).

- Find out about inert ingredients that are not fully disclosed on package labels; though "inert," they may pollute the air.
- Avoid vinyl, products with formaldehyde, and other products that off-gas.
- Remember that "environmentally friendly" does not mean that a product is safe for people.

Some states and organizations are developing purchasing guidelines based on human health and environmental criteria. Other materials are listed in the Resource List. It is worthwhile to closely investigate materials in current use and alternatives to them.

GASES

A volatile organic chemical is any carbon-containing substance that becomes airborne when it is used or that off-gasses from a product over time. Such products and substances include paint, cleaners, glues, varnishes, pesticides, formaldehyde, laminators, photocopiers, and chemicals used in science, industrial arts, welding, auto shop, or other vocational classes. Any area that uses volatile chemicals routinely, such as a science lab or art room, should have a special ventilation system that keeps fumes out of a student's breathing zone. Depending on the material, exhaust fans or local exhaust hoods may be necessary.

Formaldehyde, a colorless gas and volatile organic compound, is released from many building products (like plywood or particle-board), wood furniture, carpeting, and some consumer products. This gas has a pungent odor, irritates the lining of the nose and respiratory tract, is considered a sensitizer, and can cause cancer. Find out if formaldehyde is present in construction materials, new furnishings, computers, and other purchases proposed by the school.

Carbon dioxide is not itself a toxic gas, although at high concentrations (15,000 ppm) it does cause symptoms of asphyxia (such as reduced mental acuity). Carbon dioxide is a natural byproduct of human metabolism, so the concentration of carbon dioxide in a room is one indicator of how well the ventilation is working. The ASHRAE standards recommend 1,000 ppm as the upper limit of carbon dioxide for comfort reasons. An elevated level indicates that ventilation is inadequate or that there is contamination from a furnace, vehicle, or other combustion source.

BIOLOGICAL CONTAMINANTS

Biological sources of indoor pollution include bacteria, fungi (mold or mildew), pollens, insect parts, and other allergens. Harmful bacteria and fungi flourish in warm, moist environments, such as damp carpets, moist insulation, or leaky roofs and walls. Contaminants that grow in the ducts, cooling pans, or other air-handling system components can be circulated throughout the building. Outdoor pollen and allergens can also be drawn in through open windows and doors.

TOBACCO SMOKE

Second-hand tobacco smoke, also called environmental tobacco smoke (ETS), is a common trigger of asthma symptoms. Even in people who do not have asthma, it can cause irritation of the eyes, nose, throat and lungs. Second-hand smoke has been strongly implicated in thousands of cancer deaths each year. People who are chronically exposed to secondary smoke are at increased risk of developing asthma and experience greater severity of asthma problems. Many communities have banned smoking in school buildings and on school grounds. Effective implementation of this policy protects the health of all school occupants, especially students and staff with asthma.

CONSTRUCTION, RENOVATION AND REPAIR

Construction creates dust from all kinds of materials, ranging from irritants to known carcinogens. In addition, glues, varnish, stripping chemicals and cleaners used in construction present potential health hazards. These contaminants can provoke airway inflammation and symptoms in an individual with asthma who is sensitive to them, and can sensitize individuals who were not previously affected. Any construction, repair or renovation work done to the school must be sealed off and vented outside and away from the renovation site to prevent the introduction of unhealthy materials into occupied spaces. If students or staff can see dust in spaces they are using (outside of the construction zone), it means that they are being exposed to small particles that can be inhaled into the lungs. Demolition, renovation, and new construction are hazardous activities and should be handled as such.

In Summary

You can work with your child's school to promote policies and practices that make it a safe and healthy environment for all children. As a concerned parent, you share many goals with other parents and school staff. Seek out your allies; you can't do the job alone. Build a team approach that deals with problems throughout the school, not only in your child's classroom. No student should have to take extra medicine because a building is poorly ventilated. No student should be denied medicine because the school administration has not worked out a responsive and responsible policy. Tools and resources exist to help your school meet the needs of your child with asthma.

Chapter Ten

Family and Travel

To keep asthma from disrupting your family's life, involve every family member in its treatment. A support group is often helpful. "Be prepared" is a good motto for traveling with asthma.

Asthma Is a Family Affair

Asthma is not fair to parents. Sometimes you do everything right, yet an episode disrupts a family trip or forces you to leave work to care for your sick child. Asthma is not fair to children. They must be more responsible than their friends in monitoring their bodies and taking their medicines.

But asthma does not need to stop your family from having a normal life. Parents can go out and confidently leave a child with asthma in someone else's care. A child can go on an overnight trip without running into asthma trouble. Siblings can understand that just because asthma is part of the family its presence does not need to overshadow them and their needs.

Asthma affects every member of the family: parents, brothers, sisters, and sometimes grandparents and other relatives. For asthma care to proceed smoothly, everyone in the household should be directly and positively involved. When both parents know the basics of asthma and the medicines used to treat it, they are much less likely to overreact or underreact to an asthma episode. Communication is easier if all family members have the same understanding and expectations. When this happens, the demands of asthma care are less likely to pull a family apart.

Some of my patients with asthma live in single-parent families. Most single mothers and fathers do an excellent job in caring for their children with asthma. But having a child with chronic asthma is a heavy burden to carry alone. To provide effective care, divorced parents need to coordinate the care in their different households. Parents frequently benefit from the support of other people in similar situations. Through support groups they cooperate to find practical solutions to problems.

In my experience with families, the mother usually has taken on the major responsibility for managing a child's asthma. I have also worked with some fathers who were more involved and knowledgeable about asthma management than their wives. In these scenarios, one parent ends up giving medicine, taking the child to the doctor, or staying with the child when hospitalization is necessary. One person invests the time in reading about asthma, observing the child closely, and becoming competent in providing care. And as one parent becomes more skilled and confident, it often seems easier for the family to continue in that behavior rather than teaching the spouse how to participate. This may be true in the short run, but it certainly is not true in the long run. It is really helpful if a spouse can take over some treatments in the middle of a difficult episode. It is not reasonable to expect one parent to work three shifts a day taking care of an asthma episode. Everybody needs to get some rest. The family will function better if both parents can stay healthy.

Ideally, both parents are engaged in the difficult task of learning about asthma and working out a daily plan to keep their child healthy. Both parents should read about asthma, especially reports sent home from doctor's visits and specialist consultations. Both parents should know how to use the important asthma management tools: the peak flow meter, metered dose inhaler, the holding chamber, and the compressor driven nebulizer. Both parents should know how to record asthma signs or peak flow scores in an asthma diary and understand what the zones mean. Both parents should know how to follow a Home Treatment Plan. Working together eases the burden on all family members and helps bring them together as they work toward a common goal.

▶ **TRAVEL CHECKLIST**

Before you head out on a trip, check this list to make sure you have the items you need.

- ❏ medicines
    - ❏ inhaled steroid
    - ❏ other controllers
    - ❏ quick relief
- ❏ holding chamber
- ❏ compressor driven or ultrasonic nebulizer
- ❏ peak flow meter
- ❏ asthma diary sheet
- ❏ home treatment plan
- ❏ brief summary of your history
- ❏ HEPA air cleaner
- ❏ Your doctor's phone number so you can:
    - • call for advice
    - • ask the doctor to call in a prescription
    - • have an emergency room doctor consult with your doctor

TWO MOTHERS' STORIES ABOUT LIVING WITH ASTHMA

Mike
Kathy Bowler
First visit in the 1970s

The main effect of Mike's asthma on our family is time. When Michael was young and frequently ill, he required a lot of time and attention quite often. I felt I could not go back to work since he was sick during so much (it seemed almost 50 percent) of the fall and winter. When sick, he needed a good deal of attention to keep him calm (some medicines made him awfully shaky), tempt his appetite, keep track of progress and medicines, scratch and rub his back (he would get quite itchy), keep him relatively happy (not being able to play with friends is sad), and in general to soothe, comfort, nurse, and get him well.

All this attention and special food and drink for Mike drove his sister into fits of jealousy. The sicker he was, the more attention he required, and the more concern I showed, the more attention she demanded, or tried to demand. For example, we left the children with my mother for a few days. Mike got sick, something my mother was quite competent to handle. She comforted and treated him, and in general was "nurse" for the day. She finally had him settled and quiet in our bed watching television. She got to the dishes, suds up to the elbows, and Cassandra appeared with "Let's bake."

Mother naturally replied, "Not now, dear." After some wheedling, the healthy child went and conned the sick one out of bed. Grandmother turned around to see Michael snaking on his stomach, head on pillow, wheezing away, going to play with sister-dear. When I spoke to my mother, she said she could handle Michael; but

Cassie, the one she always thought sweet and close to perfect, was driving her mad.

Michael also has numerous food allergies, which require his having different meals occasionally, ones his sister considers special, better. Maybe they could be considered special because, if you're making a substitute meal for someone, it's silly to make something they don't like. Well, if you cook special for one, why won't you cook special for two? Why does Cassie have to eat things she doesn't particularly like when Michael doesn't? No amount of talking would convince her that he can't eat it, it will make him sick, but it's good for her. So, I would cook special for her, too, sometimes.

Another difference I noted with Michael was that he wasn't invited for dinner or overnight as often as a well child. Other mothers were nervous; they did not know what to feed him or what to do if he got sick. I tried to make it clear that he's just a little boy who is sometimes sick, not a sickly child. He wanted to do, and could do, the same things as other little boys. He was just as strong and healthy, when not wheezing, as anyone else. Kids with asthma have a bad image. This seemed to straighten out as he got older.

With specialists, allergy shots, preventatives, emergency visits, check-ups, and medicines for attacks, asthma is not cheap. This also has some effect on the family. Some priorities have to be down-shifted to slip these expenses up on the list.

On the positive side, as Michael has gotten older a good preventive treatment program has been established. I've become aware of the do's and don'ts, and he has also. He's aware of the early signals and is able to initiate early treatment. He is less often ill and requires less time and less special treatment. He's happier because he's not missing out on things. This eases some of the jealousy from Cassandra, too.

■

Joey
Gail Platz
First visit in the 1980s

My son Joseph is 5 years old and has had occasional asthma episodes since he was one and a half. In August he had a mild episode, and as usual it woke us up at 3:00 A.M. My first response was, maybe it's just croup again, so we steamed up the bathroom for fifteen minutes and tried to read through the fog. Unfortunately that didn't stop the cough or slow his breathing rate down to normal, but he did manage to get back to sleep for a while. I have in my medicine chest an array of medicines but I wasn't sure which one to use or how much. Since it was still the middle of the night I didn't want to wake the doctor, whom I had just met the week before. At last Joey went back to sleep. The following day we took him in to see the doctor and got his medicine straightened out and his asthma episode under control.

In October we attended the Parents' Asthma Group. Finally, we were learning what was going on and how to deal with it effectively. One of the worst things about the asthma had always been not understanding it. We learned about the various medicines — which are used, how to use them, and perhaps most important, what their effects are. We got a practice inhaler and Joey has now mastered the technique for getting metaproterenol directly into his lungs. We also have a peak flow meter he can now use correctly, although it took him a while to learn.

Perhaps the most valuable part of the Parents' Asthma Group was finally getting to ask all those questions that arise, but that you don't feel there is time for in an office visit, or that get forgotten until the next episode. I learned a lot from other people's experiences and how they handled their situations. Another important element was involving my husband in the treatment. This has helped me to share the responsibility that I had felt was primarily mine.

In November, Joey had a moderate asthma episode and my husband was the first to notice it. This time everything was easier to deal with since we had a better understanding of what was going on with our son. We were able to bring the episode under control fairly quickly, and with much less anxiety. Joey was soon off to bed and slept peacefully all night.

Role of Family Members

PARENTS

If you are a parent of a child with asthma, you need to know a great deal. Talking with your doctor and the office staff and reading this book are good places to start. Learn the four signs of asthma or how to measure peak flow on a peak flow meter. By recording scores in an asthma diary and learning how to interpret them, you learn the individual details of your child's asthma, and deepen your understanding of asthma and medicines. Learn how to give medicines and what the effects of each medicine are. Then you can apply all of this learning and observation to helping your child's doctor work out an effective asthma management plan. The written Home Treatment Plan guides you in providing care at home. You can also use it to teach someone else how to care for your child.

Sometimes parents make assumptions based on their own experiences with asthma. For example, a parent may have had asthma as a child and been forced to "tough it out." This parent learned to ignore or downplay the importance of symptoms and needs to learn that these days a child with asthma can feel good and be fully active. I have found that parents are able to learn this much more easily for their children than for themselves. Then, after they see their children achieve excellent control, some parents with asthma realize that they can improve their own situation, too.

Sometimes parents have had very bad experiences with asthma as a child or have relatives who have suffered for decades with poorly controlled asthma. When these parents hear the diagnosis "asthma," they feel great fear that their child will follow a similar path. These experiences can be put in perspective as a parent gets reliable information about asthma. Discussion with members of an asthma support group can help, too.

TEENAGERS

Teenagers don't like to be bugged by their parents. Several of my teenage patients have worked out a system with their parents that lets them take on as much responsibility as they can handle safely. The teenager is in charge of asthma management in the green and high yellow zones. The parents agree not to ask the teenagers about symptoms or medicines in these zones. However, they can ask their child to blow a peak flow at any time. If the score is in the low yellow zone, the parents take over management.

BROTHERS AND SISTERS

Brothers and sisters are also involved in asthma care. Older siblings often remind a child to take medicine and serve as advisors to babysitters. They report symptoms to their parents and can also help younger siblings take an inhalation treatment or use a peak flow meter.

But asthma can also be hard on siblings. It can feel like the child with asthma is the center of attention or gets special treatment. Just as with adults, the more siblings understand and

can be actively involved in the asthma care, the more likely that they will feel in control of how asthma affects their lives.

I often recommend that parents read *Winning Over Asthma* to their children (see Resource List). In addition to being full of accurate information about 5-year-old Graham, the book has large illustrations of a compressor driven nebulizer, a peak flow meter, and a holding chamber. My young patients have become excited when they see these everyday asthma devices from their lives in the book.

Many of the families I work with have two children with asthma. They generally find that the experience and learning they had with the first child puts them in a good position to take care of the second. They also come to realize that asthma differs with each child and the treatment plan is individual. But they have the basic skills — they can score signs, measure peak flow, record in a diary, give medicines, and follow a plan — and this makes it much easier. Most importantly, they have learned from their first child to expect excellent asthma control.

OTHER CAREGIVERS

Many children spend a lot of time with other adults, such as grandparents, other relatives, teachers, and day-care providers. These adults need to know enough about asthma and your child so they can keep her healthy and safe. They would benefit from an asthma education session. Here are the minimum requirements I would recommend for an adult who will take care of your child:

- Read *One Minute Asthma: What You Need to Know.* This 56-page pamphlet covers the basics of asthma, medicines, peak flow, asthma signs, diaries, and treatment plans. It takes only half an hour to read, and later can serve as a quick reference.

Clear line drawings make the learning easy.

- Learn to score the four signs of asthma or measure peak flow. After caregivers learn these skills from the booklet, you should check to make sure their observations and techniques are accurate.
- Understand the asthma diary and how to record information in it. It should be clear what the zones mean and how scores are assigned to a zone.
- Understand how to follow the Home Treatment Plan and what to do if the child's asthma status changes.
- Learn to deliver medicines, including controller medicines, which are given each day, and quick relief medicines, which are needed if the child drops below the green zone.

This may sound like a lot for a person to learn, but remember how much you have learned. All the tools these adults need are at their fingertips, and they have you and your doctor to guide them. A written treatment plan based on the zone system takes the guesswork out of asthma care. It helps a caregiver make prudent decisions based on simple observations. With experience, they will solidify their understanding of your child's asthma.

BABYSITTERS AND OTHERS

It is often hard for parents to leave their child in a babysitter's care. However, with proper preparation, you should be able to go out and not worry. Most babysitters, neighbors, and relatives have little knowledge of asthma. The amount of information you need to give them will depend on the severity and frequency of asthma episodes, the amount of time your child spends with the babysitter, and the availability of other people who can help in case of a problem.

A babysitter should have some general knowledge about asthma, such as the information presented in *One Minute Asthma: What You Need to Know.* She can read it during the hour before you leave. The sitter should also have specific information about quick relief medicine: when and how it is given, desired effects, and adverse effects. She shouldn't need to give controller medicines, since these can be scheduled when you are at home. The babysitter will need to know the four signs of asthma, or how to measure peak flow scores, and what to do if your child's condition changes. Provide your babysitter with the Home Treatment Plan and explain how to follow it. Give instructions about whom to call in case of an asthma emergency. This foundation should prepare your babysitter fully for any asthma situation that might arise during your absence.

Sometimes in the midst of a particularly difficult episode, parents want (and need) a quick break. But they hesitate, even though they have a well-trained babysitter. This is when a cooperative babysitting service that has been organized through an asthma support group can be a lifesaver. Another parent of a child with asthma can give you the break you need without the worry. The service can be started during a support group meeting by signing up anyone who is willing to babysit or would like to trade babysitting, then sending a copy of the sign-up sheet to all who are interested.

Neighbors and children who are in contact with your child, but not responsible for her, should understand that asthma does not usually interfere with normal activity. Make *One Minute Asthma* available to interested adults. After they spend half an hour reading it, you can have an informed discussion with them.

Divorce

In families of divorce, both parents need to know about asthma and the medicines used to treat it. Both need a written copy of the Home Treatment Plan used in the management of their child's asthma. In my practice, the two divorced parents and sometimes their partners often attend office visits together. Doctors should do their best to communicate fully with both sets of parents and sent a report of the office visit to each.

Sometimes divorced parents do not see eye-to-eye on asthma care for their child. Often, one parent has more day-to-day experience with the child and thus a greater opportunity for learning than the other. Sometimes the noncustodial parent may feel left out or does not take the management of asthma seriously. This parent may fail to recognize significant triggers or may neglect to give medicine. On occasion, the custodial parent tries to use asthma as a tool to deprive an ex-spouse of visiting privileges.

It may take one or more educational sessions with me before both parents agree to follow the asthma plan I have worked out for their child. However, I have found that almost all parents eventually do what is best for their child. Your child's doctor can provide objective information to you and your ex-spouse and also help facilitate communication in the interest of your child's health.

Here is the story of how Helen Chesney and her ex-husband, Robert, resolved a substantial difference of opinion about managing 3-year-old Susan's asthma. Helen sent me this letter:

■

I would appreciate your advice and assistance in an important matter regarding Susan's asthma. Susan, now a few months past her third birthday, had a severe asthma attack during a Christmas vacation trip with her father. Because he did not follow the written medical plan, Susan became much sicker than on recent occasions when the plan was followed. I would be grateful for your recommendations regarding future vacations and extended visits Susan has with her dad. Here is what transpired, from my perspective:

Susan and her brother William spent a week over Christmas vacation with their dad, Robert, visiting Robert's brother in San Diego. This visit had been carefully planned and many precautions regarding Susan's asthma had been taken. The house where Susan was to stay was thoroughly cleaned and a cat that had been staying there was boarded out. I spoke to my former sister-in-law regarding other possible asthma triggers in the environment such as pollen and dust. I also explained that I was sending a detailed medication plan with Susan's dad but that if she had any questions or concerns during the visit, she should be sure to call me. Robert also knew I was home and reachable in case of a medical problem. I provided Robert with both your phone number and our regular pediatrician's twenty-four hour on-call number. I sent Susan's peak flow meter, since it forms the basis of our treatment routine. (She has been blowing peak flows for ten months, and her personal best is 105.)

In spite of the above precautions, a serious asthma episode occurred. I received a phone call from Robert on December 29, 1992 at 8 A.M. (5 A.M. San Diego time). This was the day Susan, William, and Robert were scheduled to fly back to New York. Robert, however, was calling to report that Susan was "breathing very poorly." He said Susan had started wheezing the preceding day following a trip to the zoo. Robert felt the zoo animals triggered the problem.

Susan was in acute respiratory distress by the time of this phone call. Robert reported that Susan's respiration rate was very high. She was having trouble drawing a breath and could not move the marker on the peak flow meter when she tried. He said Susan didn't even want to take a drink of water because she "couldn't breathe." Robert observed that Susan was having skin retractions. So far, Robert's response to these serious, clearly "red zone" symptoms was to give Susan one dose of albuterol with her nebulizer. This treatment had not caused the symptoms to abate. Robert had not followed the treatment and medication plan and did not give Susan prednisolone or seek medical attention prior to our telephone conversation.

I suggested that Robert immediately give Susan prednisolone and an additional dose of albuterol while I called our pediatrician in New York. He felt that Susan needed to be seen in California prior to getting on an airplane. I recontacted Robert, and his sister-in-law was able to make arrangements with a local pediatrician who is a neighbor and friend of theirs.

The California pediatrician (I don't know his name) recommended yet another dose of albuterol and said while Susan's lungs were still not "clear," she was able to move air well enough to fly home safely that same day. Robert did not administer any more medication during the next eight hours. When Susan arrived with Robert at JFK airport she was in poor shape. I took her at once to see our pediatrician, who was waiting for her at the office.

We spent the next two hours in the pediatrician's office trying to assess whether Susan could be stabilized without a hospitalization. She was retracting badly and her respirations were rapid (between 45 and 55 breaths per minute) and shallow. She was not moving air well. Our pediatrician gave her an oral steroid and administered two treatments of albuterol by compressor driven nebulizer. He allowed Susan to go home with the stipulation that I continue to administer albuterol every four hours through the night and continue to check her respiration regularly. If her respiration rate started to climb, I was to bring her at once to the emergency room. Susan continued to wheeze throughout the night; however, her respiration rate did not increase.

Two days later Susan was seen again by our pediatrician. Her left lung was still very congested. An X ray confirmed the diagnosis of pneumonia in the left lung. Her doctor continued prednisolone and albuterol and treated the pneumonia with amoxicillin. Susan improved significantly over the next four days.

My major concern regarding the above incident is that Susan's father did not follow the asthma medication plan I had given him. After he assessed that "something was wrong with Susan's breathing" he was slow to intervene. His interventions did not relieve Susan's symptoms. He did not seek medical advice in a timely fashion. The delay in administering medicine and seeking assistance allowed a mild problem to develop into a serious one. This caused Susan distress and almost required her to be hospitalized.

Certainly I would like Susan to continue to spend time with her father, but not at the risk of her health and physical well-being. I am not sure how best to protect Susan's health and would appreciate suggestions and guidelines for future visits and vacations. For example, as we discussed, would you suggest Robert restrict his vacations with Susan to places within an hour of a major metropolitan area medical facility? Could Robert receive additional education and training from you?

I am particularly concerned that now that the December crisis has passed and Susan is once again in good health, Robert views my continued concern about future possible travel plans as unnecessary. He has already indicated that he thinks that my reaction was "blown out of proportion." Any thoughts, recommendations and ideas to assist with the management of Susan's asthma will be deeply appreciated.

■

I sent this reply to Helen:

I have received your letter describing the course of a serious asthma episode that occurred several months ago. From your account, it appears that Susan's father did not follow the asthma treatment plan that you and I had worked out in August. Namely, he did not give albuterol when her asthma signs first appeared and did not give prednisolone when treatment with albuterol was ineffective. Robert failed to treat Susan promptly. In addition, he did not correctly interpret Susan's asthma signs or her inability to move the peak flow marker.

I agree with you that Susan should be allowed to vacation with her father. This can be done safely only after he becomes completely familiar with:

- the four signs of asthma trouble
- how to measure a peak flow score
- the function and use of Susan's asthma medicines, including their names, doses, how they work, and how long the effects last
- how to record Susan's condition on the Asthma Signs Diary or the Asthma Peak Flow Diary (to be decided)
- when to call for help

I believe that all of this could be accomplished with one office visit and some follow-ups by phone and letter. I have sent a copy of this letter to Robert.

■

Three months later, Robert came in with Susan to review her asthma treatment plan and to make sure he knew how to assess her status. He learned that when Susan is using the compressor driven nebulizer, she must breathe less often than 20 times per minute if possible, and her inhalation should take longer than exhalation.

After instruction, Robert understood how to monitor peak flow and asthma signs and keep an adequate record. We reviewed the purpose of giving the medicine listed on the treatment plan and when to intensify treatment. I told him that I would be available to answer any questions he had regarding asthma routines while he was out of the state on vacation. He agreed to keep Susan's record on the Asthma Signs Diary or the Asthma Peak Flow Diary twice a day and to read the 120 pages of *Children With Asthma: A Manual for Parents* that I suggested.

Two weeks after this educational consultation, Susan went on a three-day vacation with her dad without incident. During vacation the following year, Susan developed asthma symptoms, and her peak flow score was stuck in the low yellow zone. Her dad gave her prednisolone, extra albuterol, and arranged a visit to the doctor. She recovered without further difficulty. In the five years since, Susan has had no significant asthma problems while vacationing with her dad.

Asthma Education Groups and Asthma Support Groups

All asthma groups will be educational for you, but some focus more on asthma information, while others spend more time sharing experiences and supporting their members during difficult times.

People often attend asthma education groups because they haven't received enough information about asthma during visits with their doctor. In fact, it would take many hours for a doctor to convey the information that you need to manage your asthma. Reading a book and attending an asthma group are more effective and inexpensive ways to get much of this information. Many people also attend support groups to share their own experiences and learn how others have handled common problems with families, schools, work, doctors, and insurance.

Asthma groups have been launched in many ways. They are usually started by parents, patients, doctors, organizations, or a combination of these. One mother began a group because she knew she needed support in dealing with her son's newly diagnosed asthma. Another decided to start a group so she could share the knowledge she had found useful in the care of her daughter. National organizations, like the Asthma and Allergy Foundation of America (AAFA), provide free startup materials and guidelines. Hundreds of groups already exist around the country; AAFA can tell you if one exists near you. Some local affiliates of the American Lung Association (ALA) sponsor asthma groups. Many of these groups combine education and support missions.

In my pediatric practice, I started an asthma education group so parents of my patients could jump-start their asthma knowledge rather than picking it up bit by bit during office visits. The goals of the program were:

- to increase parents' knowledge of facts and myths about asthma, its treatment, and the prevention of episodes
- to provide a comfortable setting for sharing feelings about the ways in which asthma affects the child, parents, and others

- to build the family's skills in monitoring the child with asthma, recognizing the onset of episodes, and making appropriate decisions about using medicine, contacting doctors, and dealing with schools, friends, and babysitters

During the two two-hour sessions (one week apart), filled with information, demonstrations, practice, and discussion, parents had an opportunity to consolidate their knowledge of asthma and its treatment. They also discussed their feelings with parents who have had similar experiences. We worked to create a positive attitude by demonstrating that parents can manage various practical problems. Parents learned from each other how to cope with sleepovers, problems with teachers, dealing with doctors, and the fright of an acute episode. This learning among parents helped them feel less dependent on me and more ready to handle many problems on their own.

Parents who participated in the asthma group become more capable of monitoring their child's asthma and of handling episodes. Their increased knowledge and skills resulted in a more confident attitude and less of a tendency to restrict the child. The children increased their participation in sports and social activities. Families as a whole functioned better because the stress on them was reduced. Some of these changes are illustrated by comments obtained from several parents three months after they attended a meeting of the asthma group:

- I found out Lindsay's problem is not as severe as we originally thought. I feel comfortable that my doctor has studied asthma and knows a lot about it. I feel that information before a crisis is worth its weight in gold. We are now able to anticipate and organize things.

- I feel more secure about medication, and am not worried about giving Mike an overdose and killing him. I feel more confident about when he should be seen by physician. The Asthma itself is unchanged.
- am much more comfortable with Josh's asthma. Recently he started wheezing at wilderness camp 100 miles away. The nurse called, frantic, at 7:00 A.M. and asked me to come and get him right away. I assessed the situation on the phone and gave instructions to the nurse for treatment. Josh remained at camp with his class. I was able to go to work.

For the past few years, I have presented the basic asthma information to parents and patients in a single two-hour session. Each person receives a copy of *One Minute Asthma: What You Need to Know.* The booklet serves as the outline for the talk and a place to take notes, and it can be used as a reference long after the session is over.

Knowledge of asthma and the medicines used to treat it is essential if you want to manage your child's asthma at home. But knowledge isn't enough. You need to develop the skills to make accurate observations of your child's breathing, to interpret peak flow readings, to keep an accurate asthma diary, and to deliver medicines properly. Besides attaining these skills, you must develop the confidence to apply them. An asthma group can be a huge help.

Feelings

Asthma is nobody's fault, yet you may be angry that it happened to your family.

An asthma episode is always inconvenient and often disruptive. If you don't know how to take care of it, the episode can also be very frightening. When your child has trouble breathing and you don't know what to do, you may become anxious and scared. Your distress has an unsettling effect on your child. The only thing you can think of is to get help as fast as possible.

Your child misses school. You have to miss work to care for her or to take her to the doctor. You feel you are not in control of events. You have less energy to spend on other members of the family. Plans are disrupted. You have to cancel or cut short family outings. Your child misses a basketball game or has to cancel an overnight visit.

During the first session of the parents' asthma group (taught with my partner, Emlen H. Jones, M.D., in the 1980s), parents received basic information about asthma and the medicines used to treat it. Although the goal of the group was to present facts and demonstrate skills, it also gave parents a chance to talk about their feelings. Between the two sessions they filled out a feelings sheet, which we discussed at the second session.

Parents realized that they have a lot in common. In a group of twelve parents, several came up with the same words and phrases when asked how they, their child, and others felt about their child's asthma. For example:

What frightens you most about your child's asthma?
- She may not always be able to participate in any activity she wants.
- I won't know when or what to do.
- Possible ill effects of long-term medication.
- The possibility of not being able to reverse an episode.
- That the breathing would become so difficult he'd not be able to.
- I don't feel frightened anymore; we understand how to handle it.

What frightens you most during an episode?
- The medication is not bringing it under control and her breathing becomes more labored.
- He coughs and can't keep his medicine down.
- She has to be hospitalized.
- He becomes gaunt, frightened.
- I think that I am losing control.

During an asthma attack, I wish I were able to:
- Know why it's happening and judge the severity better.
- Help her relax, and have a well-thought-out plan of action.
- Feel sure about what I am doing right.
- Console him, encourage him.
- Breathe for him!
- Reverse it immediately.

I feel angry when:
- I have to miss a lot of sleep because of her asthma.
- An episode interferes with family activities for a prolonged duration.
- I sit here and feel that I'm dumb and don't know enough about what's going to happen.
- He won't help himself until the episode gets more severe.
- He does not take his medication and I know he needs it.
- He uses his allergies and asthma for attention or as an excuse.
- He forgets his medicine at a friend's house.
- I can't do anything to help him.

What makes you feel guilty about asthma?
- I don't.
- Not knowing enough when she has an episode.

- Not detecting earlier signs.
- Getting angry when he's sick.
- The fact that the asthma comes from my side of the family.

Do you treat your child differently because of asthma?
- I don't, except to check how she feels before she starts something strenuous.
- I overprotect sometimes, worrying about him more.
- I don't let him play as hard.
- I watch her too closely.
- I don't believe I do.
- I encourage him to learn methods to cope with asthma.

How does your child feel when an asthma episode occurs?
- Scared and angry that it's happening.
- Frustrated — "What, again?"
- Unhappy and sometimes frightened.
- Likes sticking very close to mom and familiar surroundings.
- Sick.

How does asthma make your child feel about him or herself?
- Different.
- Different from other kids and often angry.
- Frustrated that he cannot do everything he'd like to.
- Frightened, anxious, tired.
- Cautious.
- Like most other kids.
- Haven't noticed a difference.

Do others treat your child differently because of the asthma?
- They don't.
- They worry about medicine time.

- They let him take a break when he is playing sports. Otherwise, others don't treat him differently.
- They wonder how asthma affects her.
- They are overprotective.

I have found that parents' level of concern about their child with asthma depends on the age of the child, the severity of the child's asthma, and the ability of the parents to manage the child's asthma.

■

Starting an Asthma Group
Barbara Westmoreland

In the fall of 1989 my fourth (and last) child had just started school. I had relinquished my position as cochairman of the PTA and was ready for a little rest and relaxation. For the first time in years I saw new horizons. I would have time to pursue those things I had been putting off for years. The anticipation was wonderful! Then my 6-year-old son, Gary, was diagnosed with asthma. In a span of twenty-four hours my life was changed forever.

I was transformed into a fearful, anxious mother of a very sick child. My dreams of rest and relaxation were turned into sleepless nights and anxious days. I lived in fear. I needed help. I looked but could not find an asthma support group north of Boston. I leaned heavily on our school nurse, Ellen, for strength and support. She has a son with asthma and could understand enough to help me over the rough spots. I can't count the number of days I ended up in her office just for a few reassuring words. I pursued my asthma education by studying reams of books bought at the local mall. I sent for and re-

ceived wonderful materials from the major asthma organizations.

The thought of creating a support group came to mind, but I was not ready to make that commitment. I finally found peace when I made the decision to proceed. I felt I had an opportunity to help others who were in that horrible place between diagnosis and control, even though I still had trouble getting through some days. As a nurse, asthma mother and active school parent, I felt I was qualified to tackle this project.

The night of our first meeting will be with me forever. Four of us had planned the meeting and were we scared! What if no one shows up? What if too many come and we run out of room? How do you prepare for a totally unknown number of people? This is when top-gun support is required. Nancy Sanker, coordinator of support services for the Asthma & Allergy Foundation, provided me with a lot of guidance and answered questions as they came up.

Forty-five people attended. Their interest and enthusiasm carried us through the next months, during some discouraging times as we scheduled regular meetings and launched our newsletter. Three years later we're still going strong. Fifteen to fifty people attend each meeting and our newsletter goes out to four hundred people. The group has given me support even as I nourish it. When Gary is having a bad asthma day, I can talk with people who really understand. Their empathy is such a comfort. With their help, I can work through my asthma struggles calmly.

The group has given my life added purpose. I glow when I am able to help a kindred soul in need. My joy in helping others has lessened my anger as I confront my son's asthma.

Travel

PREPARE FOR THE SPECIAL CHALLENGES OF TRAVELING

Traveling with asthma often follows Murphy's Law: "Anything that can go wrong will go wrong." But there are many things you can do to prevent Murphy's Law from operating: hold to your usual routine, have a written treatment plan, and anticipate triggers that will burden your breathing so you can act promptly. Of course, managing asthma away from home often presents special challenges. You may find it harder to:

- avoid polluted air, especially cigarette smoke and cat dander.
- arrange prescription refills (although most out-of-state pharmacies will accept prescriptions over the phone from your doctor).
- remember to take daily medicines and keep track of medicines and devices.
- replace devices that were left at home.
- see a doctor if you need one, because most practices don't take walk-ins.
- get a doctor to understand your problem without your record.

Even so, you can travel with little difficulty, provided you have worked out an effective treatment plan, bring all of your medicines and devices, and keep clear of triggers. It is easier to prevent an asthma episode than to treat one, so it is important to keep taking your controller medicine daily just as you do at home. This is more manageable if you have worked out a schedule with your doctor which calls for taking medicine only once or twice a day.

It is important to bring your asthma medicines on a trip, even if you have had no asthma trouble for several months, even a year. Several years ago, the mother of a 4-year-old child called me at 3:00 A.M. from Ohio. Her son was having serious trouble breathing. She was on vacation with her family and needed my advice. She had brought no medicine with her, and the nearest hospital was sixty miles away. What should she do?

The only safe advice I could give her was to have her son evaluated and treated at the hospital. When she returned from vacation, I asked her why she had traveled without her son's asthma medicines. She said that he hadn't had symptoms for a year and she thought he'd outgrown his asthma. If this mother had contacted me before this trip, I would have advised her to come in for a visit before traveling. We would have updated her son's written treatment plan. I would have written prescriptions so that she would have medicines available in case of an unexpected episode.

A short trip or outing calls for planning, just as vacations do. Some doctors will recommend that a person who is allergic to animal dander take an oral steroid before visiting the zoo or a house that has cats. This is usually effective but should be done infrequently and only if there is no better way to deal with the problem.

One of my patients hesitated to visit his in-laws because their house contained smokers, a cat, a dog, and a carpet. He had developed asthma symptoms on each visit to their house, but he was able to avoid symptoms by pretreating with prednisone the day before and the day of the visit, as well as using albuterol according to his Home Treatment Plan. This routine is safe a few times per year, but certainly an alternative method should be found for situations that occur more often. It is best to avoid contact with significant triggers instead of taking more medicine, but that may not always be possible.

Bring a one- or two-paragraph summary of your asthma history with you on your vacation. Consider taking your HEPA air cleaner with you if you have the space. It can change a dusty room into a sleepable room. Sometimes the hardest task you face on the road is finding a healthy place to sleep. A friend wrote this account of her family's vacation.

Our main difficulty on last year's trip was finding a safe place to spend the night at a reasonable price. I stopped at a few places and checked the prices. One place seemed clean and was reasonable. Before signing, I decided I had better check the room. Good thing I did. It smelled musty. In my mind, mustiness equals mold, which is a major allergen for my son. When I asked if they had a fresher room, the receptionist asked which one of us had asthma. They must have had this problem before. It took two more tries before we found an acceptable room.

■

Emily: The Thanksgiving Disaster
Gail Hall
First visit in the 1980s

When my brother phoned to ask me and the two girls to join his family for Thanksgiving dinner, I was delighted. I was very ready to take a break from combining work, school, and single parenthood, even if it was only for two days. I think I would have been glad to go anywhere as long as it took me out of Amherst, but I was especially happy for a chance to enjoy my sister-in-law's fantastic cooking and to visit their new baby. Yet I couldn't help feeling some misgiving. On our last visit to New York City my 6-year-old daughter, Emily, had an asthma reaction to my brother's cats and we spent Easter dinnertime in the emergency room.

Emily had been diagnosed as having asthma three years earlier. Most of her trouble occurred as a result of infection; when she got a cold, she got asthma. Trouble with allergies was something fairly new. I'd learned a lot about keeping Emily well in my own home, but I hadn't really become comfortable with travel and the demands it made on me. One of the things I liked the least was imposing the asthma situation on other people's lives. I knew that in preparation for our visit my brother and sister-in-law would do a lot of extra vacuuming and cleaning to try to get rid of the cat hairs. They told me on the phone that they had kept the cats out of the guest room since summer. But even with these preparations, I knew I would still have to pay constant close attention to Emily, and hoped my monitoring wouldn't dominate everyone else's experience of the visit.

I planned for trouble as best I could. I let my brother know that I wouldn't make the final decision about coming until the last minute. If Emily developed a cold we would have to cancel our trip since I knew that a cold would send her over the edge if she were with cats. Three days before we were scheduled to leave I put her on the metaproterenol inhaler. I increased her dose gradually, from one day to the next, until she was using it three times a day, two whiffs each time. This gradual approach helps prevent adverse effects. I decided to use the inhaler, even though I knew it was likely that I would be getting up two or three times during the night, because she doesn't sleep well when she's taking it. That was just part of the deal. I also let my brother know that it was likely to be a very brief trip.

On Thanksgiving Day we took the bus to New York and arrived at my brother's before noon. After lunch and a turn holding my baby niece, I helped Emily with her midday medications. We were able to tell fairly quickly that things might not go as smoothly as we wanted. I didn't have a peak flow meter, but had developed my own system of gauging Emily's ability to breathe. It's important to hold your breath after using the inhaler so that the medication gets absorbed. But if you are heading into trouble with asthma, your breathing gets faster and holding your breath gets harder and harder. Emily took the first whiff from the inhaler and tried to hold her breath while I counted out loud, "One green elephant, two green elephants . . ." We only made it to four. After the second whiff, we got as far as six. The difficulty she had holding her breath let me know that Emily was reacting to the environment.

So I knew we were having some difficulty. I could have tuned into the situation more clearly at that point and decided it was time to leave, but I really didn't want to. I told myself that perhaps I had miscounted, or perhaps the inhaler would see us through anyway, along with the long-acting theophylline that she took twice a day. My brother and sister-in-law had washed the guest room walls and vacuumed the rugs within an inch of their lives. The rest of the house was also spotless, as always, and the turkey's aroma was filling the house with its promise of an irreplaceable family feast. It was definitely not the time to go home.

The rest of the day was the kind of balancing act I had feared it would be. When I took the suitcases upstairs to the guest room, it was indeed moist and clean, right down to the tenacious cat hairs which my all too wary eye detected. I kept an eye on Emily, shooed her away from the cats, and tried to limit her time with the dog she adored. After a while I sent her upstairs to the guest room to watch television. After our Thanksgiving dinner, the second use of the inhaler told me things were a little worse. When asked, Emily said she was fine. As far as Emily is concerned, what is ignored will go away. I began to think of ways to stay out of the house the next day.

The next morning Emily was having so much trouble breathing that even my sister-in-law knew Emily was fibbing when she said she was fine. As we worked on the second round of the Thanksgiving dishes, we devised a plan for getting everyone out of the house and on the road, in hopes of giving Emily's breathing a chance to get back to normal. The weather was nice enough to go to the Bronx Zoo, so we got people fed and left for the day. We'd be outside, and everyone, including Emily's 11-year-old sister, Adrianne, could have a good time.

I was being a little too optimistic, however. Emily was having so much trouble breathing that she had difficulty walking up the hills the zoo provided. My brother carried her while Adrianne limped along behind in the leg brace she was wearing for a troublesome but not serious knee problem. I watched the clock, trying to decide whether to leave enough time for a trip to my sister's pediatrician if things didn't improve. But we were having a good time and I figured the worst that could happen if we stayed was an evening trip to the emergency room as we had done last Easter. On that trip she received a shot of Sus-Phrine, a long-acting form of epinephrine which got us through the night.

At five o'clock everyone was tired. We used the inhaler again, but things weren't getting better. In fact, they were getting worse. The inhaler ceased being useful because Emily could no longer hold her breath long enough to let the medication stay in the bronchial tubes and have its effect.

From then on events progressed pretty quickly. I let my brother know that things were definitely not okay and we left for his house, not really sure what to do. When we arrived, I sent Emily up to the guest room. I wanted a minute to rest and think and I thought this room was the best place in the house for her to be. But I was wrong.

Unbeknownst to me, Emily was allergic to

more than just cat hairs. There were other things in the room to which she reacted. Within minutes she was in severe distress. Adrianne came downstairs and told me Emily was really sick. I said I knew she was sick and I was planning to come upstairs in a few minutes. Her real concern for her sister came through as Adrianne made it totally clear that we were needed upstairs NOW. I wrapped Emily in a blanket while my brother got the car started. We drove to the hospital with Emily lying in the back seat, gasping short breaths, no longer pretending she was okay.

We drove to the hospital in Bronxville where we had been at Easter. The same doctor who was there in April was not there now, of course. I brought Emily in and after the usual insurance procedures I told the nurse that Emily was having trouble with asthma, that I thought she needed an injection, that we had been there before, that she took theophylline, a 200 mg tablet twice a day, and that she used a metaproterenol inhaler, but it was no longer useful to us because she was unable to hold her breath.

The nurse spoke with the intern or resident and he came over and asked me what I thought the problem was. I repeated what I had said to the nurse and added that it felt that, given Emily's previous experience with asthma, the situation warranted an injection of adrenaline. "I think she needs a shot because the medication we've been using is no longer working," I said.

"I think you need to calm down," was his response.

I had entered the emergency room aware that I had to play a low-key role because I knew some physicians find it difficult to deal with parents who have a lot of information, and, God help them, an opinion. I understood that it was important to avoid acting as if I were going to be the one to make a decision. Instead, it was my role to simply feed information, and very slowly at that. I understood it was important not to irritate the people who had the drug my kid needed. In retrospect, I see that I should have followed this insight more closely and not suggested the shot. At any rate, I was not prepared for the level of hostility that I met, partly because it was not there on my last visit, and partly because I am never prepared for hostility.

We had to wait another fifteen minutes for the physician who was on duty. He was moving from bed to bed and it seemed that he had spoken with the nurse and the intern or resident. The fact that it was hard to tell who was who or who had talked with whom illustrates a device that I think people either consciously or subconsciously use in emergency rooms. That is, no one identifies themselves in terms of rank or name. They simply move at you and away from you without letting you know who they are, who is making decisions, what's going on, or what the plan is.

He finally came over and listened very briefly to Emily's chest. His diagnosis was, "This isn't an asthma attack." As he walked away with an air of disdain, he remarked over his shoulder, "She's hyperventilating."

I was amazed that he did not notice her retractions or that her inhale to exhale ratio was reversed, two signs of real trouble with breathing which occur with asthma but not with hyperventilation. I knew why he said she wasn't having an asthma attack. It was because she wasn't wheezing. But wheezing isn't an essential part of an asthma attack; in fact, you can only wheeze if some air goes through the windpipes. Emily wasn't wheezing because many of her windpipes were completely closed.

I started to stay something but he was gone. I was trying to hold out for a rational explanation for what was going on, but it was difficult. Perhaps the emergency room was truly overloaded with emergencies; however, all I had heard were two discussions of how to apply Ace bandages and where to go for a throat culture. While the physician was gone, the nurse gave Emily some oxygen through a nasal device. He returned, after another fifteen minutes, and took the device off Emily, saying, "We don't need this." He started firing questions at me about her medications and interrupting me every time I tried to answer. Finally he said, "We'll give her an injection. We can X ray her, too." After more delays and confusion she got the injection and X rays. To no one's surprise, she did not have pneumonia. As we left, I said to myself that even though it had been a truly unpleasant experience, it was over. We were home free. She would sleep through the night as she had done at Easter and we would leave right away in the morning.

We went back to my brother's house and I put Emily to bed. Soon thereafter, I went to sleep in the room with her. What I thought would be a night of much-needed sleep turned into a nightmare. Emily woke at midnight in real distress and beginning to panic. She was struggling to catch her breath with little success. The inhale to exhale ratio was reversed. She was exhaling with such difficulty that it sounded like somebody was punching her in the stomach every time she tried to exhale. I was becoming upset because I couldn't help her and things weren't making any sense. Also, I was going to have to get my brother out of bed and go back out in the cold.

When we got back to the emergency room, the intern, I could see, was not pleased to see us but was somewhat softened in his response. The other physician was gone for the night. The nurses were solicitous as usual and trying to be useful. I came with the fear that the intern would decide that the next step would be to give Emily more injected medication. On several occasions when she had had more than one shot in one day she had developed severe side effects. While most kids get cranky and nervous, Emily gets paranoid. She imagines that she is in danger, that everything around her is rotting. Her legs shake.

She has fits of anger. It usually starts with headache, pain in her chest and vomiting, and lasts for an hour or more. In short, a bad drug trip. I had gotten used to the vomiting — vomiting on the sidewalk is part of living with asthma — but I had never gotten used to that terror.

I went into the emergency room thinking about how I would have to deal with people who really didn't want to see me again. Last time, I just had to wait it out until they gave her the medicine. This time I was going to have to try to change their minds. I wanted them to admit her to the hospital, and give her medicine intravenously. She had been hospitalized once before. Oxygen and intravenous medication had brought the breathing under control and there had been no side effects. Also, if she were in the hospital she would be away from the cats, which had been the source of the problem. Even though at that time I didn't know how her allergy situation had changed, I knew something had changed. I knew I couldn't go back to my brother's house.

I presented my case to the intern: "I don't think she should have another injection. I know from my experience with injections that it might cut the symptoms in half at best, and — I don't know for sure — but she may have severe side effects which, given how uncomfortable she is now, seem like a bad idea."

"Well, who's the doctor here?" shouted the resident or intern or whoever he was.

I said, "I can tell you from my experience that we're not going to have any success with just injection. I can't go home. I either have to go to a motel room in the middle of the night, or she has to spend the night in the hospital."

"Well," he said, "we'll have to call in the pediatrician who is on call." I felt bad, I don't know why, about getting somebody else out of bed on a cold night.

The pediatrician came in about half an hour later and said, "Have you had this child desensitized?" It was 1:00 A.M. and a lecture on how he thought asthma should be dealt with was not of interest to me. I wanted my kid to be relieved of her distress. He ordered an injection, she got it and we waited to see if she would respond. I hadn't fought about it anymore, since I didn't see any other way to make progress and she needed something to help her breathe right away. The pediatrician was reluctant to hospitalize her. "I can't just hospitalize someone; she would have to stay for the whole day. We would have to do a lot of blood tests." What he really meant was he couldn't hospitalize her just because her mother wanted it. After her second injection, Emily was much better.

I leaned down to hug her and said, "You're being a real trooper."

"That's enough compliments for now," she said, ever articulate. The decision was made not to hospitalize her, so my brother and I headed for Yonkers Holiday Inn. Miraculously, the side effects never occurred.

The doctors, for all their obnoxious attitudes, had followed standard protocol for the treatment of asthma. As far as they were concerned, I was a crazy woman off the street, hysterical, and with a hysterical child. I don't know that I would have had much more luck in dealing with anyone, my sister-in-law's pediatrician or anybody else. It's difficult to talk anyone into skipping standard protocol for the treatment of asthma, and that's the dilemma of being away from home. As we arrived at the Holiday Inn, I seriously considered giving up traveling forever.

My brother left us and Emily and I quickly went to sleep. But at 4:30 A.M. she woke again, this time in severe distress and panicky. I spent half an hour trying to get her to breathe calmly, but again the inhale to exhale ratio was reversed, and her breathing was shallow, rapid and

out of control. The interval gave me time to think. I considered going to Montefiore Hospital, which Emily's pediatrician had suggested in case of emergency. Now I was sorry I hadn't followed his advice. But the fact was, I had gotten her away from the cats, the injections were now part of a pattern lasting four hours and she wasn't having side effects. We would be going back to Amherst soon. I might as well go back and get another adrenaline shot.

I called my sister-in-law, just to touch base with the world of the sane, and then called the cab company. We arrived in a taxi at 5:30 A.M. The nurse who had been there the whole time stared at us sadly as we came in. Emily went to the bed she had been on before. Her tears fell on the floor as she told the nurse that she could never go back to her uncle's house to play with the dog. The intern looked sympathetic. I wasn't angry or interested in proving that I had been right. At this point I felt as if were sleepwalking, going through the motions I had gone through before. She got the shot and they didn't record it. We were not billed for that visit but the other two visits came to $156. The motel room was $62.

I had asked the taxi to wait outside. Emily vomited on the sidewalk, and we got back in the cab for another $5 ride across Yonkers as the sun began to rise over New York. Emily said, "This is a big cab, Mom." I said, "Yeah, well, you probably wouldn't get to ride in a big yellow cab with jump seats unless we were doing this, so let's think of it that way." Back at the Holiday Inn, I called my brother to let him know we were back and I called the bus station to find out when we could get a bus. So far I'd had three hours of sleep. I was on automatic pilot. I'm glad my kid didn't vomit in the back seat of the cab, I thought to myself, but frankly, I didn't care.

I fell asleep for a couple of hours. At 10:30 A.M. I called my brother and said, "Things are better, but we'll have to move fast to catch the 12:30 P.M. bus." My brother picked us up and we drove to his house. Emily waited in the car while I ran in and threw everything in suitcases. My sister-in-law, as always, had the turkey sandwiches and celery sticks and ginger ale packed for us and my brother took a picture of Emily with her beloved friend Peaches, the golden retriever. We all piled into the car and headed for the George Washington Bridge Bus Terminal. When we got there, found a parking space and the ticket window, they said, "Sorry, that bus is filled. That's the express bus, you know."

The bus ride back was not bad: five hours on the local route, eating turkey sandwiches. I got several cans of soda into Emily and she actually ate some bits of turkey, to my surprise. We got back and it was 7:00 P.M. before everyone was settled at home. I managed to get a little more food into Emily before the post-asthma-attack complaining session began. She had behaved like a soldier through the worst of it, but safe at home, she began to whine and cling. There is a closeness between mother and child in a severe illness that's like infancy; so much attention must be paid to the child's body that long periods of time are spent in close quarters. Then suddenly it's over. I was totally exhausted. Adrianne was edgy, and Emily wanted to sit on my lap. But this was part of the deal. Somehow we got through the evening and Emily went to bed and slept well.

The next day it was hard to tell she had ever had an asthma episode. I sent her to a baby-sitter's and went to work. But Monday night she had a bad time trying to sleep, apparently a delayed reaction to the whole event: three or four nightmares, restless sleeping, waking up, and talking in her sleep. But that was the end of it, at least for her. I needed about a week of sleep.

Could any of it have been changed? When I talked with Emily's pediatrician, he was disappointed that I hadn't called him from the hospital. I had indeed thought about it but it seemed like a crazy idea. But in thinking about it more, I realized that he could have talked to the ER staff, and they might have listened. He could have given them a sense of her history and they might have been able to treat her more effectively. Doctors talk to doctors when they don't talk to civilians — that's the way it is.

■

Emily had a terrible asthma experience during the Thanksgiving visit to her uncle's family. The change in treatment that her mother and I had agreed upon — increasing the use of her quick relief medicine — was not adequate to prevent symptoms with the triggers she encountered. In addition, her mom denied the obvious signs that Emily's asthma was worsening.

After this trip, Emily's mom told me she did two things that changed her ability to manage Emily's asthma. She learned more about asthma in general and she changed her attitude toward it. She wrote to me about the trip.

On our ill-fated trip, I kept hoping that things would take care of themselves. I assumed that nothing new would happen and that I had seen the worst that asthma could do. In fact, hoping instead of acting on the problem ruined the trip. Nowadays, I start out prepared for the worst and begin treatment at the first sign of trouble.

With Emily's story clear in my mind I was able to work out a more effective asthma plan with her mother. The next year her family returned to her uncle's house for Thanksgiving. This time she brought a peak flow meter, a very specific treatment plan, a compressor driven nebulizer, all of her asthma medicines (including prednisone), and a letter from me to the emergency room doctor. She stayed in a motel and had no trouble at all.

Because of Emily's experience, I now make a point of suggesting a review visit for my patients to plan for any strenuous or distant travel. I update their daily plan and review the procedure for handling a red zone emergency. Patients or their parents carry an individualized Home Treatment Plan, keep an asthma diary, and know to start treatment early. They use a holding chamber (or a nebulizer) to take their inhaled medicines. (A doctor or medical supply house might be able to lend or rent you a portable nebulizer to gain more freedom of movement.) They have a supply of prednisone to use in case their peak flow scores get stuck in the low yellow zone. In addition, I give them prescriptions for an adequate supply of their daily medicine, quick relief medicine, and prednisone in case they need more during their travels. By the end of the review visit, they know how to identify problems early, to treat symptoms or a drop in peak flow promptly, and to call for help if improvement does not occur.

JESSE'S TRIP TO THE GRAND CANYON

My patient Jesse had been diagnosed with exercise-induced asthma when she was 11 years old. A couple of years later she complained she was "winded after half an hour of tennis and dying after running one mile." She continued her strenuous activities, controlled symptoms by pretreating with albuterol and at other times taking medicine in the middle of a strenuous activity.

In 1995, two weeks before a four-week trip of cycling, climbing, and hiking, Jesse came in to work out a treatment plan for her travels. Before strenuous activities she was to pretreat with albuterol. If she had symptoms that did not clear with 4 puffs of albuterol she was to take 30 mg of prednisone.

Shortly after the visit, she called from the Grand Canyon. That day she had pretreated with albuterol, hiked seven miles into the canyon, and then took another two puffs before heading up. She had a lot of difficulty on her ascent, wheezing if she went at more than a snail's pace. This difficulty was unusual, as she had exerted herself more in the past without any breathing trouble. Perhaps it was because grasses and flowers were blooming in the lower canyon. I suggested that she pretreat with two puffs of albuterol and 30 mg of prednisone before hiking the next two days. She followed this advice and had no further trouble during her next three weeks of strenuous activity.

In Summary

Everyone in the family can help to create an asthma-friendly environment by reducing triggers and helping the person with asthma follow the treatment plan. When both parents are involved in the care of a child with asthma, the work of achieving excellent control is less of a burden. With excellent control, both parents and children can lead fully active lives.

Asthma does not need to keep your child home from overnights or day trips or stop your family from traveling. Just make sure you have anticipated your needs and are prepared for emergencies. Asthma groups provide an opportunity for learning about asthma, sharing experiences and supporting members through difficult times.

Resource Section

Asthma Management Tools for
Your Personal Use

Feel free to copy these forms to bring to doctor's visits and to use at home in monitoring, tracking, and managing your asthma. The following forms are included:

- Asthma Peak Flow Diary, front and back (two pages)
- Asthma Signs Diary, front and back (two pages)
- Peak Flow Based Home Treatment Plan (one page)
- Signs Based Home Treatment Plan (one page)

You can use an asthma diary to collect and analyze information, to help you learn about asthma, to know when to adjust treatment, and to provide important asthma information to your doctor during visits or over the phone. A Home Treatment Plan should be filled out by your doctor to guide your asthma treatment.

ASTHMA DIARY
PEAK FLOW

For adults, teens & children
five years of age and over

O - Before quick relief
X - After quick relief

Name: _____

Triggers, Comments

Date

See back for instructions. Please bring to each visit.

Signs

◆ **Wheeze**

None	0
End of exhale	1
Throughout exhale	2
Inhale and exha e	3

◆ **Cough in past 5 minutes**

None	0
Less than one per minute	1
One to four per minute	2
More than four per minute	3

◆ **Activity**

Fully active	0
Can run short distance	1
Can walk only	2
Missed work or school or stayed indoors	3

◆ **Sleep**

Fine	0
Slight wheeze or cough	1
Awake 2-3 times because of wheeze or cough	2
Awake most of the night	3

Peak Flow Rate

Green Zone	100%
	90%
	80%
High Yellow Zone	70%
	65%
Low Yellow Zone	60%
	50%
Red Zone	

Medicines

* Inhaled steroid
* Other controller
* Quick-relief
* Oral steroid

Signs

Wheeze
Cough
Activity
Sleep

* Fill in the brand name of your medicine, dose, and number of times per day you take it.

From *Dr. Tom Plaut's Asthma Guide for People of All Ages* © Pedipress, Inc. All rights reserved. May be copied for personal or individual office use but not for sale or commercial use. Pedipress, 125 Red Gate Lane, Amherst, MA 01002 publishes *Children with Asthma: A Manual for Parents*, *One Minute Asthma*, *El asma en un minuto* and *Winning Over Asthma*. (800) 611-6081. http://www.pedipress.com

INSTRUCTIONS FOR USING THE ASTHMA PEAK FLOW DIARY
For adults, teens and children five years of age and over

This asthma diary can help you learn about asthma and asthma medicines. With this information, you and your doctor can work out a written plan that will help you care for your (child's) asthma at home.

❶ DATE: Fill in date above the grid.

❷ ASTHMA CARE ZONES:

- *Green Zone:* Your current treatment plan is effective.
- *High Yellow Zone:* Avoid triggers and change your medication routine.
- *Low Yellow Zone:* Intensify treatment if your peak flow score does not increase into the high yellow zone within 10 minutes after inhaling a quick-relief medicine, or if it falls back into the low yellow zone within four hours.
- *Red Zone:* Take emergency medicine and see your doctor or go to the Emergency Room if your peak flow score does not increase into the low yellow zone within 10 minutes after inhaling a quick-relief medicine, or if it falls back into the red zone within four hours.

Put your (child's) personal best peak flow score here: _____. This is the top of the *Green Zone.* Find your (child's) personal best score on the table below. List it and the numbers below it on the front of this sheet.

If your (child's) personal best peak flow score has not yet been determined, use the average peak flow score for your (child's) height from a standard chart, e.g., *Children with Asthma,* page 100.

If your (child's) personal best peak flow score reaches a higher level on two separate days, start a new section by drawing a thick vertical line to indicate the change. Enter the new numbers from the chart below.

❸ DAY/NIGHT COLUMNS: Use the clear column for daytime scores (7 a.m. - 7 p.m.) and the shaded column for nighttime scores (7 p.m. - 7 a.m.).

❹ PLOT PEAK FLOW SCORE: Use an "O" to plot scores blown before taking an inhaled bronchodilator and an "X" to plot scores blown after taking an inhaled bronchodilator. Estimate placement of mark between zone lines.

❺ PEAK FLOW TREND: Connect the O's with a line to illustrate a trend. Do the same thing for the X's.

❻ MEDICINES: Enter the name, dose, and number of doses per day for each medicine. Put one check mark (✓) in the box for each dose given.

❼ SIGNS: Sign scores are listed on the right side of diary. Enter each score by time of day. Cough is assessed during a five minute period.

❽ COMMENTS: Enter comments above the date such as *"Exposed to cigarette smoke," "Had cold," "Rabbit in school"* and *"Painting bedroom."*

◆ RELATIONSHIPS: Try to see connections between triggers, medicines and signs. For example, did peak flow drop after contact with a cat or a rabbit? Does peak flow always change with a cold? If not, why not? Any time there is a change in peak flow, you should look for a trigger.

◆ ILLNESS: If you (or your child) are sick, and you want to record peak flow more often, use several sections to record each day.

SAMPLE DIARY:

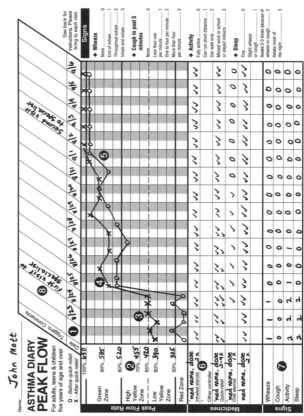

Personal Best - 100%	100	110	120	130	140	150	160	170	180	190	200	210	220	230	240	250	260	270	280	290	300	310	320	330	340	350	360	370	380	390	400	420	440	460	480	500	520	540	560	580	600	620	640	660	680	700	720	740	760	780
90%	90	100	110	120	125	135	145	150	160	170	180	190	195	205	215	225	235	240	250	260	270	280	285	295	305	315	325	330	340	350	360	375	395	415	430	450	465	485	505	520	540	555	575	595	610	630	645	665	685	700
80%	80	90	95	105	110	120	130	135	145	150	160	170	175	185	190	200	210	215	225	230	240	250	255	265	275	280	290	295	305	310	320	335	350	370	385	400	415	430	450	465	480	495	510	530	545	560	575	590	610	625
70%	70	75	85	90	95	105	110	120	125	130	140	145	155	160	165	175	180	190	195	200	210	215	225	230	235	245	250	260	265	270	280	295	305	320	335	350	365	375	390	405	420	435	445	460	475	490	505	515	530	545
65%	65	70	80	85	90	100	105	110	115	125	130	135	145	150	155	160	170	175	180	190	195	200	210	215	220	230	235	240	245	255	260	275	285	300	310	325	340	350	365	375	390	405	415	430	440	455	470	480	495	505
60%	60	65	75	80	85	90	95	105	110	115	120	130	135	140	145	150	160	165	170	175	180	185	190	200	205	210	215	225	230	235	240	250	265	275	285	300	310	325	335	345	360	370	385	395	405	420	430	445	455	465
50%	50	55	60	65	70	75	80	85	90	95	100	105	110	115	120	125	130	135	140	145	150	155	160	165	170	175	180	185	190	195	200	210	220	230	240	250	260	270	280	290	300	310	320	330	340	350	360	370	380	390

ASTHMA DIARY
SIGNS

For children under five years of age

O - Before quick relief
X - After quick relief

Name: _____

Date

Triggers, Comments

SIGNS

SIGNS
- Cough
- Wheeze
- Chest skin
- Breathing faster

TOTAL:

ZONES

Green Zone	0
	1
High Yellow Zone	2
	3
	4
	5
Low Yellow Zone	6
	7
	8
Red Zone	9

MEDICINES

* Cromolyn
* Inhaled steroid
* Quick relief
* O'ral steroid

DAILY

- Activity
- Sleep

See back for instructions. Please bring to each visit.

SIGNS

◆ **Cough in past 5 minutes**
- None 0
- Less than 1 per minute 1
- 1 - 4 per minute 2
- More than 4 per minute 3

◆ **Wheeze**
- None 0
- End of exhale 1
- Throughout exhale 3
- Inhale and exhale 5

◆ **Sucking in chest skin**
- None 0
- Barely noticeable 1
- Obvious 3
- Severe 5

◆ **Breathing faster**
- None 0
- Slight increase 1
- Up to 100% increase 2
- Over 100% increase 3

DAILY ROUTINE

◆ **Activity**
- Fully active 0
- Runs less 1
- Plays quietly 2
- Sleeps during day 3

◆ **Sleep**
- Fine 0
- Slight wheeze or cough 1
- Awake 2 - 3 times because of wheeze or cough 2
- Awake most of the night ... 3

---

* Fill in the brand name of your medicine, dose, and number of times per day you take it.

From *Dr. Tom Plaut's Asthma Guide for People of All Ages* © Pedipress, Inc. All rights reserved. May be copied for personal or individual office use but not for sale or commercial use. Pedipress, 125 Red Gate Lane, Amherst, MA 01002 publishes *Children with Asthma: A Manual for Parents*, *One Minute Asthma*, *El asma en un minuto* and *Winning Over Asthma*. (800) 611-6081. http://www.pedipress.com

INSTRUCTIONS FOR ASTHMA SIGNS DIARY
For children under five years of age

This asthma diary can help you learn about asthma and asthma medicines. With this information you and your doctor can work out a written plan that will help you care for your child's asthma at home.

❶ DATE: Fill in the date at the top of the chart.

❷ DAY/NIGHT COLUMNS: Use the clear column for daytime scores (7 a.m. - 7 p.m.) and the shaded column for nighttime scores (7 p.m. - 7 a.m.). See also "Charting Before and After Quick Relief Medicine."

❸ SCORING ASTHMA SIGNS: Before giving medicine, determine the score for each asthma sign using the guide on the right side of the diary. Enter your child's asthma score for each of the four signs. Add up scores and place sum in the *"Total"* row.

Graph the total score obtained by placing an "O" in the *"Zones"* section of the graph.

❹ ASTHMA CARE ZONES:

- *Green Zone:* Your current treatment plan is effective.
- *High Yellow Zone:* Avoid triggers and change medication routine.
- *Low Yellow Zone:* Intensify treatment if your child's total asthma signs score does not increase into the High Yellow Zone within 10 minutes after inhaling a quick relief medicine, or if the score falls back into the Low Yellow Zone within four hours.
- *Red Zone:* Give emergency medicine and see your doctor or go to the Emergency Room if your child's total asthma signs score does not increase into the Low Yellow Zone within 10 minutes after inhaling a quick relief medicine, or if the score falls back into the Red Zone within four hours.

❺ ASTHMA SIGN PATTERN: Connect the O's to determine a pattern.

❻ MEDICINES: Enter the name, dose and number of doses per day for each medicine. Put a check mark (✓) in the box for each dose given. Use blank spaces to record additional medicines, symptoms or comments.

❼ DAILY: Score sleep and activity according to guide on right side of diary. Put numbers in columns daily.

❽ COMMENTS: Enter comments above the date, such as *"Exposed to cigarette smoke," "Had cold," "Rabbit in day care"* and *"Painting bedroom."*

◆ RELATIONSHIPS: Try to see the connections between triggers, medicines and symptoms. For example, do sign scores increase after contact with a cat or rabbit? Do sign scores change with a cold? If not, why not? Any time there's a change in sign scores, you should look for a trigger.

◆ ILLNESS: If your child is sick and you want to record signs more often, use several sections to record each day.

◆ CHARTING BEFORE AND AFTER QUICK RELIEF MEDICINE: You can use the diary to monitor your child's progress during an asthma episode.

In this case, use the clear column for before giving quick relief medicine and the shaded column for after. In the *"Zones"* section, use an "O" to plot total score before giving a quick relief medicine and an "X" after.

◆ FREQUENCY: Many parents plot asthma scores twice a day for two or three months until their child is in the green zone daily for a full month. Then they reduce the frequency.

SAMPLE DIARY:

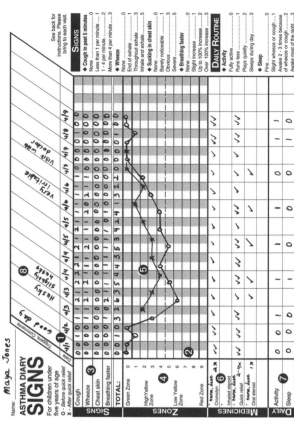

Name: Maya Jones

From *Dr. Tom Plaut's Asthma Guide for People of All Ages* © Pedipress, Inc. All rights reserved. May be copied for personal or individual office use but not for sale or commercial use. Pedipress, 125 Red Gate Lane, Amherst, MA 01002 publishes *Children with Asthma: A Manual for Parents, One Minute Asthma, Asma en un minuto* and *Winning Over Asthma*. (800) 611-6081. http://www.pedipress.com

For Adults, Teens and Children Age 5 and Over
PEAK FLOW BASED HOME TREATMENT PLAN
Do not guess. Call the doctor If you have any questions about this plan.

Name: _____   Date: _____   Best Peak Flow: _____

GREEN ZONE: peak flow between _____ and _____.

- **Normal activity.**
  - ❑ Quick relief medicine _____ : 1 or 2 puffs 15 minutes before exercise.
  - ❑ Nedocromil or cromolyn _____ : 2 puffs before contact with cat or other allergens.
- **Medicine to be taken every day:**
  - ❑ Inhaled steroid _____ : ____ puffs by holding chamber ____ times a day.
  - ❑ Other controller medicine _____ : _____ .
  - ❑ Quick relief medicine _____ : ____ puffs before taking inhaled controller medicine for the first month.

HIGH YELLOW ZONE: peak flow between _____ and _____.

- **Eliminate triggers and change medicines. No strenuous exercise.**
- **Medicines to be taken:**
  - ❑ Quick relief medicine: ____ puffs ____ to ____ times in 24 hours. Continue until peak flow is in the Green Zone for 2 days.
  - ❑ Double dose of inhaled steroids to ____ puffs ____ times per day. Continue until peak flow is in the Green Zone for as long as it was in the Yellow Zone.
  - ❑ Continue other controller medicines as instructed in the Green Zone.

LOW YELLOW ZONE: peak flow between _____ and _____.

- ✓ Take 4 puffs of quick relief medicine.
- ✓ Check your peak flow again 10 minutes after inhaling quick relief medicine.

  If your score has increased into the High Yellow Zone, follow the High Yellow Zone plan and continue to check peak flow every 1 to 2 hours.

  If your score is still In the Low Yellow Zone, or falls back into the Low Yellow Zone in less than 4 hours, follow the Low Yellow Zone plan (below):
  - ❑ Continue treatment with High Yellow Zone medicines as above.
  - ❑ Add oral steroid* ____ mg immediately. Continue daily until peak flow scores are in the Green Zone for at least 24 hours.
  - ❑ Please call the office before starting oral steroid.

  * If your condition does not improve within 2 days after starting oral steroid, or if peak flow does not reach the Green Zone within 7 days of treatment, see your doctor.

RED ZONE: peak flow score less than _____.

- ✓ Take 4 puffs of quick relief medicine.
- ✓ Take oral steroid ____ mg immediately.
- ✓ Check your peak flow again 10 minutes after inhaling quick relief medicine.
  - If your peak flow score has increased into the Low Yellow Zone, follow the Low Yellow Zone plan and continue to check peak flow every 1 to 2 hours.
  - If your peak flow score is still in the Red Zone, or falls back into the Red Zone within 4 hours, visit your doctor or **GO TO THE EMERGENCY ROOM NOW**.

Green Zone

High Yellow Zone

Low Yellow Zone

Red Zone

For Children Under Age 5
SIGNS BASED HOME TREATMENT PLAN
Do not guess. Call the doctor if you have any questions about this plan.

Name: _____   Date: _____

Green Zone

GREEN ZONE: absolutely no cough, wheeze, breathing faster or sucking in of the chest skin.

- **Normal activity.**
- **Medicine to be taken every day:**
  - ❏ Cromolyn _____ : _____ ampules _____ times a day.
  - ❏ Inhaled steroid _____ : _____ puffs _____ times a day by holding chamber with mask.
  - ❏ Quick relief medicine _____ : 0. _____ cc by compressor-driven nebulizer with each cromolyn dose for the first month OR give _____ puffs from MDI by holding chamber with mask before each inhaled steroid dose for the first month.

High Yellow Zone

HIGH YELLOW ZONE: total asthma signs score 1 to 4 measured before inhaling quick relief medicine.

- **Eliminate triggers and add medicines. No strenuous exercise.**
- **Medicine to be taken:**
  - ❏ Cromolyn: as above.
  - ❏ Double dose of inhaled steroid to _____ puffs _____ times a day. Continue until signs score is in the Green Zone as long as it was in the High Yellow Zone.
  - ❏ Quick relief medicine 0. _____ cc by compressor-driven nebulizer with each cromolyn dose OR give _____ puffs from MDI by holding chamber with mask before each inhaled steroid dose. Give _____ to _____ times in 24 hours.* Continue until signs score is _____ for 2 days.
  - * If you need to give more than 6 treatments of quick relief medicine in 24 hours, start the Low Yellow Zone plan.

Treatment Plan based on total score of all 4 signs:

Cough in past 5 minutes
None..0
Less than 1 per minute 1
1 - 4 per minute 2
More than 4 per minute 3

Wheeze
None 0
End of exhale.........................1
Throughout exhale 3
Inhale and exhale 5

Sucking in the chest skin
None..0
Barely noticeable 1
Obvious 3
Severe 5

Breathing faster
None..0
Up to 50% increase 1
Up to 100% increase 2
Over 100% increase 3

Low Yellow Zone

LOW YELLOW ZONE: total asthma signs score 5 to 8.

- ✓ **Give 0.____cc of quick relief medicine by compressor-driven nebulizer OR give _____ puffs from MDI by holding chamber with mask.**
- ✓ **Check your child's total signs score again 10 minutes after giving quick relief medicine.**

  If your child's total score has improved into the High Yellow Zone, follow the High Yellow Zone plan and continue to check signs every 1 to 2 hours.

  If your child's total score is still in the Low Yellow Zone, or falls back into the Low Yellow Zone in less than 4 hours, continue with High Yellow Zone treatment and:
  - ❏ Give oral steroid† _____ mg, _____ cc immediately. Continue once daily until total signs score is _____ for at least 24 hours.
  - ❏ Please call the office before starting oral steroid.
  - † If your child's condition does not improve within 2 days after starting oral steroid, or does not reach the Green Zone within 7 days of treatment, see your doctor.

Red Zone

RED ZONE: total asthma signs score 9 or more.

- ✓ **Give 0.____ cc of quick relief medicine by compressor-driven nebulizer OR give _____ puffs from MDI by holding chamber with mask.**
- ✓ **Give oral steroid _____mg, _____ cc immediately.**
- ✓ **Check your child's total asthma signs score again 10 minutes after giving quick relief medicine.**

  If your child's total score has improved into the Low Yellow Zone, follow the Low Yellow Zone plan and continue to check signs every 1 to 2 hours.

  If your child's total score is still in the Red Zone, or falls back into the Red Zone in less than 4 hours, visit your doctor **OR GO TO THE EMERGENCY ROOM NOW.**

Food and Drug Administration
Approval of Drugs

The Food and Drug Administration carries a mandate from Congress to regulate the evaluation, manufacture, distribution, labeling, and advertising of prescription medicines and devices. Under FDA regulations, a drug company must conduct clinical trials to document the safety and effectiveness of a new medicine for specific uses. These trials produce data based on the age of the patients, as well as on the dose and the route of administration of the medicine (inhaled, oral, or injected). The FDA staff then evaluates these data.

Manufacturers have not yet supplied the FDA with enough data on some medicines to determine whether they are safe and effective in young children. Therefore, some asthma medicines carry the statement, "The safety and effectiveness in children under [number] years of age have not been established for this product." The three medicine formulations I use most often in the treatment of asthma in children under 2 years of age have not been specifically approved for this age group. This does not mean that these medicines are dangerous, only that sufficient data to establish their safety and effectiveness in children have not been provided to the FDA by the manufacturers. A doctor may prescribe these medicines for use in untested age groups. This use is called an "unlabeled indication."

The FDA commented on such usage in *The FDA Drug Bulletin* of April 1982, as follows:

Use of Approved Drugs for Unlabeled Indications

The appropriateness or the legality of prescribing approved drugs for uses not included in their official labeling is sometimes a cause of concern and confusion among practitioners.

Under the Federal Food, Drug and Cosmetic (FD&C) Act, a drug approved for marketing may be labeled, promoted, and advertised by the manufacturers only for those uses for which the drug's safety and effectiveness have been established and which the FDA has approved. These are commonly referred to as "approved uses." This means that adequate and well-controlled clinical trials have documented these uses, and the results of the trials have been reviewed and approved by the FDA.

The FD&C Act does not, however, limit the manner in which a physician may use an approved drug. Once a product has been approved for marketing, a physician may prescribe it for uses or in treatment regimens or patient populations that are not included in approved labeling. *Such "unapproved," or, more precisely, "unlabeled" uses may be appropriate and rational in certain circumstances, and may, in fact, reflect approaches to drug therapy that have been extensively reported in the medical literature.*

The term "unapproved uses" is, to some extent, misleading. It includes a variety of situations ranging from unstudied to thoroughly investigated drug uses. Valid new uses for drugs already on the market are often first discovered through serendipitous observations and therapeutic innovations, subsequently confirmed by well-planned and executed clinical investigations. Before such advances can be added to the approved labeling, however, data substantiating the effectiveness of a new use or regimen must be submitted by the manufacturer to the FDA for evaluation. This may take time, and, without the initiative of the drug manufacturer whose product is involved, may never occur. For that reason, *accepted medical practice often includes drug use that is not reflected in approved drug labeling* [emphasis added].

The prescription of a drug for a condition or an age group not included on the label is entirely proper if it is based on "rational scientific theory, reliable medical opinion, or controlled clinical studies," according to *AMA Drug Evaluations,* published in 1986. Medical journals frequently contain studies that report on the effectiveness of old drugs for new uses or new techniques for using an old drug. The FDA does not review its assessment of drugs to include new uses or techniques of administration unless a drug company or other interested party requests a change and supplies the necessary data. Often no such request is made.

The laws under which the FDA operates have protected the American public from using inadequately tested drugs. However, every drug, whether approved by the FDA or not, can cause adverse effects. Physicians and patients share the responsibility of monitoring their asthma carefully and in a timely manner to be sure that each drug is having the intended beneficial effect and not causing serious adverse effects.

U.S., Canadian and U.K. Drug Names*

Quick Relief Medicines	U.S.†	Canada†	U.K.
Beta$_2$-agonists	albuterol	salbutamol	salbutamol
	Ventolin	Ventolin	Ventolin
	Proventil		
	levalbuterol		
	Xopenex		
	metaproterenol	orciprenaline	orciprenaline
	Alupent	Alupent	Alupent
	pirbuterol		pirbuterol
	Maxair		Exirel
	terbutaline	terbutaline	terbutaline
	Bricanyl	Bricanyl	Bricanyl
Anticholingerics	ipratropium	ipratropium	ipratropium
	Atrovent	Atrovent	Atrovent

Controller Medicines	U.S.†	Canada†	U.K.
Inhaled Steriods	beclomethasone	beclomethasone	beclomethasone
	Beclovent	Beclovent	Beclovent
	Vanceril	Aldecin	
	budesonide	budesonide	budesonide
	Pulmicort	Pulmicort	Pulmicort
	flunisolide	flunisolide	flunisolide
	Aerobid	Bronalide	Syntaris
	fluticasone	fluticasone	fluticasone
	Flovent	Flixotide	Flixotide
	triamcinolone	triamcinolone	
	Azmacort	Azmacort	

(Continued)

Food and Drug Administration Approval of Drugs

Controller Medicines, continued	U.S.†	Canada†	U.K.
Cromolyn and Nedocromil	cromolyn Intal	cromolyn	cromolyn Intal
	nedocromil Tilade	nedocromil Tilade	nedocromil Tilade
Beta₂-agonists, long-acting			
inhaled	salmeterol Serevent	salmeterol Serevent	salmeterol Serevent
oral	albuterol Volmax Proventil Repetabs	salbutamol Volmax	salbutamol
Leukotriene Modifiers	montelukast Singulair		
	zafirlukast Accolate	zafirlukast Accolate	zafirlukast Accolate
	zileuton Zyflo	zileuton Zyflo	
Theophylline, long-acting	theophylline Slo-bid	theophylline Slo-bid	theophylline
	Theo-Dur	Theo-Dur	
	Theo-24		
	Uniphyl	Uniphyl	Uniphyllin
	Uni-Dur		
Oral Steroids‡	prednisolone Pediapred Prelone	prednisolone Pediapred	prednisolone Pediapred
	prednisone	prednisone	prednisone
	methyl- prednisolone	methyl- prednisolone	methyl- prenisolone

*Blanks indicate that the medicine is not available or is available under a different name. Brand names are capitalized.

†Medicine doses in the United States are stated as the dose that leaves the mouthpiece. Canadian and European doses are stated as the dose that exits the canister (some will then be trapped in the mouthpiece). Therefore, the dose listed in the United States is smaller, even though the amount of medicine per puff inhaled by the patient is the same.

‡An oral steroid may be used as a controller medicine for people with severe persistent asthma. More commonly, it is taken for a short period of time to treat severe asthma episodes.

Resource List

Materials from Pedipress

Pedipress, Inc.
125 Red Gate Lane
Amherst, MA 01002
Toll free: (800) 611-6081
Fax: (413) 549-4095
www.pedipress.com

Dr. Tom Plaut's Asthma Guide for People of All Ages
Thomas F. Plaut, M.D., with Teresa B. Jones, M.A.
336 pages, with 120 illustrations, tables, and forms.
1999, $25.00

Comprehensive, accurate, and current guide for people who want to understand and control their asthma. Includes complete discussion of the basics of asthma and the medicines used to treat it. Provides detailed description of inhalation devices, peak flow monitoring, and the use of asthma diaries and home treatment plans. Includes first-person stories by patients who gained control over their asthma. Addresses asthma issues faced in the school, the family and in travel. Includes a resource section, medical bibliography, glossary, and index.

One Minute Asthma: What You Need to Know
Thomas F. Plaut, M.D.
56 pages, 1998, $5.00

An ideal guide for adult patients, parents, and others who are just starting to learn about asthma. Accurate, clear, and illustrated with line drawings and charts. One Minute Asthma covers the basics of asthma and the medicines used to treat it. This easy-to-read guide will help keep adults and children with asthma out of the emergency room, out of the hospitals, and as active as everyone else.

El asma en un minuto: lo que usted necesita saber
Thomas F. Plaut, M.D.
46 pages, 1998, $5.00

Spanish-language edition of One Minute Asthma.

Children With Asthma: A Manual for Parents
Thomas F. Plaut, M.D.
Pocket-size edition, 300 pages, revised 1995, $10.00

Known as the "asthma bible" by parents and physicians alike, this book emphasizes the importance of the parent's role in asthma management. It teaches the basics of asthma, how medicines work, and when to call for help. Has sections on infants, children, and teenagers. Contains stories by parents and patients as well as illustrations, tables, and instructions.

Winning Over Asthma
Eileen Dolan Savage
40 pages, 1996, $7.00

Good reading for parent and child, this picture book presents asthma facts while telling the story of 5-year-old Graham. It describes the asthma reaction, mentions several triggers and medicines, and emphasizes teamwork between parents and physicians. Demonstrates that childhood asthma can be controlled.

Asthma Peak Flow Diary
Thomas F. Plaut, M.D.
A pad of 25 three-color sheets, revised 1999, $3.00
Also available in Spanish.

A powerful tool for helping adult patients, teens, and parents of children age 5 and older track and understand asthma and thus manage it more effectively. It gives patients and professionals the information they need to monitor step down treatment with inhaled steroids.

Asthma Signs Diary
Thomas F. Plaut, M.D.
A pad of 25 three-color sheets, 1999, $3.00

This diary helps parents of children under 5 years of age understand asthma and how triggers, signs, symptoms, and medicines interact. It gives professionals the information they need to monitor step down treatment with inhaled steroids.

Asthma Charts & Forms: For the Physician's Office and Managed Care
Thomas F. Plaut, M.D.
80 pages, 1999, $95.00

Templates, charts, diaries, Home Treatment Plans, questionnaires, and letters for office visits that save time and improve patient compliance. Computer disk is provided so you can customize forms for your practice. Requires Microsoft Word for either Windows or Macintosh. Full refund in 30 days if not completely satisfied.

Other Recommended Materials

Asthma Magazine
3 Bridge Street
Newton, MA 02458
800-527-3284
Six issues per year, $19.95

Provides appropriate information about all levels of asthma to interested readers. Includes patient pointers, expert opinions, and first-person stories.

Asthma Update
David Jamison, Editor
123 Monticello Avenue, #100
Annapolis, MD 21401
e-mail: dcjamison@toad.net
Four to six pages per issue. $15.00 per year
(410) 267-8329

Quarterly newsletter for adult patients, parents, and professionals. Includes annotated abstracts from current medical journals and perspectives on asthma by asthma experts.

Asthma & Exercise
Nancy Hogshead and Gerald Couzens
239 pages, 1990, $19.95
Henry Holt and Company

Nancy Hogshead has asthma, yet she won four medals in swimming in the 1984 Olympics. She offers clear and detailed advice and instruction on how adults and children with asthma can safely participate in exercise and sports activities.

The Asthma Self-Help Book
Paul J. Hannaway, M.D.
272 pages, 1992, $12.95
Prima Publishing

This revised edition covers many areas important to asthma patients, including diagnosis, medicine treatment, environmental controls, air pollution, and the guidelines established by the National Heart, Lung and Blood Institute in 1991. Dr. Hannaway's style is conversational and easy to follow.

Athletic Drug Reference '96: Compliance with
NCAA and USOC Rules
Robert J. Fuentes, Jack M. Rosenberg, Art Davis, eds.
498 pages, 1996, $14.95
Glaxo Wellcome, Inc.

Provides essential information for coaches, doctors and athletes.

Breathe Easy: Getting the Most From Your
Asthma Medication
Gary Rachelefsky, M.D., and Colleen Lum Lung,
R.N., M.S.N., C.P.N.P.
30 minutes, 1996
Key Pharmaceuticals, Inc.

This excellent videotape presents clear and accurate descriptions of asthma, the goals of treatment, and peak flow monitoring. Giving medicine by MDI, holding chamber and compressor driven nebulizer are discussed in detail.

Complete Book of Children's Allergies
B. Robert Feldman, M.D., with David Carroll
352 pages, 1986, $17.95
Times Books

This is a good guide for parents of children with allergies. The evaluation of allergy problems is reviewed in a no-nonsense fashion. Contains comprehensive sections on specific allergic conditions, including asthma, chronic rhinitis, hives, insect stings, and food allergies.

Practical Guide for the Diagnosis and
Management of Asthma
52 pages, 1997, $5.00
National Institutes of Health Publication No. 97-4053
National Asthma Education and Prevention Program

A must-read. This guide presents the information that you, your doctor, and your nurse should consider in treating your asthma.

A Parent's Guide to Asthma
Nancy Sander
264 pages, 1994, $10.95
Plume/Penguin

Friendly and easy to read. Helps families overcome the physical and emotional effects of asthma on the family. Includes discussion of sibling rivalry, schools, vacations, smoking, and pet allergies.

Taking Charge of Asthma
Betty B. Wray, M.D.
232 pages, 1997, $14.95
John Wiley & Sons

A very readable book. Discusses the causes of asthma and the ways it is diagnosed and treated. Describes the connection between allergies and asthma, occupational hazards, relaxation breathing, and alternative treatments.

Taming Asthma and Allergy by Controlling
Your Environment: A Guide for Patients
Robert A. Wood, M.D.
164 pages, 1995, $19.95
Asthma and Allergy Foundation of America,
Maryland Chapter

An excellent discussion of allergies and asthma. Includes chapters on allergen avoidance and environmental control, indoor air pollution, and non-allergic triggers, and a review of products you can use to improve your environment.

Organizations

Allergy and Asthma Network/Mothers of
Asthmatics, Inc.
2751 Prosperity Ave., Suite 150
Fairfax, VA 22031
(800) 878-4403
www.aanma.org

Publishes *MA Reports*, a monthly newsletter, along with booklets and videos for people with asthma.

American Academy of Allergy, Asthma and Immunology

611 East Wells Street
Milwaukee, WI 53202
(800) 822-2762
www.aaaai.org

Organization of allergists, asthma specialists, and allied health professionals with a special interest in the research and treatment of allergic disease. Publishes a variety of educational materials for the public.

American Academy of Pediatrics

141 Northwest Point Boulevard
Elk Grove Village, IL 60007
(800) 433-9016
www.aap.org

Organization of pediatricians. Publishes a variety of educational materials for the public.

American Association for Respiratory Care

11030 Ables Lane
Dallas, TX 75229
(972) 243-2272
www.aarc.org

Organization of respiratory therapists. Offers *Peak Performance, USA,* a free, peak flow based program for schools.

American College of Allergy, Asthma and Immunology

85 West Algonquin Road, Suite 550
Arlington Heights, IL 60005
(800) 842-7777
www.allergy.mcg.edu

Association of allergists and related health-care professionals. Publishes a variety of educational materials and sponsors regional asthma educational conferences and asthma screening programs for the public.

American Lung Association

1740 Broadway
New York, NY 10019
(800) LUNG-USA (connects to your local association)
www.lungusa.org

More than three hundred local and state lung associations provide many asthma education services.

Some chapters sponsor support groups, newsletters, and asthma camps.

Asthma and Allergy Foundation of America

1233 20th St. NW, Suite 402
Washington, DC 20036
(800) 7-ASTHMA
www.aafa.org

A number of chapters throughout the country offer patient and public education programs, support groups, school programs, community workshops, and conferences. Special programs include "Meeting in a Box" for support groups, "Asthma Care Training" for children, and "Power Breathing" for teenagers.

Association of Asthma Educators

15322 Ripplestream Drive
Houston, TX 77068
281-444-6737
www.cwagner@flash.net

Organization of health professionals dedicated to improving asthma education materials and services available to the public and professionals.

Asthma Consultants

Thomas F. Plaut, M.D.
125 Red Gate Lane
Amherst, MA 01002
(413) 549-3918

Offers consultation for individuals, health maintenance organizations, group practices, hospitals, support groups, and government agencies committed to improving the care of people with asthma.

Food Allergy Network

10400 Eaton Place, Suite 107
Fairfax, VA 22030-2208
(800) 929-4040
www.foodallergy.org

Provides information on food allergy and anaphylaxis to patients, health professionals, and the public through a newsletter, product alerts, videos, and cookbooks. Works to educate government agencies, health professionals, food manufacturers, restaurant associations, and schools about the needs of food-allergic individuals.

Healthy Kids: The Key to Basics
Educational Planning for Students with Asthma
and Other Chronic Health Conditions
79 Elmore Street
Newton, MA 02459-1137
(617) 965-9637
erg_hk@juno.com

Ellie M. Goldberg, M.Ed., directs this consulting service dedicated to promoting health and educational equity for students with asthma and other chronic health conditions. Works with families, schools, health professionals and organizations to promote policies and practices that enable students to attend school safely and successfully.

National Asthma Education and Prevention Program

NHLBI Information Center
P. O. Box 30105
Bethesda, MD 20824-0105
(301) 251-1222
www.nhlbi.nih.gov

The NAEPP publishes information for health professionals, schools, and the public. See medical bibliography. Order the *Practical Guide for the Diagnosis and Management of Asthma* and other resources by phone, or download from the Web: www.nhlbi. nih.gov/nhlbi/lung/asthma/prof/ practgde.htm.

National Institute of Allergy and Infectious Diseases

31 Center Drive, Room 7A50
MSC 2520
Bethesda, MD 20892-2520
(301) 496-5717
www.niaid.nih.gov

Publishes a variety of educational materials on allergies and related topics for the public.

National Jewish Medical and Research Center

1400 Jackson Street
Denver, CO 80206
(800) 222-LUNG
www.njc.org

Provides information on asthma and lung disease via the LUNG LINE, (800) 222-LUNG. Engaged in treat-

ment, research, and education in chronic respiratory disease. Accepts patients through physician or self-referral.

Equipment Vendors

Allergy Asthma Technology, Ltd.

8224 Lehigh Avenue
Morton Grove, IL 60053
(800) 621-5545
www.allergyasthmatech.com

Informative catalogue includes mattress encasings, HEPA air filters, holding chambers, nebulizers, and peak flow meters.

Allergy Control Products

96 Danbury Road, P.O. Box 793
Ridgefield, CT 06877
(800) 422-DUST
www.allergycontrol.com

Informative catalogue includes mattress encasings, HEPA air filters, holding chambers, nebulizers and peak flow meters.

Clement Clarke, Inc.

5500 Courseview Dr.
Mason, OH 45040
(800) 848-8923
www.clement-clarke.com

Mini-Wright peak flow meter, Windmill Trainer, Sonix ultrasonic nebulizer

Devilbiss Company

P.O. Box 635
Somerset, PA 15501
(800) 333-4000
(814) 443-4881
www.sunrisemedical.com

Pulmo-Aide compressor driven nebulizer

Dey, L.P.

2751 Napa Valley Corporate Drive
Napa , CA 94558
(800) 869-9005
www.deyinc.com

Astech peak flow meter

Ferraris Medical, Inc.
9681 Wagner Road, P.O. Box 344
Holland, NY 14080
(800) 724-7929
www.ferrarismedicalusa.com

PocketPeak peak flow meter

Glaxo Wellcome, Inc.
5 Moore Drive
Research Triangle Park, NC 27709
(888) 825-5249
www.glaxowellcome.com

Serevent Diskus, Flovent Rotadisk, Ventolin Rota-haler

Key Pharmaceuticals, Inc.
2000 Galloping Hill Road
Kenilworth, NJ 07033
(800) 222-7579
www.myhealth.com

InspirEase holding chamber, Breathe Easy video

Meditrack
433 Main Street
Hudson, MA 01749
800-863-9633
www.doser.com

Doser, a device that displays dose remaining in a metered dose inhaler

Monaghan Medical Corporation
P.O. Box 2805
Plattsburgh, NY 12901
(800) 833-9653

AeroChamber holding chamber and AeroChamber with mask; TruZone peak flow meter

National Allergy Supply, Inc.
1620-D Satellite Blvd.
Duluth, GA 30097
(800) 522-1448

Informative catalogue includes mattress encasings, HEPA air filters, holding chambers, nebulizers, and peak flow meters

Pari Respiratory Equipment, Inc.
13800 Hull St. Rd.
Midlothian, VA 23122
(800) 327-8632

ProNeb and Dura-Neb compressor driven nebulizers, Pari LC Plus, and Pari LC Star reusable nebulizer cups, and Space Chamber holding chamber

Pedipress, Inc.
125 Red Gate Lane
Amherst, MA 01002
(800) 611-6081
Fax: (413) 549-4095
www.pedipress.com

Asthma books: *Dr. Tom Plaut's Asthma Guide for People of All Ages, Children With Asthma: A Manual for Parents, One Minute Asthma: What You Need to Know, El asma en un minuto: lo que usted necesita saber, Winning Over Asthma, Asthma Charts & Forms: For the Physician's Office and Managed Care,* the Asthma Peak Flow Diary and the Asthma Signs Diary

WE Pharmaceuticals, Inc.
P.O. Box 1142
Ramona, CA 92065
(760) 788-9155
(800) 262-9555
www.weez.com

E-Z Spacer holding chamber

Medical Bibliography

Books and Reports

Bierman, C.W., Pearlman, D.S., Shapiro, G.G., Busse, W.W., eds. *Allergy, Asthma, and Immunology from Infancy to Adulthood.* 3rd ed. 1996. Philadelphia: W.B. Saunders Co. 805 pages.

A comprehensive, practical text that covers all the major aspects of asthma and allergy of concern to the primary care physician. The writing is clear and easily understood by a layperson using a medical dictionary.

National Asthma Education and Prevention Program. National Heart, Lung, and Blood Institute. Bethesda, MD (http://www.nhlbi.nih.gov):

Practical Guide for the Diagnosis and Management of Asthma. 1997. 52 pages. National Institutes of Health Publication No. 97-4053 (Download from http://www.nhlbi.nih.gov/nhlbi/lung/asthma/prof/practgde.htm.)

A must-read. This guide presents the information you, your doctor, and your nurse should consider in treating your asthma. Easier to digest than the full *Expert Panel Report 2.*

Expert Panel Report 2: Guidelines for the Diagnosis and Management of Asthma. 1997. 86 pages. National Institutes of Health Publication No. 97-4051.

This full report includes many tables, forms, and an extensive bibliography.

Executive Summary: Guidelines for the Diagnosis and Management of Asthma. 1991. 44 pages. National Institutes of Health Publication No. 91-3042A

A clear summary of the original NHLBI report on asthma.

The Pharmacotherapy of Asthma During Pregnancy: Current Recommendations and Future Research. *J Allergy Clin Immunol* 1999; 103(2): S329-S376.

The Physician's Desk Reference, ed. 52. 1998. Montvale, NJ: Medical Economics Company, Inc. 3223 pages.

Gives indications, effects, dosages, routes, methods, frequencies, and durations of administration of medicines, as well as any relevant warnings, hazards, contraindications, side effects, and precautions. The text is the same as the medicine package inserts approved by the FDA.

Plaut, T. *Asthma Charts and Forms for the Physician's Office and Managed Care.* 1999. 80 pages, with Windows or Mac disk. Amherst, MA: Pedipress, Inc.

Charts, diaries, questionnaires, and letters for health professionals to use with patients who have asthma. These tools improve communication, save time, increase efficiency, and improve asthma care.

The United States Pharmacopeial Convention, Inc. *Drug Information for the Health Care Professional*, ed 18. 1998. The United States Pharmacopeial Convention, Inc., 3360 pages.

Information is more comprehensive, readable, and current than that found in most package inserts. Updated regularly by experts who base their descriptions on the current medical literature and practice. Contains many tables comparing the traits of several medicines in the same class. Covers prescription and nonprescription medicines.

Journal Articles by Chapter

The Basics of Asthma

Elliott, D.H., Ed. *Are Asthmatics Fit to Dive.* 1996. Kensington, MD.: Undersea and Hyperbaric Medical Society.

Martinez, F.D., Cline, M., Burrows, B. Increased Incidence of Asthma in Children of Smoking Mothers. *Pediatrics* 1992;89:21–6.

Plaut, T., Westby, L. A Minimal Response to Albuterol Challenge Does Not Exclude a Diagnosis of Asthma. *J Asthma* 1997;34(3):255–56.

Storms, W.W., Joyner, D.M. Update on Exercise-Induced Asthma: A Report of the Olympic Exercise Asthma Summit Conference. *The Physician and Sportsmedicine* 1997;25(3): 45–55.

Turkeltaub, P.C., Gergen, P.J. Prevalence of Upper and Lower Respiratory Conditions in the U.S. Population by Social and Environmental Factors: data from the second National Health and Nutrition Examination Survey, 1976–1980 (NHANES II). *Ann Allergy* 1991;67:147–54.

Asthma Medicines

Agertoft, L., Pedersen, S. Effects of Long Term Treatment with an Inhaled Corticosteroid on Growth and Pulmonary Function in Asthmatic Children. *Respir Med* 1994;88:373–81.

Beasley R., Fishwick D., Miles J.F., Hendeles L. Preservatives in nebulizer solutions: risks without benefit. *Pharmacotherapy* 1998;18(1):130–9.

Boushey, H.A. Effects of Inhaled Steroids on the Consequences of Asthma. *J Allergy Clin Immunol* 1998;102:S5–16.

Creticos, P., Burk, J., Smith, L. The Use of Twice-Daily Nedocromil Sodium in the Treatment of Asthma. *J Allergy Clin Immunol* 1995;95(5): 829–36.

Drazen, J.M., Israel, E., Boushey, H.A., et al. Comparison of Regularly Scheduled with As-Needed Use of Albuterol in Mild Asthma. *N Engl J Med* 1996;335:841–7.

Garbe, E., LeLorier, J., Boivin, J., Suissa, S. Inhaled and Nasal Glucocorticoids and the Risks of Ocular Hypertension or Open-Angle Glaucoma. *JAMA* 1997;277(9):722–27.

Greening, A.P., Wind, P., Northfield, M., Shaw, G. Added Salmeterol versus Higher-Dose Corticosteroid in Asthma Patients with Symptoms on Existing Inhaled Corticosteroids. *Lancet* 1994; 344:219–24.

König, P. Asthma in Childhood. 1983. In Conn, H.F., Saunders, W.B. (eds). *Current Therapy*, pp. 580–87.

Martin, R., et al. A Comparative Study of Extended-Release Albuterol Sulfate (Volmax) and Long-Acting Inhaled Salmeterol Xinafoate (Serevent) in the Treatment of Nocturnal Asthma. *Ann Allergy, Asthma Clin Immunol* 1999 (in press).

Nelson, H.S., et al. Improved bronchodilation with levalbuterol compared with racemic albuterol in patients with asthma. *J Allergy Clin Immunol* 1998;102:943–52.

O'Hickey, S.P., Rees, P.J. High-Dose Nedocromil Sodium as an Addition to Inhaled Corticosteroids in the Treatment of Asthma. *Respir Med* 1994;88:499–502.

Sears, M.R., Taylor, D.R., Print, C.G., et al. Regular Inhaled Beta-Agonist Treatment in Bronchial Asthma. *Lancet* 1990;336:1391–6.

Silverstein, M.D., Yunginger, J.W., Reed, C.E., Petterson, T., Zimmerman, D., Li, J.T.C., O'Fallen, W.M. Attained Adult Height after Childhood Asthma: Effect of Glucocorticoid Therapy. *J Allergy Clin Immunol* 1997;99:466–74.

Szefler, S.J., Nelson, H.S. Alternative Agents for Anti-Inflammatory Treatment of Asthma. *J Allergy Clin Immunol* 1998;102:S23–35.

Szefler, S. Leukotriene Modifiers: What is Their Position in Asthma Therapy? Editorial. *J Allergy Clin Immunol* 1998;102:170–2.

Tal, A., Levy, N., Beaman, J.E. Methylprednisolone Therapy for Acute Asthma in Infants and Toddlers: A Controlled Clinical Trial. *Pediatrics* 1990;86(3):350–56.

Toogood, J.H. Side Effects of Inhaled Corticosteroids. *J Allergy Clin Immunol* 1998; 102:705–13.

Weinberger, J., Hendeles, L. Theophylline in Asthma. *N Engl J Med* 1996;334(21):1380–88.

Welch, M.J. Inhaled Corticosteroids and Growth in Children. *Ped Annals* 1998;27(11):752–58.

Woolcock, A., Yan, K., Lundback, B., Ringdal, N., Jacques, L.A. Comparison of Addition of Salmeterol to Inhaled Steroids with Doubling of the Dose of Inhaled Steroids. *Am J Respir Crit Care Med* 1996;153: 1481–88.

Woolcock, A.J. Effect of Therapy on Bronchial Hyperresponsiveness in the Long-Term Management of Asthma. *Clin Allergy* 1988;18:165–76.

Devices for Inhaling Asthma Medicine

Newhouse, M.T. Pulmonary Drug Targeting with Aerosols. *Amer J Allergy Asthma Ped* 1993;7(1): 23–35.

Newman, S.P., Pavia, D., Clarke, S.W. How Should a Pressurized Beta-Adrenergic Bronchodilator Be Inhaled? *Eur J Respir Dis* 1981;62:3–21.

Loffert, D.T., Ikle, D., Nelson, H.S. A Comparison of Commercial Jet Nebulizers. *Chest* 1994;106: 1788–93.

Finlay, W.H., Stapleton, K.W., Zuberbuhler, P. Variations in Predicted Regional Lung Deposition of Salbutamol Sulphate Between 19 Nebulizer Types. *J Aerosol Med* 1998;11(2):65–80.

Peak Flow

Hsu, K., Jenkins, D., Hsi, B., Bourhofer, et al. Ventilatory Functions of Normal Children and Young Adults — Mexican-American, White, and Black. *Journal of Pediatrics* 1979;95:192–96.

Leiner, G.C., et al. Expiratory Peak Flow Rate. Standard Values for Normal Subjects. Use as a Clinical Test of Ventilatory Function. *Am Rev Resp Dis* 1963;88:644.

Asthma Treatment

Allen, D.B., Mullen, M.L., Mullen, B. Clinical Aspects of Allergic Disease: A Meta-Analysis of the Effect of Oral and Inhaled Corticosteroids on Growth. *J Allergy Clin Immunol* 1994;93:967–76.

Pincus, D.J., Humeston, T.R., Martin, R.D. Chronotherapeutic Effect of Inhaled Steroids on Asthma at 8:00 A.M. or 5:30 P.M. *J Allergy Clin Immunol* 1997;99:S319.

School Resources

Asthma at School

Healthy Kids: The Key to Basics
Ellie Goldberg, M. Ed., Director
79 Elmore St.
Newton, MA 02459-1137
(617) 965-9637
e-mail: erg_hk@juno.com

Articles by Ellie Goldberg Referenced in Chapter 9:

"Asthma at School: A Comprehensive Care and
Advocacy Plan," 1992
"Advocacy for Students with Food Allergies,"
1996
"Integrating Students with Chronic Illness,"
1996, workshop handout
"School Liability Waivers," 1994

Additional Healthy Kids Titles:

"Individual Health Plans: A Strategy for Achiev-
ing Educational Equity, Information for Parents
about Using IHPs to Plan For Students with
Asthma, Allergies and Other Chronic Health
Conditions"
"Why School Nurses?"

For the brochure "Educational Planning for Students
with Chronic Health Conditions" and a complete
Healthy Kids resource list, send $1.00 and a self-
addressed, stamped business envelope to the above
address.

The School Environment and Indoor Air Quality
Building Air Quality: A Guide for Building Owners and Facility Managers
229 pages, 1991, $24.00
U.S. Environmental Protection Agency
Information Resource Center
(202) 260-5922
Or order from:
U.S. Government Printing Office
Superintendent of Documents
P.O. Box 371954
Pittsburgh, PA 15250-7954
(202) 512-1800
Fax: (202) 512-2250

The Healthy School Handbook: Conquering the Sick Building Syndrome and Other Environmental Hazards In and Around Your School, $24.95
National Education Association professional library.
(800) 229-4200

Indoor Air Pollution: An Introduction for Health Professionals
U.S. Environmental Protection Agency
Indoor Air Qualty Clearinghouse
(800) 438-4318 (free)

Indoor Air Quality Management Program.
1987. **Maintaining Acceptable IAQ During the Renovation of a School,** 1995. **The Maintenance of Heating, Ventilating and Air Conditioning Systems and Indoor Air Quality in Schools,** 1994
Maryland Department of Education
School Facilities Branch
200 W. Baltimore St., 2nd floor
Baltimore, MD 21201-2595
(410) 767-0098

More than a dozen environmental-quality manuals on a variety of topics. Call for list of resources.

Indoor Air Quality: Tools for Schools
Binder, 1995, $22.00
U.S. Environmental Protection Agency
Superintendent of Documents
(see above for contact information)

Helps participants develop a current indoor air quality profile on their school, formulate an air quality management plan to prevent problems, and diagnose and solve air quality problems that may already exist. Includes background information, sample memos, checklists, logs. Lists government, organizational, informational, and other resources.

School Health/Individualized Health Plans (IHP)

Massachusetts Comprehensive School Health Manual
1995, $44.65 plus handling
Department of Public Health
State House Bookstore, Room 116
Boston, MA 02133
(617) 727-2834

Guidelines for Serving Students with Special Health Care Needs, 1992
Utah State Office of Education
250 East 500 South
Salt Lake City, UT 84111

School Health Alert
P.O. Box 150127
Nashville, TN 37215
(615) 370-7899
Ten issues, $34.00

Monthly newsletter of authoritative medical and scientific research, commentary, and advice.

The School Nurse's Source Book of Individualized Health Care Plans
Marykay B. Haas, et al.
1993, $39.95
Sunrise River Press
(800) 551-4754

Serving Students with Special Health Care Needs, 1992
Connecticut Dept. of Education
Special Education Resource Center
(860) 632-1485

Also discusses legal aspects. Free.

Legal Aspects

The Civil Rights of Students with Hidden Disabilities under Section 504 of the Rehabilitation Act of 1973 (free pamphlet)
U.S. Department of Education
Office for Civil Rights
Washington, D.C. 20202-1328
(800) 421-3481

Educational Rights of Children with Disabilities: A Primer for Advocates
Eileen L. Ordover and Kathleen B. Boundy
Center for Law and Education
(202) 462-7688 (for publications)

Free Appropriate Public Education for Students with Handicaps
U.S. Department of Education, Office for Civil Rights
(see above for contact information)

Materials Safety

The Artist's Complete Health and Safety Guide
Monona Rossol
343 pages, 1994, $19.95
Allworth Press
(800) 247-6553

The Healthy Household: A Complete Guide for Creating a Healthy Indoor Environment
Lynn Marie Bower, 1995
The Healthy House Institute
(812) 332-5073

Guide to less toxic products and techniques for cleaning, personal care, and other purposes.

Materials Safety Data Sheets
http://www.msdssearch.com/

Pesticides

Getting Pesticides Out of Our Schools
Becky Riley, 1994
Northwest Coalition for Alternatives to Pesticides
P.O. Box 1393
Eugene, OR 97440
(541) 344-5044

Pest Control in the School Environment: Adopting Integrated Pest Management
Office of Pesticide Programs, 1993
U.S. Environmental Protection Agency Information Resource Center
(202) 260-5922

Organizations

Arts, Crafts and Theater Safety (ACTS)
181 Thompson Street, #23
New York, NY 10012
(202) 777-0062 (hotline)

Provides a variety of health and safety services, educational materials, referral to health services, and other resources. Also publishes a monthly newsletter.

Center for Law and Education
197 Friend Street, 9th floor
Boston, MA 02114
(617) 371-1166
www.cleweb.org

National Asthma Education and Prevention Program
4733 Bethesda Ave., Suite 530
Bethesda, MD 20814-4820
(301) 251-1222
www.nhlbi.nih.gov/nhlbi/nhlbi.htm

Selected publications for schools:
  Managing Asthma: A Guide for Schools
  Asthma Awareness Curriculum for the Elementary Classroom
  Asthma and Physical Activity in the School
  Making a Difference: Asthma Management in the School (video)

National Information Center for Children and Youth with Handicaps
(800) 695-0285

Provides free reprints of articles on special education laws, related services, the individualized education program, and due process procedural safeguards.

National Institute for Occupational Safety and Health (NIOSH)
4676 Columbia Parkway, Mail Stop C-13
Cincinnati, OH 45226-1998
(800) 35-NIOSH
(800) 356-4674
www.cdc.gov/niosh

New York Coalition for Alternatives to Pesticides
P.O. Box 6005
Albany, NY 12206-0005
(518) 426-8246 or 9331

Ask for information on the Healthy Schools Campaign.

New York Healthy School Network
96 South Swan Street
Albany, NY 12210
(518) 462-0632
www.hsnet.org

Clearinghouse for information and resources on environmentally safe and healthy schools. The *Parent's Guide to School Indoor Air Quality* is available for $3.00.

Occupational Safety and Health Administration (OSHA)
Ten regional offices, consultation offices in every state.
(800) 321-OSHA (6742)
www.osha.gov

U.S. Dept. of Education — Office for Civil Rights
Customer Service Team
Mary E. Switzer Building
330 C Street, S.W.
Washington, D.C. 20202-1328
(800) 421-3481
http://www.ed.gov/offices/OCR

U.S. Environmental Protection Agency
Indoor Air Quality Information Clearinghouse
P.O. Box 37133
Washington, D.C. 20013-7133
(800) 438-4318
www.epa.gov/iaq

Ten regional EPA offices are spread around the country. The regions and addresses are available from the national office or on the Web site, and are listed in *Indoor Air Quality: Tools for Schools.*

Glossary

acceptance: agreement by patient to a treatment routine they understand

Accolate: brand name for zafirlukast, a leukotriene modifier (oral)

acute: sudden

adrenal insufficiency: inability of the body's adrenal glands to produce an adequate amount of cortisol, the hormone needed to respond to stress

adrenaline (epinephrine): a quick relief medicine, produced by the body and available in synthetic form

adrenergic: adrenaline-like medicine

adverse: undesirable

Aerobid: brand name for flunisolide, an inhaled steroid medicine, controller

AeroChamber: brand of holding chamber

Air Watch: airflow monitoring device with electronic link to the doctor

airflow: the rate at which you can blow air out of your lungs

albuterol: generic name of Proventil and Ventolin; beta$_2$-agonists, quick relief medicines

allergen: any substance that can induce an allergy

allergist: doctor who specializes in understanding and treating allergies

allergy: condition in which the body has an immune reaction to a substance that is normally harmless

alveoli: air sacs located at the end of the tiniest airways

ampule (ampoule): small, sealed vial containing medicine in liquid form

anaphylaxis: severe allergic reaction throughout the body which can be fatal if not treated immediately; commonly includes respiratory symptoms, itching, hives, and fainting

antibody: protein that develops in the body in response to a foreign substance (antigen)

anticholinergic: type of inhaled quick relief medicine that acts through a different mechanism than beta$_2$-agonists

antihistamine: generic name for medicine that blocks the actions of histamine, such as swelling and itching

antiinflammatory: medicine that counteracts inflammation

asthma: inflammatory disease of the airways characterized by airways that are hyperresponsive and symptoms that can be reversed

Asthma Peak Flow Diary: an individual record of peak flow scores, medicines, asthma signs, and triggers; helps in monitoring peak flow trends in people 5 years and older

asthma signs: physical indicators of asthma that can observed by another person

Asthma Signs Diary: an individual record of asthma signs scores, medicines, and triggers that helps in monitoring the trends in asthma signs in children under 5 years of age

asthma treatment zone: a range of peak flow scores or total scores of asthma signs that calls for following a particular treatment plan

asymptomatic: without symptoms

atopic: allergic

Atrovent: brand name for ipratropium bromide, an inhaled quick relief medicine

attack: a dramatic term for an episode of asthma

Azmacort: brand name for triamcinolone, an inhaled steroid medicine, controller

beclomethasone: generic name for Vanceril, Beclovent, and Qvar, inhaled steroid medicines, controller

Beclovent: brand name for beclomethasone, an inhaled steroid medicine, controller

beta-blockers: medicines that block the action of beta-agonist medicines, and responses of the sympathetic nervous system

beta$_2$-agonist: a class of quick relief medicine

b.i.d.: a dosing schedule calling for medicine to be taken twice a day

blood concentration: amount of a substance in a given quantity of blood expressed as weight per unit volume (e.g., mg/ml)

blow-by technique: a low-efficiency method for administering inhaled medicines

book: to leave quickly (slang)

breath-activated: method for triggering the release of medicine from a device by inhalation

breathing cycle: total time it takes to breathe in and out once

breathing rate: number of breaths per minute

Brethaire: brand name for terbutaline, an inhaled beta$_2$-agonist, quick relief medicine

Brethine: a brand name for terbutaline, an inhaled beta$_2$-agonist, quick relief medicine

Bricanyl: a brand name for terbutaline, an inhaled beta$_2$-agonist, quick relief medicine

bronchi: large air passages or airways

bronchiolitis: inflammation of the smallest airways (bronchioles); caused by a virus

bronchitis: inflammation of the large airways (bronchi)

bronchoconstriction: narrowing of the airways caused by contraction of the smooth muscles encircling them (same as bronchospasm)

bronchodilator: medicine that causes the airways to open

bronchospasm: narrowing of the airways caused by contraction of the smooth muscles encircling them (same as bronchoconstriction)

budesonide: generic name for Pulmicort, an inhaled steroid medicine, controller

candidiasis: yeast infection in the mouth or vagina; same as moniliasis

capillary: tiniest blood vessel

cartilage: strong, flexible tissue that supports the large airways

cc: abbreviation for cubic centimeter; equivalent to a milliliter or $^1/_{1000}$ of a liter. This metric measurement is equal to $^1/_5$ of a measuring teaspoon.

CDN: compressor driven nebulizer

CFC: chlorofluorocarbon; propellant used in most metered dose inhalers

chemical mediator: class of chemical that plays a role in the asthma reaction; includes histamine and leukotrienes

chronic: continuous or long-term

cilia: tiny hairlike projections from the surface of the cells that line the airway

closed mouth technique: a method for inhaling medicine from an MDI; open-mouth technique is preferred

compliance: doing exactly what the doctor says, whether or not you understand it

compressor: machine that produces air under pressure

compressor driven nebulizer (CDN): electric- or battery-powered device that uses compressed air to create a medicine mist

consultation: full review of a patient's asthma history, physical exam, and other information; leads to the creation of a written asthma management plan

controlled-release: same as long-acting, sustained-release, or slow-release; applies to some theophylline and albuterol preparations

controller: medicine that prevents or reduces the frequency and severity of asthma episodes, taken daily

corticosteroid: another term for a steroid or cortisone-like medicine

coughing asthma: form of asthma in which coughing is the only symptom

cromolyn: generic name for Intal, controller medicine that prevents mast cells in the airways from releasing asthma-causing chemicals

croup: illness usually produced by a virus, in which the larynx and trachea are inflamed; produces a barking cough

dander: scales of dead skin

decongestant: a medicine that reduces congestion (swelling)

discard date: date when an MDI should be thrown away because it will no longer deliver a full puff of medicine

Diskus: brand name for dry powder inhaler device

diurnal variation: change within a day

DPI: dry powder inhaler

dry powder inhaler: device for inhaling asthma medicines in powder form; dependent on the force of inhalation to disperse medicine into the lungs

EasiVent: brand of holding chamber

eczema: a skin rash, also known as atopic dermatitis

effort monitor: part of a holding chamber which indicates the effort a person is making when inhaling medicine

electrostatic air precipitator: air cleaner

eosinophils: white blood cells involved in inflammation

ephedrine: oral adrenergic medicine, bronchodilator; no longer commonly used because of its adverse effects

epinephrine (adrenaline): a quick relief medicine, produced by the body and available in synthetic form

EpiPen: brand name for epinephrine for intramuscular use (injection); used to treat anaphylaxis

episode (flare): period of time when asthma signs or symptoms occur, peak flow scores drop, breathing is changed, or additional asthma medicine is needed

exacerbation: worsening

exercise induced asthma: a form of asthma in which exercise is the only trigger

exhale: to breathe out

expiration: act of breathing out

extended-release: medicine preparation that acts over a longer period of time than the standard preparation; also called slow-release, sustained-release

E-Z Spacer: brand of holding chamber

family practitioner: primary care physician who sees patients of all ages

FEV$_1$: forced expiratory volume in one second. This measurement of airflow is done using a spirometer. It provides information about the status of the large and small airways

flare (episode): period of time when asthma signs or symptoms occur, peak flow scores drop, breathing is changed, or additional asthma medicine is needed

Flovent: brand name for fluticasone, an inhaled steroid medicine available in MDI or DPI, controller

flow monitor: part of a holding chamber which makes a sound if inhalation is too fast

flunisolide: generic name for Aerobid, an inhaled steroid medicine, controller

fluticasone: generic name for Flovent, an inhaled steroid medicine, controller

gastroesophageal reflux: backward flow of material from stomach to the esophagus; causes irritation which can lead to bronchospasm

green zone: asthma treatment zone in which there are no symptoms and peak flow is 80 to 100 percent of the personal best

growth retardation: slowing of rate at which height increases

Gyrocap: capsule containing Slo-Phyllin, a slow-release theophylline preparation, controller

hay fever: allergic condition of the nose and eyes brought on mainly by ragweed or other pollen

HEPA filter: abbreviation for a "high-efficiency particulate air" filter; removes tiny particles from the air

HFA propellant: hydrofluoroalkane, a propellant used in MDIs which does not destroy ozone in the stratosphere (upper atmosphere)

high yellow zone: asthma treatment zone in which there are only mild symptoms and peak flow is 65 to 80 percent of personal best

histamine: one of the chemical mediators of the asthma reaction

hives: itchy swellings of skin usually due to allergy

holding chamber: inhalation device used with a metered dose inhaler that holds the medicine mist to improve medicine effect

home care company: organization that provides many aspects of asthma care in the home, including teaching, monitoring, and review of environment and treatment

hyperresponsive: refers to airways that overreact to various asthma triggers

hyperventilation: excessive rate and depth of breathing

IAQ: indoor air quality

I/E ratio (I/O ratio): in/out ratio, or relative length of inspiration compared to expiration

IgE: immunoglobulin E, an antibody that reacts with an allergen, initiating the asthma reaction

immunotherapy: synonymous with allergy shots, injection treatment, hyposensitization, desensitization

indication: reason to use

indoor air quality (IAQ): overall healthfulness of the air inside a building

inflammation: a response of the body to physical or chemical triggers; includes swelling due to movement of cells, fluid, and chemicals into the area

inhalation device: apparatus for inhaling asthma medicine

inhaled steroid: inhaled medicine that prevents inflammation in the airways and reduces inflammation that already exists; the most commonly

prescribed type of controller medicine for people with persistent asthma

inhaler: also metered dose inhaler (MDI). Device that uses propellant to create a medicine mist that can be breathed into the airways

I/O ratio (I/E ratio): in/out ratio, or relative length of inspiration compared to expiration

inspiration: act of breathing in

InspirEase: brand of holding chamber

inspiration-expiration ratio: see in/out (I/O) ratio

Intal: brand name for cromolyn, controller

intermittent flow director: a vent in the nebulizer tubing that, when covered, allows production of mist

internist: primary care physician who sees adult patients

intradermal: into the skin

intravenous: into a vein

intubation: placing a tube into the trachea to enable artificial breathing; can be a lifesaving procedure during a severe asthma episode

ipratropium: generic name for Atrovent, an anticholinergic medicine, quick relief medicine

irritant: a nonallergenic substance that may provoke a reaction in the airways

kg: kilogram; 1,000 grams or 2.2 pounds

levalbuterol: generic name for Xopenex, a beta$_2$-agonist; quick relief medicine

leukotriene: chemical mediator involved in the asthma reaction

leukotriene modifier medicine: class of medicine that blocks the formation or action of leukotrienes in the airways, thereby blocking part of the asthma reaction, controller

liter (L): metric measurement, slightly more than a quart

liters/minute (L/min): a flow rate, applied to peak flow or oxygen delivery

long-acting: synonymous with slow-release or sustained-release when referring to a theophylline or beta$_2$-agonist preparation

low yellow zone: asthma treatment zone in which symptoms are moderate and peak flow is 50 to 65 percent of personal best

malingering: pretending to be ill

mask: a device that fits snugly over the nose and mouth; used to help deliver inhaled asthma medicines

mast cell: one of the cell types that contain chemicals which can produce the asthma reaction

Maxair: brand name for pirbuterol, a beta$_2$-agonist, quick relief medicine

Maxair Autohaler: brand name for an MDI with a special "breath-activated" release mechanism; contains pirbuterol (quick relief medicine)

mcg: microgram, 1/1,000,000 (one millionth) of a gram

MDI: metered dose inhaler

mean (average) peak flow score: the average peak flow score for people of a certain height, expressed in liters per minute

mediator: a chemical that is the middleman or go-between in the asthma reaction

medicine retaining valve: valve in the exit port of a holding chamber which holds medicine until a person begins to breathe in

Medrol: brand name of methylprednisolone, an oral steroid

metabolize: to change chemically or physically in the body

metered dose inhaler (MDI): device that creates medicine mist for inhalation by using propellant to expel liquid medicine

metaproterenol: generic name for beta$_2$-agonist, quick relief medicine

methylprednisolone: generic name for Medrol, oral steroid medicine

methotrexate: immunosuppresive drug used to treat severe asthma that does not respond to usual treatment; also used to treat cancer

micron: micrometer, 1/1,000,000 (one millionth) of a meter

mg: milligram, 1/1,000 (one thousandth) of a gram

mite: tiny arachnid (spiderlike animal); skeleton and feces are found in house dust

ml: milliliter, 1/1,000 of a liter; same as a cubic centimeter (cc)

moniliasis (candidiasis): yeast infection in the mouth or vagina

monitoring: keeping track of

montelukast: generic name for Singulair, a leukotriene modifier medicine, controller

mouthpiece: part of an asthma device which is put in the mouth

mucus: protective and cleansing material produced by glands in the airways, nose, sinuses, and elsewhere in the body

nebulizer (nebulizer cup): device that converts liquid medicine into a mist for inhalation

nedocromil: generic name for Tilade, an antiinflammatory medicine, controller

normal (tidal) breath: usual breathing volume when no extra effort is made

objective sign: something that can be seen and scored by an observer

onset of action: time span from when a medicine is inhaled or swallowed until it starts to work

open mouth technique: effective method for inhaling medicine from a metered dose inhaler, as compared to closed-mouth technique

osteoporosis: decrease in bone density causing increased bone fragility

ozone: a form of oxygen (O_3) that is a respiratory irritant; one component of smog; see ozone layer

ozone layer: layer of ozone in the upper atmosphere which encircles the Earth, protecting the surface from harmful effects of cancer-causing ultraviolet light

palate: roof of mouth

peak expiratory flow rate (PEFR): speed at which air exits the lungs when you give your fastest blast for a fraction of a second; also known as peak flow

peak flow meter: a device used to measure peak expiratory flow rate

peak flow score: the best of three attempts blown on the peak flow meter, expressed in liters per minute

peak flow zone: one of the four treatment zones of asthma management as defined by peak flow scores

Pediapred: brand name of prednisolone, an oral steroid

pediatrician: primary care physician for children

persistent asthma: condition in which a person experiences asthma symptoms two or more times a week (when taking no asthma medicine)

personal best peak flow score: highest peak flow score that an individual has blown on two separate days when the airways are completely clear and technique is good

pirbuterol: generic name for Maxair; beta$_2$-agonist, quick relief medicine

pollen: potent allergen shed during a plant's flowering season

pollutant: impurity or substance that contaminates the air

postbronchodilator: occurring after inhaling a quick relief medicine

ppm: parts per million. Number of molecules of a particular substance (e.g., a pollutant) found in a million molecules of air, water, etc.

prebronchodilator: score occurring before inhaling a quick relief medicine

prednisone: generic name of oral steroid medicine; many brand names

prednisolone: generic name for Prelone and Pediapred; oral steroid medicine

Prelone: a brand name for prednisolone, an oral steroid

prick test: type of skin test for allergy

Proventil: brand name for albuterol; beta$_2$-agonist, quick relief medicine

Proventil HFA: brand name for albuterol with non-CFC propellant in the MDI; beta$_2$-agonist, quick relief medicine

Proventil Repetabs: brand name for long-acting albuterol preparation; oral

puffer: another word for inhaler or MDI

Pulmicort Turbuhaler: brand name for a dry powder inhaler containing budesonide; inhaled steroid, controller

pulmonary function test: a test or series of tests used to measure various aspects of lung function and capacity

pulmonologist: doctor specializing in the care of people with lung diseases

q.i.d.: four times per day dosing schedule

quick relief medicine: inhaled medicine that acts to open constricted airways within minutes (e.g., inhaled beta$_2$-agonists)

Qvar: brand name for beclomethasone, an inhaled steroid medicine; controller

RAST: radioimmunosorbent test, an allergy test that measures IgE (antibody) to a specific antigen

RAD: abbreviation for reactive airway disease, a name for asthma

red zone: asthma treatment zone in which symptoms are severe and peak flow is less than 50 percent of personal best; requires immediate treatment

relative humidity: amount of water in the air compared to the total amount of water the air can hold at a given temperature

rescue medicine: quick relief medicine

respiratory therapist: health professional who provides assessment, treatment, and education for people with lung disease

respirable range: size of particles that can be inhaled into the small airways (1 to 5 microns in diameter)

retraction: "sucking in" of the chest or neck skin

ROAD: reversible obstructive airway disease, a term that is sometimes used to describe the asthma condition

Rotacap: capsule containing albuterol in powder form for use in a Rotahaler; beta$_2$-agonist, quick relief medicine

Rotadisk: brand name for dry powder inhaler device containing fluticasone; an inhaled steroid, controller

Rotahaler: dry powder inhaler device for inhaling Rotacaps, which contain albuterol; quick relief medicine

runout time: length of time it takes for the effect of a medicine to disappear after the last dose; may be minutes, hours, or days

salmeterol: generic name for Serevent; inhaled long-acting beta$_2$-agonist, controller

sensitization: process of becoming sensitized to an allergen

sensitizer: allergen or irritant that primes the asthma reaction

Serevent: brand name for salmeterol, controller

serum: the liquid portion of the blood

serum level: the amount of medicine in a quantity of serum

shake test: shaking the MDI canister, an unreliable method for determining whether the MDI can deliver a full puff of medicine

side effect: undesired or adverse effect of medicine

sign: a physical indication of asthma that can be noted by an observer

Singulair: brand name for montelukast, a leukotriene modifier medicine, controller

sinuses: one of the eight bone-enclosed cavities surrounding the nose

sinusitis: inflammation of one or more paranasal (around the nose) sinuses

Slo-bid: brand name for a theophylline preparation, controller, oral

Slo-Phyllin: brand name for a theophylline preparation, controller, oral

small airways: airways less than 2 mm in diameter; bronchioles

Space Chamber: brand of holding chamber

spacer: device used with an MDI to improve effectiveness; also known as "holding chamber" or "extender"

Spinhaler: brand name for dry-powder device containing cromolyn; controller medicine; no longer available in the U.S.

spirometer: device used in a doctor's office to measure various components of airflow

spirometry: the act of using a spirometer

step down: method for bringing asthma under control quickly, then gradually decreasing medicines to the lowest effective dose

steroid burst: a short treatment with oral steroids, usually lasting for seven days or less

steroid: type of hormone produced by the adrenal cortex which has antiinflammatory effects. Also, medicine similar to this hormone that is given by inhalation or orally to help control asthma

subcutaneous: under the skin

sustained-release: synonymous with long-acting or extended-release; refers to theophylline and beta$_2$-agonist preparations

sympathomimetic: produces the same effect as epinephrine injection or stimulation of sympathetic nervous system

symptoms: anything you feel that is different from usual; for example, a tight chest or shortness of breath

terbutaline: generic name for Brethaire, Brethine, Bricanyl; beta$_2$-agonist, quick relief medicine

Theo-24: brand name for a long-acting theophylline preparation, controller, oral

Theo-Dur: brand name for a long-acting theophylline preparation, controller, oral

theophylline: slow-acting brochodilator medicine; controller, oral

tidal breathing: normal, relaxed breathing

Tilade: brand name for nedocromil, controller

toxicity: quality of being poisonous; the adverse effect(s) of a medicine

triamcinolone: generic name for Azmacort, inhaled steroid preparation (controller)

trigger: instigator; precipitating factor in causing airway inflammation and asthma symptoms

twitchy: overreactive, hyperresponsive; used in reference to airways

ultrasonic: sound waves above the range that humans can hear; can cause a medicine solution to turn into a mist

ultrasonic nebulizer: device that uses sound waves to create medicine mist; usually small, light, and portable

unit dose: medicine in liquid or pill form that is packaged in individual doses

Uni-Dur: brand name for a long-acting theophylline preparation, controller, oral

Uni-Phyl: brand name for a long-acting theophylline preparation, controller, oral

USN: ultrasonic nebulizer

valve: device that regulates the flow of air or other substance

Vanceril: brand name for beclomethasone; an inhaled steroid medicine, controller

vent: tube that can be uncovered to interrupt the flow of air into a compressor driven nebulizer cup

Ventolin: brand name for albuterol, a beta$_2$-agonist, quick relief medicine

voice box: larynx, part of the upper airways which lies between the throat and the trachea

wheeze: high-pitched whistling that occurs when air flows through narrowed airways

white blood cells: cells whose main function is to defend the body from bacteria and allergens

Windmill Trainer: a feedback device that people use to improve their ability to blow peak flow

workup: evaluation of a patient

Xopenex: brand name for levalbuterol, a beta$_2$-agonist, quick relief medicine

zafirlukast: generic name for Accolate, a leukotriene modifier; controller

zone borders: limits of the asthma treatment zones as defined by peak flow or total score of asthma signs

zileuton: generic name for Zyflo, a leukotriene modifier medicine; controller

Zyflo: brand name for the zileuton, a leukotriene modifier medicine; controller

Index

Note: An "f" after a page number denotes a figure; a "t" after a page number denotes a table.

Asthma (*cont.*)
  excellent control, steps toward, 181–186
  two stories of, 176–179
  treatment zones
    adjusting, 198
    defined, 45–46, 46f, 47t, 186–187
    and peak flow, 135–137, 137t, 155
    setting up in diary, 155, 156t, 157t
  undiagnosed, 65–67
Asthma Peak Flow Diary, 152f, 154–164
  blank, for personal use, 273–274f
  and controlling asthma, 161–163
  filling out, 154–161
  with Home Treatment Plan, 196–197
  how often and how long to use, 163–164, 164t
  steps one, two, and three of, 155–157, 158f
  step four of, 157–158, 159f
  step five of, 158–159, 160f
  step six of, 159–161, 161f
Asthma Signs Diary, 164–174, 166f
  blank, for personal use, 275–276f
  filling out, 165–170
  with Home Treatment Plan, 210
  how often and how long to keep, 170–171, 172t
  steps one through four of, 166–168, 169f
  step five of, 168, 170f
  steps six and seven of, 168–170, 171f
  usefulness of, 164–165, 185
athletics. *See* sports
atopy. *See* allergies
Atrovent. *See* ipratropium bromide
attack. *See* asthma episode
attitudes. *See* feelings
Azmacort. *See* triamcinolone

babysitters, 252–253
beclomethasone, 70, 79t, 82t
Beclovent. *See* beclomethasone
bedroom, reducing dust in, 50
beta-adrenergic medicines. *See* beta2-agonists
beta2-agonists
  long-acting, 89–93. *See also* medicines, controller
    action of, 78t, 89
    missed or extra doses of, 102t
    role of in managing asthma, 74, 77, 89–90
    table of, 89t
  names of in U.S., Canada, and U.K., 281–282t
  short-acting, 96–100. *See also* medicines, quick relief
    action of, 78t, 96
    before exercise, 54t
    missed or extra doses of, 102t
    role of in managing asthma, 77
    usual doses of, 98t, 100t
beta-blockers, 63, 71, 101
biological contaminants, as triggers, 245
blow-by technique, 111, 125, 125t
books on asthma, 283–285
breathing
  changes in, as early clue to episode, 43
  in-to-out ratio of, 124–125
  increased rate of, 38, 41–42, 47, 47t
  normal, 32–33, 42t
  slowing of, during nebulizer treatment, 124
Brethaire. *See* terbutaline
Brethine. *See* terbutaline
Bricanyl. *See* terbutaline
bronchi, 32, 33f
bronchioles, 32, 33f, 34f, 37f

bronchiolitis, 66
bronchitis, 36, 39–40, 49, 65
bronchoconstriction, 29, 37f
bronchodilators. *See* medicines, quick relief
bronchospasm, 36, 37f, 87
brothers and sisters, 251. *See also* family
budesonide, 79t, 82t, 119t

candidiasis. *See* yeast infection
capillaries, 32, 34f
carbon dioxide, 32, 34f, 237, 241, 245
caregivers (for children), 251–252
carpeting, as trigger, 182, 243–244
cataracts, 86
cats, as trigger, 48, 60–61, 177, 182
CDN. *See* compressor driven nebulizer
CFCs. *See* chlorofluorocarbons
chicken pox, 84
children under 5, treatment of, 198–199, 201, 202f, 224
chlorofluorocarbons (CFCs), 112, 119
chronic obstructive pulmonary disease (COPD), 67
cigarette smoke. *See* smoking
cilia, 33
cleaning materials, as triggers, 243–245
closed mouth technique, 111–112
cockroaches, 61
coexisting medical conditions, 76
cold weather. *See* air, cold
colds, 36, 179. *See also* viral respiratory infection
combination medicine, 10, 27
compressor driven nebulizer (CDN)
  described, 107, 122, 122f

with mask, 18, 26
proper use of, 123–126, 125t
conditioned response to triggers, 53
consultation with specialist
  as accepted medical practice, 219–220
  arranging, 220
  example of, 222–224
  overview of, 221–222
  preparing for, 220–221
  for small children, 224
controller medicines. *See* medicines, controller
COPD. *See* chronic obstructive pulmonary disease
cough
  chronic, 41, 64, 185
  at night, 23, 64
  scoring of, 47, 47t
  as sign of asthma, 5, 16–18, 38, 41, 64
cough variant asthma, 64–65
cromolyn, 87–89
  action of, 78t, 87
  with albuterol, 89, 98
  as controller medicine, 74, 77
  dosage of, 88, 88t
  before exercise, 54t
  missed or extra dose of, 102t
  by nebulizer, for children, 123, 125–127
  with pregnancy, 70
crying, as trigger, 52

dander, 60–61
day care, 231
deaths from asthma, 40, 225
delivery systems. *See* inhalation devices
Deltasone. *See* prednisone
depression, 9, 11, 86
diagnosis of asthma, 38–39, 142
diaphragm, 32–33, 33f, 35f

About the Authors

DR. TOM PLAUT is a nationally known asthma specialist and author of asthma publications for the public. These include *Children With Asthma: A Manual for Parents, One Minute Asthma: What You Need To Know,* the Asthma Peak Flow Diary, and the Asthma Signs Diary.

Dr. Plaut believes that almost everyone with asthma has the ability to manage it at home. People who learn the basics of asthma can work out an effective asthma care plan with their doctor or nurse. Using the plan as a guide they will be able to lead fully active lives and to avoid asthma emergencies.

After graduating from Yale with a degree in history, Dr. Plaut received his medical degree from Columbia University and his pediatric training at New York University–Bellevue Medical Center. He practiced pediatrics for twenty-four years in Appalachia, the South Bronx, and in Massachusetts before founding Asthma Consultants in 1988.

Dr. Plaut now devotes his full energy to helping patients and their families, and assisting organizations to improve the care of people with asthma. He serves as an asthma consultant to HMOs, government agencies, and various publications. Parents, teachers, and the general public learn of his views on asthma through lectures, seminars, and on radio and television. His research findings are available to health professionals in journal articles, workshops, and national meetings. His office is in Amherst, Massachusetts.

TERESA B. JONES is a science and medical writer who has collaborated with Dr. Plaut for six years. She has contributed to several of his books, co-authored articles about asthma for health professionals, and published a book and articles on environmental topics. Ms. Jones teaches college biology, genetics, and environmental science. She graduated from Yale University with degrees in environmental studies and history and received her Master's degree in plant biology from the University of Massachusetts.

Dear Reader,

Please let me know what you think about my book.

Did it help you improve communication with your doctor?

Did it help you work out a more effective treatment plan?

Did you find any section to be particularly helpful?

Did you have difficulty understanding any section?

Did you feel better the day you read my book?

Please write any additional comments:

May I use your words and name in promotional material? _____ yes _____ no

_____

signature

_____

Please print your name, address, city, state, zip and phone number

Please mail or fax to: Dr. Tom Plaut, c/o Pedipress, 125 Red Gate Lane, Amherst MA 01002 Fax: (413) 549-4095

Order Form

	Qty	Cost

Dr. Tom Plaut's Asthma Guide
for People of All Ages
1999, 336 pages, $25

Children with Asthma:
A Manual for Parents
1995, 304 pages, $10

One Minute Asthma:
What You Need to Know
1998, 56 pages, $5
10 copies, $2.00 each

El asma en un minuto
Spanish version of *One Minute Asthma*.
48 pages, $5

Winning Over Asthma
1996, 40 pages, $7

Asthma Peak Flow Diary
3 colors, 25 sheets per pad, $3
Please specify English or Spanish.

Asthma Signs Diary
3 colors, 50 sheets per pad. $8

Please fax 413-549-4095 or call
413-549-7798 for shipping costs
outside the lower 48 United States.

Prices and products subject to change.
For the most current information, visit
our web site at www.pedipress.com

Discounts available at 10 or more copies;
call or visit our web site for discount pricing.

Subtotal: _____

5% Sales Tax: _____
(Mass. Only)

5% Shipping: _____
($5 minimum)

Total Enclosed: _____

Name _____

Street (no PO Boxes) _____

_____

City _____ State _____ Zip _____

Telephone (required) _____

❑ Mastercard ❑ Visa # _____

Exp. Date _____ Signature _____

Send check or money order to:
Pedipress Fulfillment Center
125 Red Gate Lane
Amherst, MA 01002
Phone: 800-611-6081; Fax: 413-549-4095
www.pedipress.com